Orthopedic Emergencies

Editors

DAVID DELLA-GIUSTINA
KATJA GOLDFLAM

EMERGENCY MEDICINE CLINICS OF NORTH AMERICA

www.emed.theclinics.com

Consulting Editor
AMAL MATTU

May 2015 • Volume 33 • Number 2

ELSEVIER

1600 John F. Kennedy Boulevard • Suite 1800 • Philadelphia, Pennsylvania, 19103-2899

http://www.theclinics.com

EMERGENCY MEDICINE CLINICS OF NORTH AMERICA Volume 33, Number 2
May 2015 ISSN 0733-8627, ISBN-13: 978-0-323-37594-8

Editor: Patrick Manley
Developmental Editor: Casey Jackson

Emergency Medicine Clinics of North America (ISSN 0733-8627) is published quarterly by Elsevier Inc., 360 Park Avenue South, New York, NY, 10010-1710. Months of issue are February, May, August, and November. Business and Editorial Offices: 1600 John F. Kennedy Boulevard, Suite 1800, Philadelphia, PA 19103-2899. Customer Service Office: 6277 Sea Harbor Drive, Orlando, FL 32887-4800. Periodicals postage paid at New York, NY, and additional mailing offices. Subscription prices are $155.00 per year (US students), $315.00 per year (US individuals), $523.00 per year (US institutions), $220.00 per year (international students), $450.00 per year (international individuals), $642.00 per year (international institutions), $220.00 per year (Canadian students), $385.00 per year (Canadian individuals), and $642.00 per year (Canadian institutions). International air speed delivery is included in all *Clinics*' subscription prices. All prices are subject to change without notice. **POSTMASTER:** Send address changes to *Emergency Medicine Clinics of North America*, Elsevier Periodicals Customer Service, 11830 Westline Industrial Drive, St. Louis, MO 63146. Customer Service (orders, claims, online, change of address): Elsevier Periodicals Customer Service, 11830 Westline Industrial Drive, St. Louis, MO 63146. Tel: 1-800-654-2452 (U.S. and Canada); 314-453-7041 (outside U.S. and Canada). Fax: 314-453-5170. E-mail: journalscustomerservice-usa@elsevier.com (for print support); journalsonline support-usa@elsevier.com (for online support).

Reprints. For copies of 100 or more of articles in this publication, please contact the Commercial Reprints Department, Elsevier Inc., 360 Park Avenue South, New York, NY 10010-1710. Tel.: 212-633-3874; Fax: 212-633-3820; E-mail: reprints@elsevier.com.

Emergency Medicine Clinics of North America is covered in *MEDLINE/PubMed (Index Medicus), Current Contents/Clinical Medicine, EMBASE/Excerpta Medica, BIOSIS, SciSearch, CINAHL, ISI/BIOMED,* and *Research Alert.*

Contributors

CONSULTING EDITOR

AMAL MATTU, MD, FAAEM, FACEP
Professor and Vice Chair, Department of Emergency Medicine, University of Maryland School of Medicine, Baltimore, Maryland

EDITORS

DAVID DELLA-GIUSTINA, MD, FACEP, FAWM
Associate Professor, Emergency Medicine Residency Program Director, Chief, Section of Education, Department of Emergency Medicine, Yale University School of Medicine, New Haven, Connecticut

KATJA GOLDFLAM, MD
Assistant Professor, Associate Program Director, Emergency Medicine Residency, Department of Emergency Medicine, Yale University School of Medicine, New Haven, Connecticut

AUTHORS

PAUL L. ARONSON, MD
Assistant Professor of Pediatrics; Associate Director, Pediatric Residency Program, Section of Emergency Medicine, Department of Pediatrics, Yale School of Medicine, New Haven, Connecticut

VINCENT BALL, MD
Department of Emergency Medicine, Madigan Army Medical Center, Tacoma, Washington

JAMES BONZ, MD
Assistant Professor, Department of Emergency Medicine, Yale School of Medicine, New Haven, Connecticut

JASON BOTHWELL, MD
Residency Director, Department of Emergency Medicine, Madigan Army Medical Center, Fort Lewis, Washington

MARCO COPPOLA, DO, FACEP
University of North Texas Health Science Center, Fort Worth, Texas and P1 24 Hour Emergency Centers, Frisco, Texas

PAOLO T. COPPOLA, MD, FACEP
STAT-Health, Smithtown, New York

BRONSON E. DELASOBERA, MD
Department of Emergency Medicine, MedStar Washington Hospital Center, Washington, DC

DAVID DELLA-GIUSTINA, MD
Program Director, Emergency Medicine Residency; Chief, Education Section, Department of Emergency Medicine, Yale School of Medicine, New Haven, Connecticut

KAREN DELLA-GIUSTINA, MD
Department of Emergency Medicine, Pediatric Emergency Department, Bridgeport Hospital, Bridgeport, Connecticut

RICKY DURBIN, MD
Department of Emergency Medicine, Madigan Army Medical Center, Fort Lewis, Washington

JILL FRANKLIN, MD
Department of Emergency Medicine, Madigan Army Medical Center, Tacoma, Washington

WILLIAM FROHNA, MD
Department of Emergency Medicine, MedStar Washington Hospital Center, Washington, DC

KATJA GOLDFLAM, MD
Associate Program Director, Emergency Medicine Residency, Department of Emergency Medicine, Yale University School of Medicine, New Haven, Connecticut

DAVID HILE, MD, FAWM
Assistant Professor, Department of Emergency Medicine, Yale School of Medicine, New Haven, Connecticut

LISA HILE, MD
Clinical Instructor, Department of Emergency Medicine, Yale School of Medicine, New Haven, Connecticut

KORIN HUDSON, MD, FACEP, CAQ-SM
Department of Emergency Medicine, MedStar Georgetown University Hospital, Washington, DC

CHRISTOPHER KANG, MD, FACEP, FAWM
Department of Emergency Medicine, Madigan Army Medical Center, Tacoma, Washington

RAJDEEP KANWAR, MD
Department of Emergency Medicine, MedStar Washington Hospital Center, MedStar Georgetown University/Washington Hospital Center Emergency Medicine Residency, Washington, DC

TRISTAN KNUTSON, MD
Assistant Residency Director, Department of Emergency Medicine, Madigan Army Medical Center, Fort Lewis, Washington

MATTHEW JAMIESON STEIN, MD
Department of Emergency Medicine, Madigan Army Medical Center, Tacoma, Washington

MATTHEW D. THORNTON, MD
Section of Pediatric Emergency Medicine, Department of Emergency Medicine, Baystate Medical Center, Springfield, Massachusetts

BRADFORD TINLOY, MD
Department of Emergency Medicine, Yale School of Medicine, New Haven, Connecticut

ALINA TSYRULNIK, MD
Emergency Medicine Clinical Instructor, Yale University School of Medicine, New Haven, Connecticut

HAO WANG, MD, PhD, FACEP
Department of Emergency Medicine, John Peter Smith Health Network, Fort Worth, Texas

IAN WEDMORE, MD
Department of Emergency Medicine, Madigan Army Medical Center, Tacoma, Washington

SCOTT YOUNG, MD
Department of Emergency Medicine, Madigan Army Medical Center, Tacoma, Washington

Contents

Most spinal cord injuries involve the cervical spine, highlighting the importance of recognition and proper management by emergency physicians. Initial cervical spine injury management should follow the ABCDE (airway, breathing, circulation, disability, exposure) procedure detailed by Advanced Trauma Life Support. NEXUS (National Emergency X-Radiography Utilization Study) criteria and Canadian C-spine Rule are clinical decision-making tools providing guidelines of when to obtain imaging. Computed tomography scans are the preferred initial imaging modality. Consider administering intravenous methylprednisolone after discussion with the neurosurgical consultant in patients who present with spinal cord injuries within 8 hours.

Correct diagnosis of wrist injuries is critical in preventing prolonged pain and dysfunction. Radiographs cannot diagnose a large percentage of injuries. Wrist sprain is considered one of the most common yet most treacherous emergency department (ED) diagnoses because radiographs do not always rule out all acute injuries. Knowledge of the anatomy, normal physical examination findings, and physical examination abnormalities associated with different pathological conditions is paramount in making the correct diagnosis. This article focuses on the anatomy, diagnosis, and ED management of acute wrist injuries, including fractures and dislocations.

Shoulder injuries are among the most common musculoskeletal complaints seen in US emergency departments (EDs). ED evaluation of the shoulder must account for the broad range of potential fracture patterns seen in the clavicle, scapula, and humerus. Acromioclavicular dislocation is often encountered in the ED and treatment varies by severity. Dislocation of the shoulder is frequently seen, and the ED physician must be skilled in several reduction techniques to optimize a successful reduction. An understanding of when orthopedic consultation is appropriate and when patients can be dispositioned with timely follow-up are integral to complete patient recovery.

Back pain is a common presenting complaint to the emergency department. The key to proper evaluation is a history and physical examination focused on determining if any red flags for serious disease are present. If no red flags are present, the patient most likely has nonspecific back pain and their symptoms will resolve in 4 to 6 weeks. No diagnostic testing is required. For patients with red flags, a focused history and examination in conjunction with diagnostic laboratory tests and imaging determine whether the patient has an emergent condition such as herniated disc, epidural compression, or spinal infection.

Although the incidence of hip fractures is decreasing, the overall prevalence continues to increase because of an aging population. People older than 65 suffer fractures at a rate of 0.6% per year—2% per year for persons older than 85. One in 5 patients suffering a hip fracture will die within a year. Additionally, the emergency physician must consider entities such as avascular necrosis, compartment syndrome, and muscular disruption. This article reviews patterns and complications of acute hip and thigh injuries and clinically relevant diagnostic, anesthetic, and treatment options that facilitate timely, appropriate, and effective emergency department management.

Posttraumatic knee pain is a common presentation in the emergency department (ED). The use of clinical decision rules can rule out reliably fractures of the knee and reduce the unnecessary cost and radiation exposure associated with plain radiographs. If ligamentous or meniscal injury to the knee is suspected, the ED physician should arrange for expedited follow-up with the patient's primary care physician or an orthopedic specialist for consideration of an MRI and further management. Patients presenting after high-energy mechanisms are at risk for occult fracture and vascular injuries. ED providers must consider these injuries in the proper clinical setting.

Foot and ankle injuries are a frequent cause for a visit to the Emergency Department. A thorough evaluation and treatment of these injuries needs to be an area of in-depth familiarity for the Emergency Medicine physician. The key to proper evaluation is first a history and physical examination that focuses on determining what, if any, imaging is required. Subsequently, a focused history, physical examination, and imaging will then determine if an injury is stable or unstable, requiring operative intervention.

The hand is especially prone to traumatic injury. Some sources indicate that injuries to the hand account for somewhere between 10% and 30% of patients treated in emergency care settings. Fractures are the most common injury, followed by tendon injury, then skin lesions. Because the mechanism of injury often results in damage to multiple tissue structures, a detailed history and evaluation are vital to properly identifying and managing these injuries. This article provides the emergency physician with tools to identify and manage orthopedic injuries to the hand.

Elbow and forearm injuries result most commonly from direct blows to the area, or from fall on outstretched hand. The elbow may be injured if it is locked at the time of impact. Elbow or forearm bone dislocations may occur alone or in conjunction with fractures and generally require reduction to minimize future morbidity. The primary goal of management is to achieve anatomic reduction of any fracture or dislocation, while allowing for early range of motion to minimize future morbidity, including in particular elbow stiffness and consequently limited mobility of the joint.

Orthopedic injuries in children are unique when compared to those of adults because of the physiologic differences, especially the growth plates, stronger periosteum, and dynamic state of growth. The approach to the orthopedically injured child requires a gentle yet thorough focus, with consideration of the growth plates as a primary area of weakness and growth when the child sustains an injury. Understanding the developmental stages of bones is paramount to being able to manage any injuries. Finally, what appears to be a benign injury may portend more serious issues, because nonaccidental trauma must always be considered in the evaluation of the injured child.

Trauma is one of the leading causes of death before the age of 40 years and approximately 5% of patients with trauma who require hospital admission have pelvic fractures. This article updates the emergency department classification of pelvic fractures first described in 2000. This information is of practical value to emergency physicians in identifying the potential vascular, genitourinary, gastrointestinal, orthopedic, and neurologic complications and further assists them in the initial evaluation and treatment of patients with pelvic fractures.

EMERGENCY MEDICINE CLINICS OF NORTH AMERICA

THE CLINICS ARE NOW AVAILABLE ONLINE!
Access your subscription at:
www.theclinics.com

PROGRAM OBJECTIVE
The goal of *Emergency Medicine Clinics of North America* is to keep practicing emergency medicine physicians and emergency medicine residents up to date with current clinical practice in emergency medicine by providing timely articles reviewing the state of the art in patient care.

TARGET AUDIENCE
All practicing physicians and healthcare professionals who provide patient care utilizing findings from *Emergency Medicine Clinics of North America*.

LEARNING OBJECTIVES
Upon completion of this activity, participants will be able to:
1. Review strategies in evaluating common emergency injuries.
2. Discuss the emergency evaluation, including imaging techniques, of skeletal injuries.
3. Recognize different methods of orthopaedic injury management in emergency treatments.

ACCREDITATION
The Elsevier Office of Continuing Medical Education (EOCME) is accredited by the Accreditation Council for Continuing Medical Education (ACCME) to provide continuing medical education for physicians.

The EOCME designates this enduring material for a maximum of 15 *AMA PRA Category 1 Credit*(s)™. Physicians should claim only the credit commensurate with the extent of their participation in the activity.

All other health care professionals requesting continuing education credit for this enduring material will be issued a certificate of participation.

DISCLOSURE OF CONFLICTS OF INTEREST
The EOCME assesses conflict of interest with its instructors, faculty, planners, and other individuals who are in a position to control the content of CME activities. All relevant conflicts of interest that are identified are thoroughly vetted by EOCME for fair balance, scientific objectivity, and patient care recommendations. EOCME is committed to providing its learners with CME activities that promote improvements or quality in healthcare and not a specific proprietary business or a commercial interest.

The planning committee, staff, authors and editors listed below have identified no financial relationships or relationships to products or devices they or their spouse/life partner have with commercial interest related to the content of this CME activity:
Paul L. Aronson, MD; James Bonz, MD; Jason Bothwell, MD; Paolo T. Coppola, MD; Marco Coppola, DO; B. Elizabeth Delasobera, MD; David Della-Giustina, MD; Karen Della-Giustina, MD; Ricky Durbin, MD; Anjali Fortna; Jillian M. Franklin, MD; William Frohna, MD; Katja Goldflam, Kristen Helm; MD; David Hile, MD; Lisa Hile, MA; Korin Hudson; Christopher Kang, MD; Rajdeep Kanwar, MD; Tristan Knutson, MD; Indu Kumari; Patrick Manley; Amal Mattu, MD; Matthew Jamieson Stein, MD; Matthew D. Thornton, MD; Bradford T. Tinloy, MD; Alina Tsyrulnik, MD; Hao Wang, MD, PhD; Ian Wedmore, MD; Scott Young, MD.

The planning committee, staff, authors and editors listed below have identified financial relationships or relationships to products or devices they or their spouse/life partner have with commercial interest related to the content of this CME activity:
Vincent Ball, MD is on the speakers' bureau for Boehringer Ingelheim GmbH.

UNAPPROVED/OFF-LABEL USE DISCLOSURE
The EOCME requires CME faculty to disclose to the participants:
1. When products or procedures being discussed are off-label, unlabelled, experimental, and/or investigational (not US Food and Drug Administration [FDA] approved); and
2. Any limitations on the information presented, such as data that are preliminary or that represent ongoing research, interim analyses, and/or unsupported opinions. Faculty may discuss information about pharmaceutical agents that is outside of FDA-approved labelling. This information is intended solely for CME and is not intended to promote off-label use of these medications. If you have any questions, contact the medical affairs department of the manufacturer for the most recent prescribing information.

TO ENROLL
To enroll in the *Emergency Medicine Clinics* Continuing Medical Education program, call customer service at 1-800-654-2452 or sign up online at http://www.theclinics.com/home/cme. The CME program is available to subscribers for an additional annual fee of $235 USD.

METHOD OF PARTICIPATION

In order to claim credit, participants must complete the following:

1. Complete enrolment as indicated above.
2. Read the activity.
3. Complete the CME Test and Evaluation. Participants must achieve a score of 70% on the test. All CME Tests and Evaluations must be completed online.

CME INQUIRIES/SPECIAL NEEDS

For all CME inquiries or special needs, please contact elsevierCME@elsevier.com.

Foreword

Orthopedic Emergencies

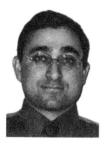

Amal Mattu, MD
Consulting Editor

Emergency orthopedics is an integral part of the practice of emergency medicine. On a routine shift this past week in the emergency department (ED), I cared for two patients who slipped on ice and sustained ankle fractures, one patient with a shoulder dislocation that occurred while he was playing basketball, an elderly patient with a spontaneous dislocation of his prosthetic hip, and another elderly patient with a hip fracture after she was involved in a motor vehicle accident. These patients were in addition to the handful of other patients with joint sprains and overuse injuries from shoveling snow, slips and falls, or manual labor. I finished the shift caring for a patient with a boxer's fracture from an altercation with another patron in a bar. Had it been summertime, the injuries would mostly have been similar, though perhaps greater in number and with more sports-related mechanisms rather than snow and ice associations.

Despite the frequency with which we see orthopedic emergencies in the ED, it seems that many training programs are often deficient in teaching the proper skills to deal with these conditions. There is always much greater emphasis during training on high-profile conditions such as multisystem trauma, acute myocardial infarction, sepsis, stroke, appendicitis, acute respiratory failure, and so on. The irony is that all these aforementioned conditions are *less common* than orthopedic emergencies. They also require admission, which, therefore, allows care to be passed on to other physicians. Many orthopedic emergencies, on the other hand, allow the emergency physician to "treat and street" the patients without requiring the immediate involvement of any consultants...IF the emergency physician is properly trained. Yet many emergency physicians, especially new graduates, are uncertain about diagnosing, treating, splinting, and providing dispositions for patients with orthopedic conditions. I'll admit that at the beginning of my career, I fit that description as well, and thankfully my senior medical colleagues and physician assistants taught me more about emergency orthopedics during my first year as an attending than I learned in all of my residency training.

Emerg Med Clin N Am 33 (2015) xv–xvi
http://dx.doi.org/10.1016/j.emc.2015.03.004
0733-8627/15/$ – see front matter © 2015 Published by Elsevier Inc.

emed.theclinics.com

For readers of *Emergency Medicine Clinics of North America* that have ever felt uncertain about how to care for some orthopedic conditions, as I did at the end of my training, this issue is written just for you. Guest editors Drs Della-Giustina and Goldflam have assembled an outstanding group of authors and they have created a fantastic curriculum in emergency orthopedics that deserves to be required reading for all emergency medicine trainees. The authors address every major and common bone and joint injury from the neck down to the foot. Detailed explanations of the proper examination techniques are provided as well as recommendations for reducing dislocations, for splinting, and for subsequent follow-up and care. They also provide a special article addressing some of the common pediatric orthopedic injuries.

This issue of *Emergency Medicine Clinics of North America* represents an invaluable resource for routine clinical practice in emergency medicine. Experienced emergency physicians as well as emergency medicine trainees will benefit tremendously from the expertise provided in the pages that follow. Our thanks to the editors and authors of this excellent work!

Amal Mattu, MD
Department of Emergency Medicine
University of Maryland School of Medicine
Baltimore, MD 21201, USA

E-mail address:
amattu@smail.umaryland.edu

Preface

The Evaluation and Management of Orthopedic Trauma and Emergencies

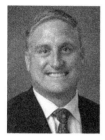 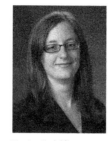

David Della-Giustina, MD,   Katja Goldflam, MD
FACEP, FAWM

Editors

The management of orthopedic trauma and emergencies is integral to the repertoire of emergency providers. Injuries range from potentially life-threatening spine and pelvic fractures to seemingly minor extremity fractures and joint dislocations. While generally less morbid, these may nonetheless result in significant disability if treated incorrectly or with delay, affecting patient quality of life and future employability. Similarly, management of acute back pain is a daily occurrence in the emergency department, where timely recognition and evaluation of red flags may significantly alter patient outcomes.

This issue of the *Emergency Medical Clinics of North America* addresses a broad range of orthopedic traumatic injuries and emergencies. Our authors address the initial evaluation and examination of the patient, imaging choices, and emergency management of the full spectrum of orthopedic traumatic emergencies. A special article is dedicated to pediatric trauma and the recognition of injury patterns affecting developing bones, including those not necessarily evident on radiographic imaging. We also highlight nomenclature and classification of bony injuries to provide a foundation for accurate communication with orthopedic consultant services.

The editors are very appreciative of the excellent contributions by our diverse group of authors. We hope this will provide an informative reference work for orthopedic

Emerg Med Clin N Am 33 (2015) xvii–xviii
http://dx.doi.org/10.1016/j.emc.2015.03.003
0733-8627/15/$ – see front matter © 2015 Published by Elsevier Inc.

emed.theclinics.com

injuries encountered in your daily clinical practice. We also thank our families for their support.

David Della-Giustina, MD, FACEP, FAWM
Section of Education
Department of Emergency Medicine
Yale University School of Medicine
464 Congress Avenue, Suite 260
New Haven, CT 06519, USA

Katja Goldflam, MD
Emergency Medicine Residency
Department of Emergency Medicine
Yale University School of Medicine
464 Congress Avenue, Suite 260
New Haven, CT 06519, USA

E-mail addresses:
David.Della-Giustina@yale.edu (D. Della-Giustina)
Katja.Goldflam@yale.edu (K. Goldflam)

Erratum

An error was made in the November 2014 issue (Volume 32, Number 4) of *Emergency Medicine Clinics* on page 830 of the article "Pressors and Inotropes." The second sentence of the first paragraph on the page should read: "Patients on β-blocking medications and unresponsive to epinephrine infusions may respond to glucagon, dosed 1 to 5 mg (0.02–0.03 mg/kg to maximum of 1 mg in children) of slow IV push over 5 minutes, then infused at 5 to 15 µg/min and titrated to clinical response."

Emerg Med Clin N Am 33 (2015) xix
http://dx.doi.org/10.1016/j.emc.2015.03.002
emed.theclinics.com
0733-8627/15/$ – see front matter © 2015 Elsevier Inc. All rights reserved.

Emergency Department Evaluation and Treatment of Cervical Spine Injuries

Rajdeep Kanwar, MD[a],*, Bronson E. Delasobera, MD[b],*,
Korin Hudson, MD, CAQ-SM[c], William Frohna, MD[a]

KEYWORDS

- Emergency department • Cervical spine • Spinal cord • Neurologic injury • Cooling
- Corticosteroid use

KEY POINTS

- Most spinal cord injuries involve the cervical spine, highlighting the importance of recognition and proper management by emergency physicians.
- Initial cervical spine injury management should follow the ABCDE (airway, breathing, circulation, disability, exposure) procedure detailed by Advanced Trauma Life Support.
- NEXUS (National Emergency X-Radiography Utilization Study) criteria and Canadian C-spine Rule are clinical decision-making tools providing guidelines of when to obtain imaging.
- Computed tomography scans are now the preferred initial imaging modality.
- Consider administering intravenous methylprednisolone after discussion with the neurosurgical consultant in patients who present with spinal cord injuries within 8 hours.

Patients who arrive at the emergency department (ED) with potential cervical spine injuries pose a common challenge for emergency physicians (EPs). EPs should be prepared to manage these patients efficiently and effectively while protecting the cervical spine to prevent additional neurologic injury during evaluation and transfers. EPs must understand the complex anatomy of the cervical spine, and the mechanism and types of injuries, as well as being comfortable recognizing and managing associated injuries. EPs must also have an understanding of the utility and limitations of available imaging

Disclosure: None.
[a] Department of Emergency Medicine, MedStar Washington Hospital Center, MedStar Georgetown University/Washington Hospital Center Emergency Medicine Residency, 110 Irving Street Northwest, NA-1177, Washington, DC 20010, USA; [b] Department of Emergency Medicine, MedStar Washington Hospital Center, 110 Irving Street Northwest, NA-1177, Washington, DC 20010, USA; [c] Department of Emergency Medicine, MedStar Georgetown University Hospital, 3800 Reservoir Road Northwest, Ground Floor CCC Building, Washington, DC 20007, USA
* Corresponding authors.
E-mail addresses: rajdeep.s.kanwar@gmail.com; Bronson.E.Delasobera@medstar.net

Emerg Med Clin N Am 33 (2015) 241–282
http://dx.doi.org/10.1016/j.emc.2014.12.002
0733-8627/15/$ – see front matter © 2015 Elsevier Inc. All rights reserved.

modalities. In addition, EPs should be aware of issues surrounding the management of specific patient populations at risk for neck and cervical spine injuries.

EPIDEMIOLOGY

The incidence of spinal cord injury remains unknown; however, in the United States and Canada, the incidence is estimated to be between 30 and 46 cases per million population.[1,2]

- Most patients with spinal cord injury (82%) are male, and aged 16 to 30 years.[3]
- The risk of cervical spine injury increases with age among children and adolescents (13.2 per 100,000 per year for those aged >11 years, compared with 1.2 per 100,000 in those younger than 11 years).[4]
- Most spinal cord injuries result from motor vehicle accidents (47%), falls (23%), gunshot wounds/violence (14%), and sports-related activities (9%).[5,6]
- Spinal cord injuries occur in 10% to 20% of patients with spinal fractures and are found in nearly 50% of patients with bony cervical vertebral injuries.[7]
- Cervical injuries occurred in 65% of the spinal cord injuries from motor vehicle collisions, 53% of the cord injuries from falls from heights, 37% of the cord injuries from gunshot wounds, and 97% of the cord injuries from diving.[8]
- It is estimated that cervical fractures occur in 1% to 3% of patients with blunt trauma.[8,9]

Significant cervical spine injuries can occur following minor trauma in the elderly[10] as well as in patients with predisposing arthritic conditions, such as:

- Ankylosing spondylitis[11,12]
- Psoriatic cervical spondyloarthropathy[13]
- Rheumatoid arthritis[14]

ANATOMY

Understanding the anatomy of the cervical spine is critical to recognizing injury patterns.

- The spinal column consists of 33 vertebrae:
  ○ 7 cervical, 12 thoracic, 5 lumbar, 5 sacral (fused), and 4 coccygeal (fused) (**Fig. 1**)
- The anterior and posterior longitudinal ligaments hold the vertebral bodies together.
- Intervertebral discs separate the vertebral bodies and provide cushioning and flexibility.
- The spinal cord is housed in a bony ring made up of 2 pedicles (or pillars) on which the roof of the vertebral canal (the lamina) rests.
- Afferent and efferent nerve roots pass through the intervertebral foramina.

The occipitoatlantoaxial complex is made up of the articulations between the base of the skull, atlas (C1), and axis (C2) (**Fig. 2**); and several strong ligaments (**Fig. 3**) with unique articular and ligamentous relationships[15] that protect the upper cervical spine while allowing a wide range of motion.[16]

- Occipital condyles articulate with the corresponding concavities in the lateral masses of the atlas to allow for flexion and extension.
- The tectorial membrane functions to stabilize extension of the occiput on the atlas.

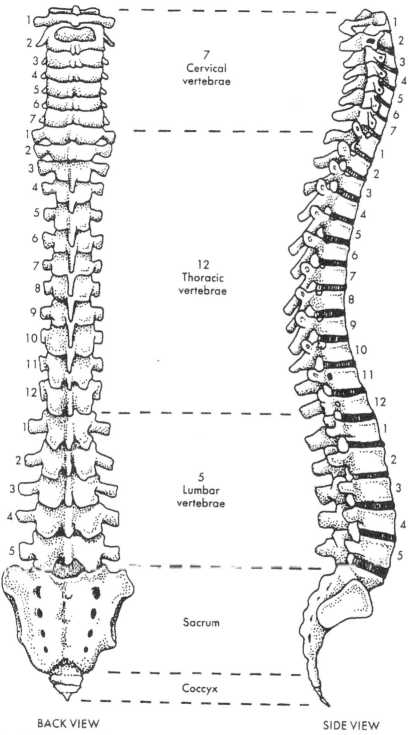

Fig. 1. Vertebral column. (*From* Hockberger RS, Kirshenbaum KJ, Doris PE. Spinal injuries. In: Rosen P, Barkin R, Danzl D, et al, editors. Emergency medicine: concepts and clinical practice. 4th edition. vol. 1. St Louis (MO): Mosby; 1998. p. 463; with permission.)

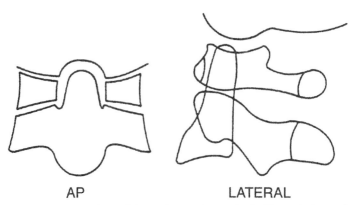

AP   LATERAL

Fig. 2. The articular relationships of the occiput, atlas, and axis. The articular surfaces of the atlas and axis are convex to each other, allowing for a great deal of rotation, flexion, and extension. AP, anteroposterior. (*From* Ellis GL. Imaging of the atlas (C1) and axis (C2). Emerg Med Clin North Am 1991;9:720.)

- Between C1 and C2, the articular surfaces of the atlas and axis are convex to each other, permitting further flexion and extension.
- Articulation between the dens process and the atlas allows for rotatory motion.
- The accessory ligaments and the alar ligaments function to limit axial rotation.
- The transverse ligament is the primary stabilizer for anterior atlantoaxial translation.
- Disruption of the transverse ligament leads to significant instability
  ○ 1 cm of potential space within the ring of the atlas allows for some displacement of the dens without cord damage.

The anatomy of the lower cervical spine is best understood in the context of mechanical stability, which can be thought of using the 2-column concept:

- Anterior column: vertebral bodies and intervertebral disks that are held in alignment by the anterior and posterior longitudinal ligaments.
- Posterior column: pedicles, laminae, articulating facets, and spinous processes, held in alignment by the nuchal ligament complex (supraspinatus, interspinous, and infraspinous ligaments), the capsular ligaments, and the ligamentum flavum (**Fig. 4**).

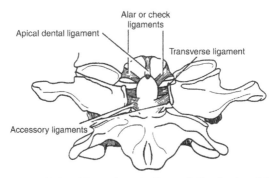

Fig. 3. The ligamentous relationships unique to the occipitoatlantoaxial region. (*From* Ellis GL. Imaging of the atlas (C1) and axis (C2). Emerg Med Clin North Am 1991;9:720.)

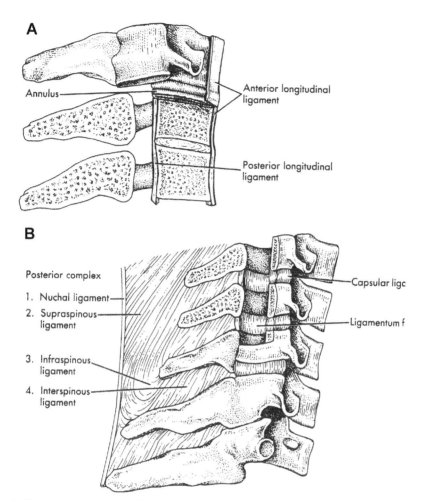

Fig. 4. Ligaments at anterior (*A*) and posterior (*B*) column. (*From* Hockberger RS, Kirshenbaum KJ, Doris PE. Spinal injuries. In: Rosen P, Barkin R, Danzl D, et al, editors. Emergency medicine: concepts and clinical practice. 4th edition. vol. 1. St Louis (MO): Mosby; 1998. p. 455; with permission.)

The injured cervical spine is considered to be mechanically unstable when both columns are disrupted at the same level.

There are 3 main spinal cord tracts, which are paired tracts that can be injured on 1 or both sides. Testing strength, sensation, and reflexes provides a rapid assessment of function of these tracts (**Table 1**).

- Corticospinal tract
  - Posterolateral segment of the cord
  - Ipsilateral motor function
- Spinothalamic tract
  - Anterolateral portion of the spinal cord
  - Pain and temperature (and some light touch) sensation from the contralateral side of the body
- Posterior columns

Table 1
Motor, sensory, and reflex examinations

Level of Lesion	Resulting Loss of Motor Function	Resulting Level of Loss of Sensation	Resulting Loss of Reflex
C2	—	Occiput	—
C3	—	Thyroid cartilage	—
C4	Spontaneous breathing	Suprasternal notch	—
C5	Shrugging of shoulders	Below clavicle	—
C6	Flexion at elbow	Thumb	Biceps
C7	Extension at elbow	Index finger	Triceps
C8	Flexion of fingers	Small finger	—

From Hockberger RS, Kirshenbaum KJ, Doris PE. Spinal injuries. In: Rosen P, Barkin R, Danzl DF, et al, editors. Emergency medicine: concepts and clinical practice. 4th edition. vol. 1. St Louis (MO): Mosby–Year Book, 1998. p. 481; with permission.

- ○ Proprioception, vibration sense, and light touch from the ipsilateral side
- ○ Sensation can be tested using light touch (posterior columns) with a cotton wisp followed by pinprick testing (spinothalamic tract) to determine the sensory dermatome involved (**Fig. 5**, see **Table 1**)

INITIAL MANAGEMENT

The important management principle for the cervical spine is protection of the spine and spinal cord with immobilization devices or by manual in-line immobilization until all injuries are fully evaluated and cervical spine injury can be ruled out. **Fig. 6** provides an approach to the management of patients with trauma with suspected cervical spine injury.

AIRWAY MANAGEMENT

Choosing the optimal technique for definitive, emergency airway management is often perceived as a clinical dilemma and many clinicians think that orotracheal intubation is hazardous in the presence of a known or potential cervical spine injury.[17]

- Several investigators have concluded that orotracheal intubation with in-line immobilization is a safe, effective method for definitive airway management.[18–20]
- Using a cadaver model, Gerling and colleagues[21] showed no significant vertebral body movement during orotracheal intubation with manual in-line stabilization.
- There is no consensus that video-assisted laryngoscopy (VAL) is safer than direct laryngoscopy. Studies on this subject have mixed results:
  - ○ Robitaille and colleagues[22] concluded that there was no significant difference between direct laryngoscopy and VAL at any level
  - ○ Turkstra and colleagues[23] found that C-spine motion reduced 50% at the C2-5 segment when VAL was used
- The current Advanced Trauma Life Support (ATLS) guidelines[24] (**Figs. 7** and **8**) list orotracheal intubation with in-line manual cervical spine immobilization as the definitive airway procedure in the apneic patients with trauma.
- A surgical airway should be considered if a definitive airway is required and cannot be established using the techniques discussed earlier and while maintaining in-line stabilization.

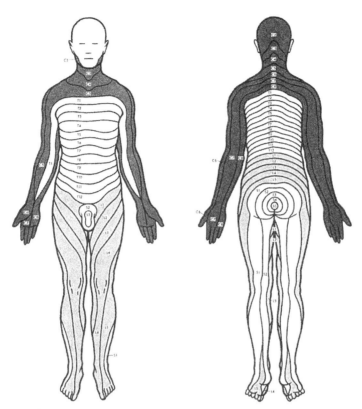

Fig. 5. Sensory dermatomes. (*From* Hockberger RS, Kirshenbaum KJ, Doris PE. Spinal injuries. In: Rosen P, Barkin R, Danzl D, et al, editors. Emergency medicine: concepts and clinical practice. 4th edition. vol. 1. St Louis (MO): Mosby; 1998. p. 482; with permission.)

Immobilization

Prehospital personnel should suspect potential cervical spine injury in all patients who have sustained significant trauma, and in any patient with altered mental status of uncertain cause.

- It is estimated that nearly 5 million patients receive spinal immobilization annually at a cost of $15 per person or $75 million a year in the United States
- The 2013 National Association of EMS Physicians and the American College of Surgeons Committee on Trauma has recommended backboard immobilization only for patients with:
  - Spinal pain or tenderness
  - Blunt trauma with altered level of consciousness
  - Neurologic complaints
  - Obvious deformity of the spine
  - High-energy impact with a distracting injury, intoxication, or inability to communicate

Patients with trauma who arrive immobilized must be evaluated quickly by EPs to determine the extent of injury, probability of cervical spine injury, and adequacy and need for ongoing immobilization.

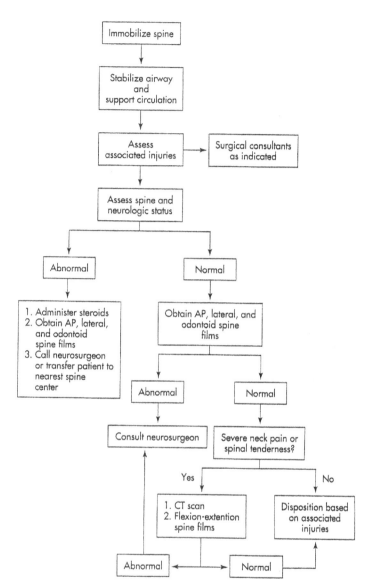

Fig. 6. Approach to patients with suspected cervical spine injury. CT, computed tomography. (*From* Kaji AH, Newton EJ, Hockberger RS. Spinal injuries. In: Marx J, Hockenberger R, Walls R, editors. Rosen's emergency medicine: concepts and clinical practice. 9th edition. St Louis (MO): Mosby; 2013; with permission.)

SHOCK

Shock (or hypotension) in multiply injured patients with trauma may have many causes, including hypovolemic, spinal/neurogenic, or (less likely) cardiogenic or distributive causes.

- Hemorrhagic shock: hypotension with tachycardia and peripheral vasoconstriction
  - Intravenous fluids while following vitals, urine output, and mental status

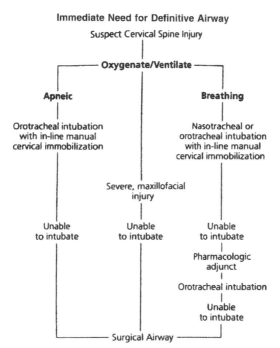

Fig. 7. Airway algorithm. Proceed according to clinical judgment and skill or experience level. (*From* Committee on Trauma. Airway and ventilatory management. In: Advanced trauma life support program for physicians. Chicago: American College of Surgeons; 1998. p. 72; with permission.)

- Neurogenic shock: hypotension, bradycardia, flaccidity, and areflexia
  - Warm, pink skin with good peripheral pulses
  - Crystalloid fluid bolus and Trendelenburg positioning

Vasopressors may be required in patients who are persistently hypotensive despite appropriate evaluation and resuscitation measures.[25]

IMAGING OF THE CERVICAL SPINE

Multiple imaging modalities are available to EPs. Plain radiographs have long been the standard initial imaging study of choice, and, in low-risk patients or those without significant mechanism of injury, they remain the first study of choice for many physicians. In patients with multiple traumatic injuries or a high suspicion for injury, many centers have moved to standard computed tomography (CT) scan of the cervical spine as part of an initial radiographic evaluation. Furthermore, MRI is becoming more widely available and many be used in cases in which there is a high level of suspicion for injury, for patients with abnormalities seen on radiograph or CT scan, or in patients for whom soft tissue or spinal cord injury are considered a part of the differential diagnosis. In addition, clinical decision rules have been developed (discussed later) to help clinicians decide which low-risk patients do not require any imaging.

Clinical Decision-making Tools

- Clinical decision-making tools have allowed EPs to make evidence-based, objective decisions about imaging, resulting in cost savings and reduced radiation exposure to patients.

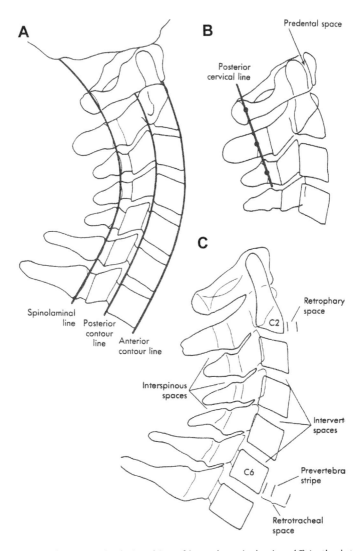

Fig. 8. (*A, B*) Normal structural relationships of lateral cervical spine. (*C*) In the lateral view, intervertebral spaces and interspinous spaces should be compared with spaces above and below for asymmetry, as important clues in flexion and extension injuries. Retropharyngeal and retrotracheal soft tissues are measured at C2 or C3 and C6 levels for swelling. (*From* Hockberger RS, Kirshenbaum KJ, Doris PE. Spinal injuries. In: Rosen P, Barkin R, Danzl D, et al, editors. Emergency medicine: concepts and clinical practice. 4th edition. vol. 1. St Louis (MO): Mosby; 1998. p. 489–90; with permission.)

- Even with low-mechanism injury (derived from dangerous mechanism in Canadian C-spine rules; **Box 2**), patients with severe osteoporosis, advanced arthritis, cancer, or degenerative bone disease have significant risk of injury and may warrant imaging even without the application of a clinical decision tool.[25]

National Emergency X-Radiography Utilization Study

- Prospectively validated in 21 EDs across the United States.[26]

- Patients who were excluded were those with penetrating trauma to the neck, or direct blows.
- In order to determine that radiographs are not necessary, a set of 5 clinical criteria must all be met (**Box 1**)[27]
  - 99.8% negative predictive value for cervical spine injury with a sensitivity of 99% and specificity of 12.9%.
    - With the low specificity, researchers were concerned that the criteria still resulted in overimaging, resulting in the development of the Canadian C-spine Rule (CCR).

Canadian C-spine Rule

- The objective of the researchers in developing the CCR was to derive a clinical rule that was highly sensitive with improved specificity to allow physicians to be more selective in the use of radiography.[28]
- Inclusion criteria: stable and alert patients with trauma who were more than 16 years of age.
- The CCR comprises 3 main questions (**Box 2**).
- By cross-validation in 10 EDs in large Canadian community and university hospitals, the CCR has 100% sensitivity and 42.5% specificity.

Comparing the Clinical Decision-making Tools

Both rules have been validated and provide useful, objective, and highly sensitive criteria that ultimately lower rates of radiographic imaging. However, much debate exists between which is superior. Inclusion criteria from the two studies differ, with the CCR not including children less than 16 years of age and patients with Glasgow Coma Scale less than 15, both of which were included in the NEXUS study. A 2003 *New England Journal of Medicine* article concluded that the CCR is superior to the NEXUS with respect to sensitivity and specificity for cervical spine injury, and its use would reduce rates of radiography.[29]

Box 1
NEXUS criteria

- No midline cervical tenderness
- No focal neurologic deficit
- Normal alertness
  - Glasgow Coma Scale of 15
  - No disorientation to person, place, time, or events
  - Ability to remember 3 objects in 5 minutes
  - Appropriate response to external stimuli
- No intoxication
- No painful, distracting injury
  - Examples: long bone fractures, visceral injury requiring surgical consultation, large lacerations, crush injuries, or large burns

Data from Hoffman JR, Wolfson AB, Todd K, et al. Selective cervical spine radiography in blunt trauma: methodology of the National Emergency X-radiography Utilization Study (NEXUS). Ann Emerg Med 1998;32(4):461.

Box 2
CCR

- Is there any high-risk factor that mandates radiography?
  - Age 65 years or older
  - Dangerous mechanism
    - Fall from 1 m (or 5 stairs)
    - Axial load to the head (eg, diving accidents)
    - Motor vehicle collisions at high speed (>100 km/h)
    - Motorized recreational vehicle accident
    - Ejection from a vehicle
    - Bicycle collision with an immovable object
  - Paresthesias in extremities
- Is there any low-risk factor that allows safe assessment of range of motion? Patients who do not have any of the following low-risk factors should be radiographed and are not suitable for range of motion testing:
  - Simple rear-end motor vehicle collision
  - Sitting position in ED
  - Ambulatory at any time since injury
  - Delayed onset of neck pain
  - Absence of midline C-spine tenderness
- Range of motion testing
  - Is the patient able to actively rotate neck 45° to the left and right (regardless of pain)? If so, imaging is not indicated

Data from Stiell IG, Wells GA, Vandemheen KL, et al. The Canadian C-spine Rule for radiography in alert and stable trauma patients. JAMA 2001;286(15):1841.

Imaging Modalities

Plain radiography

In recent years, plain radiographs have been replaced in many trauma centers by CT scan for the assessment of acute injury; however, plain films can still provide rapid assessment of alignment, fractures, and soft tissue swelling. Although there is greater detail and multiaxis reconstructions make CT examinations better suited for patients with high-risk injuries (described earlier) or high-risk patients (eg, aged 65 years or older, severe arthritis, osteoporosis), in low-risk patients with low-risk mechanisms of injury, plain radiographs may be appropriate. However, there is a paucity of large, prospective studies that focus on the utility of plain radiographs in low-risk patients.[30]

Computed tomography

The Eastern Association for the Surgery of Trauma (EAST) states that CT has supplanted plain radiography as the primary screening modality in patients who require imaging, recommending the examination scan from the occiput to T1 with sagittal and coronal reconstructions.[31]

- Holmes and Akkinepalli[32] found that the pooled sensitivity, for identifying patients with cervical spine injury, was 52% for plain radiography versus 98% for CT.

- Daffner[33] concluded that CT scan of the cervical spine takes approximately half the time taken by a 6-view cervical plain film series.
- Disadvantages of CT examination
  - Cost
    - CT may cost more than 5 times the cost of plain radiographs.
    - One study shows that CT is more cost-effective, especially in moderate-risk to high-risk patients.[34]
  - Exposure to increased ionizing radiation
    - Rybicki and colleagues[35] measured the radiation dose to the skin over the thyroid in patients undergoing cervical spine CT and plain radiography. They found that CT delivered 26.0 mGy to the thyroid versus 1.80 mGy by radiographs.
    - It is unclear what future cancer risk this single exposure to an increased radiation dose may hold.

MRI

Although the CT scan is an excellent modality for evaluating bony spine injuries, MRI may be indicated in patients who, despite a negative CT scan, have persistent midline tenderness and/or neurologic abnormalities.

- MRI provides more detailed imaging of the spinal cord, spinal canal, spinal ligaments, intervertebral discs, and paraspinal soft tissues.
- MRI may be particularly useful in the following situations:
  - Neurologic deficits caused by hemorrhage, edema, or injury to the cord
  - Determining acuity of bony injuries
  - Assessment of vascular injury (MRI and magnetic resonance arteriography)[25]
- Disadvantages of MRI
  - High false-positive rate (as high as 40% of findings are either incidental or would not change management)[36]
  - Contraindication with some cardiac pacemakers and other implanted devices or metallic objects
  - Enclosed space and duration, which makes it difficult for unstable patients

Spinal Cord Injury Without Radiographic Abnormality

Before the advent of MRI, spinal cord injury without radiographic abnormality (SCIWORA) was a term assigned to patients who had ongoing neurologic deficits despite normal imaging (radiograph and/or CT scan). With the increased use of MRI and better imaging of the spinal cord, ligaments, and vasculature, the incidence of SCIWORA has decreased dramatically.[37] Permanent neurologic injury is rare and most patients who have SCIWORA ultimately see resolution of their symptoms and return to baseline function.[38]

TYPES OF CERVICAL SPINE INJURIES

Cervical spine injuries have been variably classified according to mechanism of injury, stability, and morphology of injury. **Table 2** combines mechanism of injury with stability. **Table 3** shows the classification system developed by the Orthopedic Trauma Association. Spinal instability can be difficult to assess; therefore, **Table 4** provides a checklist to assist in the determination of subaxial stability.

Upper Cervical Spine Injuries

Common upper cervical spine injuries are described here. Note that a stable injury refers to either the anterior or posterior column being injured, but not both columns (although unstable refers to both columns being injured).

Table 2
Classification of spinal injuries

Mechanisms of Spinal Injury	Stability
Flexion	
Wedge fraction	Stable
Flexion teardrop fracture	Extremely
Clay shoveler's fracture	Stable
Subluxation	Potentially unstable
Bilateral facet dislocation	Always unstable
Atlanto-occipital dislocation	Unstable
Anterior atlantoaxial dislocation with or without fracture	Unstable
Odontoid fracture with lateral displacement fracture	Unstable
Fracture of transverse process	Stable
Flexion-Rotation	
Unilateral facet dislocation	Stable
Rotary atlantoaxial dislocation	Unstable
Extension	
Posterior neural arch fracture (C1)	Unstable
Hangman's fracture (C2)	Unstable
Extension teardrop fracture	Usually stable in extension
Posterior atlantoaxial dislocation with or without fracture	Unstable
Vertical Compression	
Bursting fracture of vertebral body	Stable
Jefferson fracture (C1)	Extremely
Isolated fractures of articular pillar and vertebral body	Stable

From Hockberger RS, Kirshenbaum KJ, Doris PE. Spinal injuries. In: Rosen P, Barkin R, Danzl DF, et al, editors. Emergency medicine: concepts and clinical practice. 4th edition. vol. 1. St Louis (MO): Mosby–Year Book, 1998. p. 481; with permission.

Atlanto-occipital dislocation

Atlanto-occipital dislocation (AOD) is typically a fatal injury secondary to severe injury to the brainstem. AOD is a general term for functional instability at the occipitocervical junction and manifests as subluxation or dislocation at the atlanto-occipital joint, the atlantoaxial joint, or both.[39]

- This injury usually results from severe hyperextension with distraction[40] but can also occur with lateral flexion and hyperflexion.[41]
- There are 3 types.[42]
  - Type I: most common type of AOD; the cranium moves anterior with respect to the atlas
  - Type II: the most common type in children; a longitudinal distraction of the occiput from the atlas
  - Type III: the cranium is displaced posteriorly with respect to the atlas
- Radiograph findings in AOD are shown in **Figs. 9** and **10**.[16,43]
- If a hanging mechanism is reported, obtain a CT scan because plain radiographs may not show all injuries.
- Acute management
  - ATLS and immobilization with a halo vest followed by occipitocervical surgical fixation is the usual treatment

Table 3
Cervical spine trauma classification of the Orthopedic Trauma Association

51	Upper cervical spine
51	AI: occipital cervical dislocation A1.1: anterior A1.2: vertical A1.3: posterior
51	A2: cervical spine, occipital condyle A2.1: type 1 A2.2: type 2 A2.3: type 3
51	A3: atlas A3.1: Jefferson A3.2: lateral mass A3.3: posterior arch A3.4: anterior arch
51	B1: cervical spine, transverse ligament B1.1: rupture midsubstance B1.2: rupture avulsion
51	B2: cervical spine, dens fracture B2.1: type 1 B2.2: type 2 B2.2.2: type 2a B2.3: type 3
51	C: cervical spine traumatic spondylolisthesis of the axis C1: type 1 C2: type 2 C2.2: type 2a C3: type 3
52	Lower cervical spine
52	A1.1: spinous process fracture A1.2: extension avulsion or teardrop A1.3: lateral mass fracture without subluxation A1.4: isolated lamina fracture A1.5: ligamentous strain
52	B1.1: facet injury B1.1.1: perched unilateral Bl.1.2: perched bilateral
52	B2.2.1: facet dislocation B2.2.1: without fracture unilateral B2.2.2: without fracture bilateral B3.3.1: with displacement unilateral B3.3.2: with displacement bilateral
52	C: severe injuries C1.1: flexion teardrop C2.1: severe ligamentous injury C3.1: compression fracture C3.2: burst fracture

From Finkelstein JA, Anderson PA. Surgical management of cervical instability. In: Capen DA, Haye W, editors. Comprehensive management of spine trauma. St Louis (MO): Mosby–Year Book, 1998. p. 146; with permission.

Table 4
Checklist for the diagnosis of clinical instability in the lower cervical spine

Element	Point Value
Anterior element destroyed or unable to function	2
Posterior element destroyed or unable to function	2
Relative sagittal plane translation >3.5 mm	2
Relative sagittal plane rotation >11°	2
Positive stretch test	2
Spinal cord damage	2
Root damage	1
Abnormal disk narrowing	1
Dangerous loading anticipated	1
Developmentally narrow spinal canal	1

Total of 5 or more indicates clinical instability.
From Finkelstein JA, Anderson PA. Surgical management of cervical instability. In: Capen DA, Haye W, editors. Comprehensive management of spine trauma. St Louis (MO): Mosby–Year Book, 1998. p. 146; with permission.

Fracture of the atlas

Fractures of the atlas are usually the result of compressive forces resulting from motor vehicle collisions, falls, or diving into shallow water.

- From 3% to 13% of all cervical spine fractures[44]
- Nearly 40% are associated with a fracture of the axis (C2)
- Accompanying neurologic injury is uncommon
- Three common patterns of atlas fractures:
  - ○ Posterior arch fractures: most common fracture pattern
    - ■ Stable fractures of the posterior arch and lateral masses
    - ■ Treatment: Philadelphia-style collar

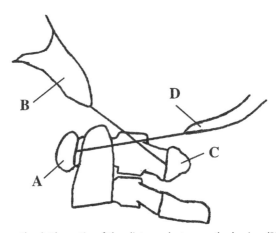

Fig. 9. The Power method. The ratio of the distance between the basion (B) and the anterior aspect of the posterior arch of C1 (C) to the distance between the opisthion (D) and the posterior aspect of the anterior arch of C1 (A), BC/DA, is normally less than 1.0. (*From* Ferrera PC, Bartfield JM. Traumatic atlanto-occipital dislocation: a potentially survivable injury. Am J Emerg Med 1996;14:294; with permission.)

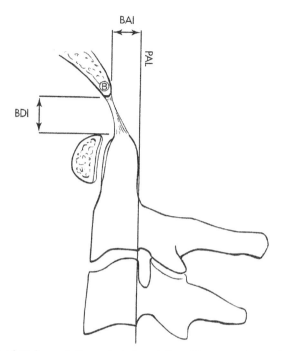

Fig. 10. The rule of 12 for occipitocervical dissociation. The posterior axial line (PAL) is the rostral extension of the posterior cortex of the axis body. The basion-axial interval (BAI) is the horizontal distance between the basion (B) and the PAL. The basion-dens interval (BDI) is the vertical distance between the basion and the tip of the dens. Values in excess of 12 mm for the BAI or BDI suggest occipitocervical dissociation. (*From* Finkelstein JA, Anderson PA. Surgical management of cervical instability. In: Capen DA, Haye W, editors. Comprehensive management of spine trauma. St Louis (MO): Mosby; 1998. p. 154; with permission.)

- ○ Jefferson or burst fracture (**Fig. 11**)
  - ▪ Disruption of both the anterior and posterior rings of C1 with displacement of the lateral masses
    - • Lateral mass displacement greater than or equal to 7 to 8 mm of instability at C1-C2
  - ▪ Treatment
    - • Stable: external immobilization
    - • Unstable: potential operative fixation
  - ○ Fractures of the lateral masses are uncommon
- • Treat as potentially unstable until evaluated by neurosurgery or orthopedics

Atlantoaxial ligamentous injuries
These injuries occur secondary to flexion or extension forces that could be combined with rotation. Recall that the transverse ligament prevents anterior movement of the atlas on the axis, and the alar ligaments prevent excessive rotation.

- • Atlantoaxial subluxation: tears of the transverse ligament widened predental space
- • Rotary subluxation: atlantoaxial subluxation plus C2 being abnormally rotated with respect to C1 (**Fig. 12**)[45]

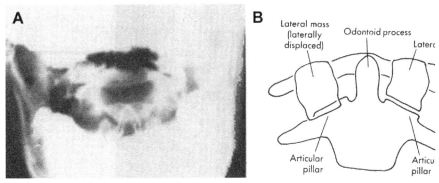

Fig. 11. Jefferson fracture. (*A, B*) Unilateral or bilateral lateral displacement of lateral masses of C1 with respect to articular pillars of C2 confirms Jefferson fracture. (*From* Hockberger RS, Kirshenbaum KJ, Doris PE. Spinal injuries. In: Rosen P, Barkin R, Danzl D, et al, editors. Emergency medicine: concepts and clinical practice. 4th edition. vol. 1. St Louis (MO): Mosby; 1998. p. 478; with permission.)

- Atlantoaxial rotatory dislocation or rotary (rotatory) fixation
  - Rotational dislocation of the articular sources of C1 on C2 owing to alar ligament injury
  - Occurs more commonly in children
  - Seen following trauma, surgery, an upper respiratory infection, or with rheumatoid arthritis
  - The open-mouth odontoid view shows an abnormal relationship between the atlas and axis that does not change on rotation of the head (**Fig. 13**)
    - Whenever ligamentous injury is suspected, MRI should be obtained
- Treatment includes cervical collar immobilization and emergency neurosurgical or orthopedic consultation

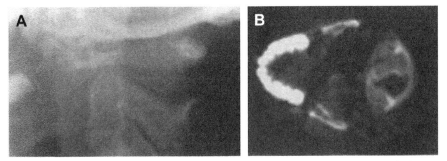

Fig. 12. Rotary subluxation. (*A*) Lateral radiograph of craniocervical junction reveals the ring of C1 to be properly oriented with respect to the base of the skull, but there is abnormal rotation between C1 and C2. (*B*) Axial CT scan of another patient who crashed into a tree on a snow sled shows that the head is oriented 90° to the cervical spine because of facet subluxation. (*From* Rothman SL. Imaging of spinal trauma pearls and pitfalls. In: Capen DA, Haye W, editors. Comprehensive management of spine trauma. St Louis (MO): Mosby; 1998. p. 52; with permission.)

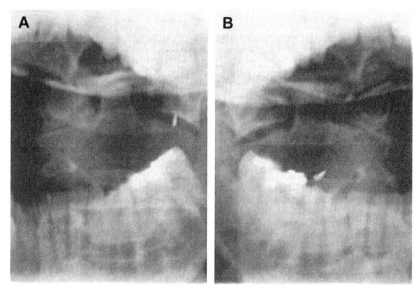

Fig. 13. Rotary fixation. Frontal radiographs of the craniovertebral junction through the open mouth with the patient's head turned to the right (*A*) and to the left (*B*) reveal consistent malposition of the dens with respect to the lateral masses of C1. The distance between the dens and the lateral mass is narrow on the same side regardless of the direction of rotation of the head. (*From* Rothman SL. Imaging of spinal trauma pearls and pitfalls. In: Capen DA, Haye W, editors. Comprehensive management of spine trauma. St Louis (MO): Mosby; 1998. p. 53; with permission.)

Fractures of the dens

Acute fractures of the axis (C2) represent 18% of all cervical fractures, and nearly 60% of these involve the dens or odontoid process. Fractures of the dens are high-energy injuries sustained in falls or motor vehicle collisions.

- Neurologic injury occurs in approximately 25% of these fractures
- There are 3 types of odontoid fractures (**Fig. 14**)[46]
  - Type I: uncommon (2%–3% of odontoid fractures) and appear as a fracture to the tip of the dens that occurs after an avulsion of the alar ligaments. This is a stable injury and is managed with external mobilization.[47]
  - Type II: most common (60%), and occurs through the waist of the dens near the attachment of ligaments
    - Most are displaced and unstable
    - Controversial management
      - High rates (30%–60%) of nonunion using external immobilization have led some clinicians to advocate surgical fixation as the primary treatment
  - Type III: occur at the very base of the dens into the body of the axis
    - Stable and managed with reduction using skeletal traction with light weight followed by immobilization with the halo vest
    - Nonunion fractures need surgical fixation

Traumatic spondylolisthesis of the axis

These injuries involve fractures through the posterior elements of C2 (**Fig. 15**).

- From 5% to 10% of all cervical spine fractures

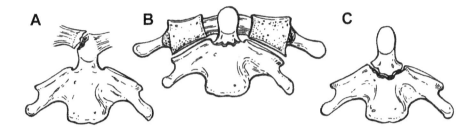

Fig. 14. Anderson-DeAlarzo classification of odontoid fractures. (*A*) Type I, avulsion fractures of the alar ligament. (*B*) Type II, fractures through the waist of the odontoid caudad to the transverse ligament. (*C*) Type III, fractures into the cancellous body of the axis. (*From* Nelson AW. Nonsurgical management of cervical spine instability. In: Capen OA, Hays W, editors. Comprehensive management of spine trauma. St Louis (MO): Mosby; 1998. p. 137; with permission.)

- Neurologic deficits are rare because the anteroposterior diameter of the spinal canal is greatest at C2 and the bilateral pedicle fractures allow decompression

The Hangman's fracture

- Occurs with extreme hyperextension (**Fig. 16**).
  - Motor vehicle collisions and diving accidents
- Consider these fractures unstable injuries and continue external immobilization

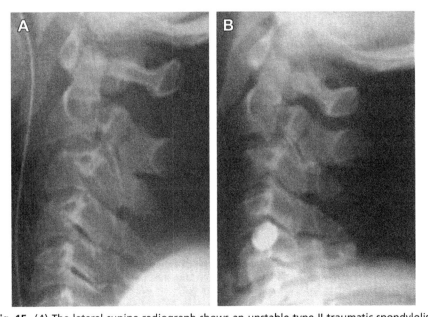

Fig. 15. (*A*) The lateral supine radiograph shows an unstable type II traumatic spondylolisthesis of the axis in a 41-year-old man. Closed reduction with traction and halo-vest immobilization was performed. (*B*) An upright radiograph showed loss of reduction with an increase in anterior translation. (*From* Finkelstein JA, Anderson PA. Surgical management of cervical instability. In: Capen DA, Haye W, editors. Comprehensive management of spine trauma. St Louis (MO): Mosby; 1998. p. 166; with permission.)

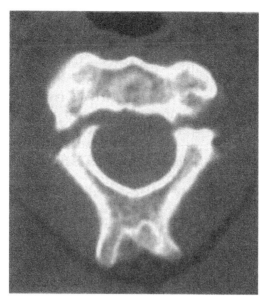

Fig. 16. Hangman's fracture. Axial CT scan shows traumatic spondylolysis of the 2 sides of the neural arch just posterior to the body of the axis. (*From* Rothman SL. Imaging of spinal trauma pearls and pitfalls. In: Capen DA, Haye W, editors. Comprehensive management of spine trauma. St Louis (MO): Mosby; 1998. p. 61; with permission.)

- Nonsurgical management is successful in more than 95% of cases

Other injuries of the atlas and axis

- Avulsion fracture of the anterior arch of the atlas
  - Rare injury caused by hyperextension forces[48]
  - The lateral radiograph reveals a horizontal fracture line through the anterior arch of the atlas with associated prevertebral soft tissue swelling
- Extension teardrop fracture
  - Avulsion of the anterior inferior corner of the body of the atlas
  - Result of hyperextension forces applied to an intact anterior longitudinal ligament
  - Risk factors: older patients with osteopenia or cervical spondylosis

Subaxial Cervical Spine Injuries

Fractures and dislocations of the subaxial cervical spine (C3–C7) are best categorized according to mechanism of injury.

- C5 is the most commonly fractured
- C5 on C6 is the most common site of subluxation
- Smaller diameter of the spinal canal leads to an increased incidence of neurologic injury at these levels

Cervical hyperflexion injuries

- Posterior ligamentous injuries:
  - Range from mild to severe
  - Focal tenderness but no focal neurologic deficits

- o Severe injuries with complete ligamentous disruption lead to cervical spine instability and anterior subluxation of the vertebral body
- o Radiographs
  - ▪ Normal or may show subtle findings (**Fig. 17**)
  - ▪ Initial radiographs and/or CT appear normal, and/or if the patient shows persistent tenderness MRI should be ordered
- o Treatment
  - ▪ Rigid cervical collar immobilization for mild, stable ligamentous injuries
  - ▪ Posterior cervical fusion for severe, unstable ligamentous injuries
- • Wedge or compression fracture
  - o Hyperflexion forces lead to impaction of one vertebra against another
  - o Diminished height and increased concavity of the anterior border of the vertebral body, increased density of the vertebral body from bony impaction, and prevertebral soft tissue swelling (**Fig. 18**)
  - o Stable without accompanying neurologic deficit
- • Flexion teardrop fracture
  - o Characterized by the presence of a triangular body fragment at the anteroinferior aspect of the involved vertebral body
  - o Often accompanied by severe ligament and intervertebral disk injury (**Fig. 19**)[49]
  - o Fragments can also be produced by downward displacement of the anterior edge of the superior endplate
  - o Unstable and often associated with severe neurologic injury

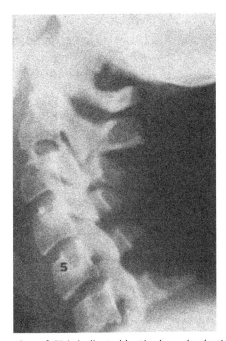

Fig. 17. Anterior subluxation of C5 is indicated by the hyperkyphotic angulation at the C5-C6 level secondary to anterior rotation and translation of C5, resulting in widening of the interspinous and interlaminar space, subluxation of the C5-C6 interfacetal joints, and posterior widening and anterior narrowing of the fifth intervertebral disk space. (*From* Harris JH, Edeiken-Monroe B, Kopaniky DR. A practical clarification of acute cervical spine injuries. Orthop Clin North Am 1986;17:17.)

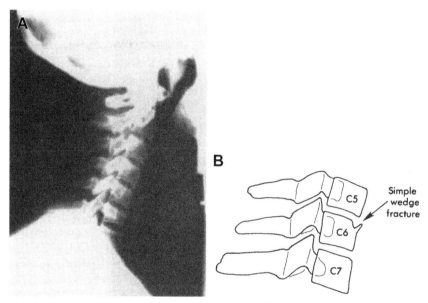

Fig. 18. (*A, B*) Lateral view of a simple wedge fracture. Note decrease in height of anterior aspect of C6 vertebral body. (*From* Hockberger RS, Kirshenbaum KJ, Doris PE. Spinal injuries. In: Rosen P, Barkin R, Danzl D, et al, editors. Emergency medicine: concepts and clinical practice. 4th edition. vol. 1. St Louis (MO): Mosby; 1998. p. 467; with permission.)

- ○ Treatment: reduction followed by surgical fixation
- Bilateral facet dislocation (**Fig. 20**)
  - ○ Severe injury characterized by 50% or greater anterior translation of the vertebral body
  - ○ Extremely unstable and often accompanied by severe spinal cord injury
  - ○ May be associated with vertebral artery injury or occlusion
  - ○ Treatment: reduction followed by surgical stabilization
- Clay shoveler's fracture (**Fig. 21**)
  - ○ Most commonly results from direct trauma to the spinous process (eg, weight lifters who drop a loaded bar onto their neck from overhead), sudden deceleration in motor vehicle collisions, or forced flexion of the neck
  - ○ Stable and not typically associated with neurologic deficits

Rotational injuries

- Unilateral facet dislocation (**Fig. 22**)
  - ○ Combined cervical flexion with simultaneous rotation
  - ○ The dislocated facet becomes wedged into the intervertebral foramen; this is a stable injury
  - ○ Radiographic findings
    - ■ Lateral view
      - From 25% to 50% anterior translation of the vertebral body
      - The bowtie sign (ie, visualization of both of the facets at the level of the injury instead of their normal superimposed position)
      - Widening of the spinous processes[50]
    - ■ Frontal view

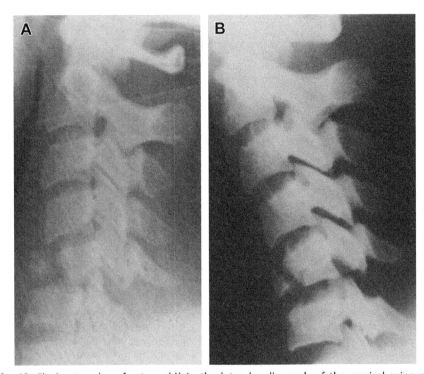

Fig. 19. Flexion teardrop fracture. (*A*) In the lateral radiograph of the cervical spine obtained immediately after the injury, the cervical spine is in the flexed attitude. A single large fragment consisting of the anteroinferior corner of the body of C5 is present. The fifth vertebral body is posteriorly displaced and, in addition, widening of the interfacetal and interspinous spaces between C5 and C6 indicates complete disruption of the posterior ligament complex and bilateral interfacetal dislocation. (*B*) In the lateral examination performed 2 weeks after the injury, the characteristic teardrop-shaped fragment is seen. In addition, the subjacent intervertebral disc space is abnormally widened, as are the interfacetal and interspinous spaces, indicating complete soft tissue disruption at the involved level. (*From* Adam A, Dixon AK, Grainger RG, et al. Grainger and Allison's diagnostic radiology. 5th edition. Philadelphia: Churchill Livingstone; 2008; with permission.)

- Spinous processes above the level of dislocation displaced to the same side as the dislocated facet
- Oblique views
  - May show the dislocated facet sitting in the neural foramen
- Unilateral facet dislocations can occur with or without associated fractures
- The patient may be neurologically intact or may show signs and symptoms consistent with nerve root injury, or incomplete or complete cord injuries
- Treatment
  - Closed reduction and halo-vest immobilization can be used for pure unilateral facet dislocations
  - Reduction with surgical management is used for fracture-dislocations and failures of closed reduction attempts

Cervical hyperextension injuries

Extension teardrop fractures, as described earlier (**Fig. 23**), may involve the axis or lower cervical (C5–C7) vertebrae. Extension teardrop and other hyperextension

A   **B**

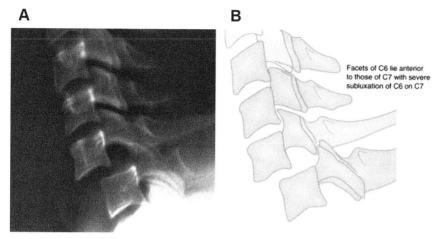

Facets of C6 lie anterior to those of C7 with severe subluxation of C6 on C7

Fig. 20. (*A, B*) Bilateral facet dislocation. Facets of C6 lie anterior to those of C7 with severe subluxation of C6 on C7. (*From* Kaji AH, Newton EJ, Hockberger RS. Spinal injuries. In: Marx J, Hockenberger R, Walls R, editors. Rosen's emergency medicine: concepts and clinical practice. 9th edition. St Louis (MO): Mosby; 2013; with permission.)

injuries are associated with variable degrees of cord injuries, including transient neurologic deficits, central cord syndrome (described later), or complete quadriplegia. Definitive management depends on imaging studies and can include reduction, decompression, and fusion.

Compression injuries
A burst fracture of the lower cervical spine (**Fig. 24**) is a comminuted fracture of the vertebral body. The nucleus pulposus is forced into the vertebral body from severe compression forces, causing the vertebral body to shatter outward from within.

- Radiographs
  - Lateral view: comminuted vertebral body fracture
  - Anteroposterior view: vertical fracture
- CT imaging
  - Obtain to show the position of the fracture fragments in relationship to the spinal canal
- Stable (all ligaments remain intact)
- Neurologic injury depends on degree of fragment retropulsion into the spinal canal
- Treatment
  - Nonsurgical treatment includes reduction with alignment and immobilization
  - Surgery is indicated for unstable injuries and inadequate closed reduction and decompression

ASSOCIATED INJURIES
Spinal Cord Injuries

A complete spinal cord injury is defined as total loss of sensory and/or motor function below a certain level. If any motor or sensory function remains (eg, sacral sparing), it is an incomplete injury and the prognosis for recovery is significantly better.

- Sacral sparing: persistent perianal sensation, rectal sphincter tone, or great toe flexor movement

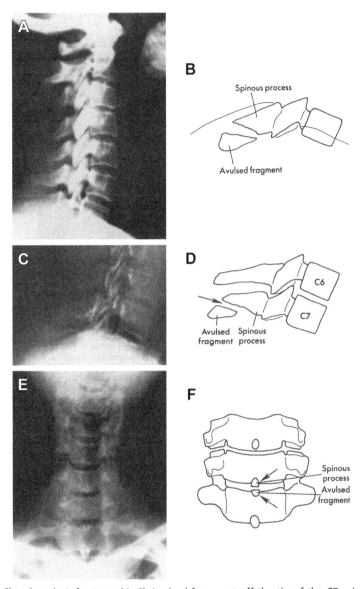

Fig. 21. Clay shoveler's fracture. (*A, B*) Avulsed fragment off the tip of the C7 spinous process in underpenetrated lateral view. (*C, D*) Avulsed fragment off the tip of the C7 spinous process in coned lateral view. (*E, F*) Vertically split appearance of the C7 spinous process confirms fracture in anteroposterior view. (*From* Hockberger RS, Kirshenbaum KJ, Doris PE. Spinal injuries. In: Rosen P, Barkin R, Danzl D, et al, editors. Emergency medicine: concepts and clinical practice. 4th edition. vol. 1. St Louis (MO): Mosby; 1998. p. 468; with permission.)

- Sensory level: most caudal segment with normal sensory function on both sides
- Motor level: lowest level providing key muscle innervation that maintains antigravity strength postinjury (see **Fig. 5, Table 1**)

Spinal shock is the flaccidity and loss of reflexes seen after a spinal cord injury.

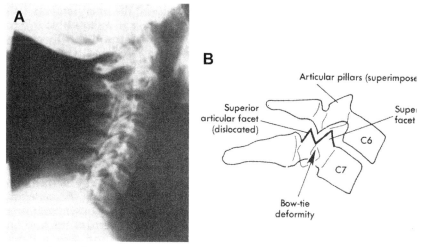

Fig. 22. Unilateral facet dislocation. (*A, B*) Dislocated superior articulating facet of C7 forms bow tie deformity with nondislocated superior articulating facet on the lateral view. C6 vertebral body is anteriorly subluxed on the C7 vertebral body. (*From* Hockberger RS, Kirshenbaum KJ, Doris PE. Spinal injuries. In: Rosen P, Barkin R, Danzl D, et al, editors. Emergency medicine: concepts and clinical practice. 4th edition. vol. 1. St Louis (MO): Mosby; 1998. p. 472; with permission.)

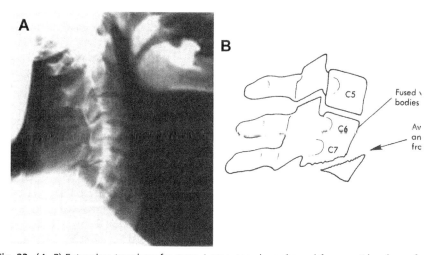

Fig. 23. (*A, B*) Extension teardrop fracture. Large, teardrop-shaped fragment has been fractured off the anteroinferior aspect of the C7 vertebral body. This avulsed fragment may be large or small and is caused by a pull on the anterior longitudinal ligament. (*From* Hockberger RS, Kirshenbaum KJ, Doris PE. Spinal injuries. In: Rosen P, Barkin R, Danzl D, et al, editors. Emergency medicine: concepts and clinical practice. 4th edition. vol. 1. St Louis (MO): Mosby; 1998. p. 476; with permission.)

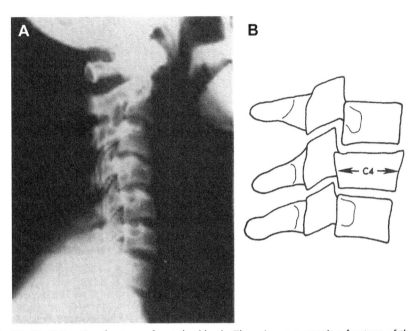

Fig. 24. (*A, B*) Bursting fracture of vertebral body. There is a compression fracture of the C4 vertebral body. During the bursting process the anterior aspect of the vertebral body protrudes anteriorly, and its posterior aspect protrudes into the spinal canal. This fracture is often associated with the anterior cord syndrome. (*From* Hockberger RS, Kirshenbaum KJ, Doris PE. Spinal injuries. In: Rosen P, Barkin R, Danzl D, et al, editors. Emergency medicine: concepts and clinical practice. 4th edition. vol. 1. St Louis (MO): Mosby; 1998. p. 477; with permission.)

- May cause an incomplete spinal cord injury to mimic a complete cord injury in the acute setting
- Concussive injury that usually lasts less than 24 hours

Neurogenic shock refers to the state produced by loss of vasomotor tone and sympathetic innervation of the heart.

- Vasodilation leads to hypotension
- No tachycardia or delayed capillary refill

Incomplete spinal cord injuries are often recognized by certain patterns of neurologic involvement, with approximately 90% of incomplete spinal injuries being classified as one of the 3 distinct clinical syndromes (**Fig. 25**).

- Central cord syndrome
  - Hyperextension injury in a patient with cervical canal narrowing secondary to degenerative arthritis
  - Ligamentum flavum is thought to buckle into the cord causing injury to central gray matter and central portions of pyramidal and spinothalamic tracts
  - Weakness in upper extremities more than in the lower extremities
  - Variable sensory loss
  - The injury can occur with or without cervical spine fracture or dislocation
- Anterior cord syndrome
  - Flexion injuries that result in cord contusion, protrusion of bony fragments, or herniated disks into the spinal canal

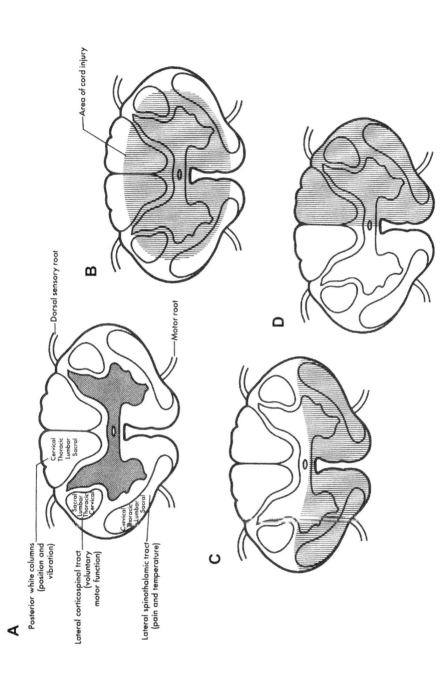

Fig. 25. Incomplete spinal cord syndromes. (*A*) Cervical spinal cord. (*B*) Anterior cord syndrome. (*C*) Central cord syndrome. (*D*) Brown-Séquard syndrome. (*From* Hockberger RS, Kirshenbaum KJ, Doris PE. Spinal injuries. In: Rosen P, Barkin R, Danzl D, et al, editors. Emergency medicine: concepts and clinical practice. 4th edition. vol. 1. St Louis (MO): Mosby; 1998. p. 483; with permission.)

Posterior white columns (position and vibration)

Dorsal sensory root

Cervical
Thoracic
Lumbar
Sacral

Sacral
Lumbar
Thoracic
Cervical

Cervical
Thoracic
Lumbar
Sacral

Lateral corticospinal tract (voluntary motor function)

Motor root

Lateral spinothalamic tract (pain and temperature)

Area of cord injury

- ○ Anterior spinal artery injury, thrombosis, or laceration causes anterior cord syndrome
- ○ Bilateral paralysis and decreased sensation to painful stimuli below the level of injury, with preservation of posterior column functions
- ○ Poorest prognosis of the incomplete spinal injuries
- Brown-Séquard syndrome
  - ○ Hemisection of the spinal cord
  - ○ Rare; usually resulting from penetrating injuries but can be seen following lateral mass fractures
  - ○ Loss of ipsilateral motor and posterior columns function associated with contralateral sensory loss beginning 1 or 2 levels below the injury
  - ○ MRI is the imaging modality of choice
  - ○ Treatment
    - ▪ Directed at the cause (eg, fracture, penetrating or blunt trauma) and recovery of function and depends on the severity and cause of injury

Glucocorticoid and Cooling: Use for Traumatic Spinal Cord Injury

Once considered standard of care, the benefit of methylprednisolone in traumatic spinal cord injury (TSCI) has limited evidence and is the subject of much debate. In animal studies, early use of glucocorticoids reduced spinal cord edema and thus improved neurologic recovery.[51] However, randomized controlled trials have shown limited efficacy and perhaps adverse outcomes in certain patient groups.

- NASCIS II (National Acute Spinal Cord Injury Studies II)[52]
  - ○ Reviewed the 1-year follow-up data of a multicenter randomized controlled trial of methylprednisolone for TSCI
    - ▪ Glucocorticoids within 8 hours of injury
      - Modest increased recovery of neurologic function
    - ▪ Glucocorticoids more than 8 hours from injury
      - Recovered less motor function than placebo
- NASCIS III[53]
  - ○ Included both complete and incomplete TSCI
  - ○ Compared the 3 treatment groups of methylprednisolone for 24 hours, methylprednisolone for 48 hours, and tirilazad mesylate (lipid peroxidation inhibitor) for 48 hours
  - ○ Treatment within 3 hours of injury
    - ▪ Methylprednisolone for 24 hours was most effective
  - ○ Treatment between 3 and 8 hours of injury
    - ▪ Methylprednisolone for 48 hours is more appropriate
- Complications of high-dose glucocorticoid therapy
  - ○ Higher risk of infection[54]
  - ○ In 2013, the American Association of Neurological Surgeons and Congress of Neurological Surgeons stated that use of glucocorticoids in TSCI is not indicated[55]
- Cooling for spinal cord injuries
  - ○ In 2011, investigators found improved spinal cord injury outcomes with mild hypothermia in a rat model[56]
  - ○ A recent prospective study was done in 20 patients with neurologically complete spinal cord injury treated with a combination of surgical decompression, glucocorticoid administration, and regional hypothermia
    - ▪ Outcomes

- Improved outcomes compared with expected outcomes for these injuries
- Unclear whether the improvements were related solely to cooling
■ Debate
  - The appropriate cooling temperature and method are unknown[57]
  - Further research is needed to determine the risks and benefits of cooling, as well as the proper timing and temperature

Vascular Injuries

Although vascular injuries (**Figs. 26** and **27**) accompanying blunt trauma to the neck are considered rare, injuries to the vertebral artery,[58] vertebrobasilar circulation,[59] cervical part of the internal carotid,[60] and distal innominate artery[61] have been reported.

- Vertebral artery injuries: 0.9% to 46% of patients with cervical spine fractures
  - Bone fragments found within the foramen transversarium are predictive for vertebral artery injury (**Fig. 28**)[62]
- Consider when a clinically apparent level of neurologic deficit does not correlate with known level of spinal injury or in the patient with cervical spine trauma and altered mental status without an identified brain injury

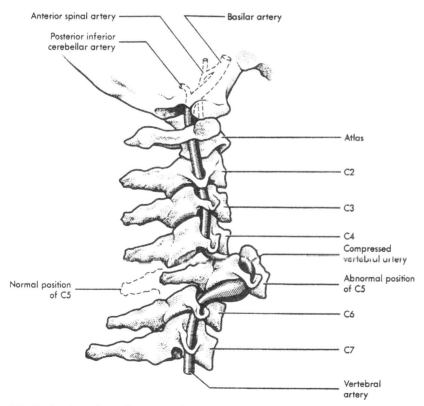

Fig. 26. Mechanism of vascular injury of spinal cord resulting from cervical vertebral injury. (*From* Hockberger RS, Kirshenbaum KJ, Doris PE. Spinal injuries. In: Rosen P, Barkin R, Danzl D, et al, editors. Emergency medicine: concepts and clinical practice. 4th edition. vol. 1. St Louis (MO): Mosby; 1998. p. 480; with permission.)

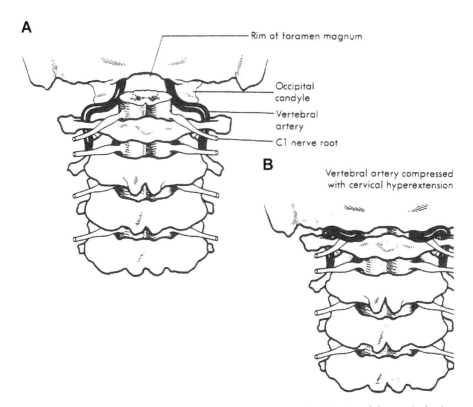

Fig. 27. (*A, B*) Mechanism of vertebral artery injury in extension injuries of the cervical spine. (*From* Hockberger RS, Kirshenbaum KJ, Doris PE. Spinal injuries. In: Rosen P, Barkin R, Danzl D, et al, editors. Emergency medicine: concepts and clinical practice. 4th edition. vol. 1. St Louis (MO): Mosby; 1998. p. 484; with permission.)

- Diagnostic imaging
  - MRI, magnetic resonance angiography, or conventional angiography

Soft Tissue Injuries

Soft tissue injuries to the neck following motor vehicle collisions are common. Motor vehicle trauma with a whiplash mechanism occurs approximately 1 million times per year in the United States.[63] The soft tissue neck injury is termed hyperextension strain, acceleration-deceleration injury, hyperextension/hyperflexion injury, cervical strain, cervical sprain, and whiplash. The symptom complex of protracted pain originates from the rich sensory innervation of cervical structures and trauma to muscle groups of this region (**Table 5**).

- Sudden acceleration-deceleration trauma
- Seat belt restraints are effective in reducing the frequency of serious injuries and death; however, cervical strain occurs more frequently in occupants using shoulder belts than in unrestrained occupants[64]
- Pathologic findings have been inconsistent,[65] but several investigators have attempted to better define the mechanism of whiplash injuries[66]
- Treatment

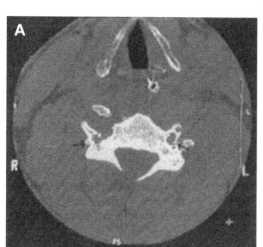
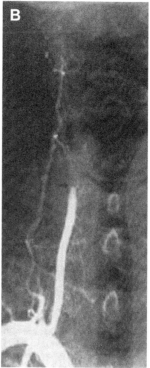

Fig. 28. (*A*) Axial CT image through C5 from a 56-year-old man who sustained a bilateral facet dislocation. He initially presented with a complete quadriplegia and a normal mental status but rapidly had deterioration in mental status. There were bilateral fractures of the foramen transversarium (*arrows*). Bone fragments are present in the right foramen. CT scan of the head was normal. (*B*) Following closed reduction using cranial tongs traction, vertebral angiography showed injury to both vertebral arteries. Complete cutoff of dye is visible in the right vertebral artery (*arrow*). (*From* Finkelstein JA, Anderson PA. Surgical management of cervical instability. In: Capon DA, Hays W, editors. Comprehensive management of spine trauma. St Louis (MO): Mosby; 1998. p. 149; with permission.)

- Rest, analgesics, nonsteroidal antiinflammatory drugs, sedatives, muscle relaxants, and physiotherapy
- Borchgrevnik and colleagues[67] found that patients who were instructed to return to normal preinjury activities had better outcomes than those who received soft neck-collar immobilization and sick leave for 14 days

INJURED ATHLETE

Injuries to the cervical spine can occur in any contact or collision sport or recreational activity.[68] The most common sports associated with vertebral column injury in the United States are football and wrestling, with C5 being the most commonly injured level.[69] Neurologic deficit from cervical spine trauma most commonly occurs in football, wrestling, and gymnastics (**Table 6**). Whether functioning as a team physician, providing sideline coverage for a competition, or evaluating athletes with cervical spine injuries in the ED, EPs should be familiar with particular issues related to on-field evaluation, special immobilization techniques, protective equipment, and return-to-play criteria.

Table 5
Cervical spine musculature

Movement	Muscle
Flexion	Sternomastoid Longus colli Longus capitis Rectus capitis anterior
Extension	Splenius capitis and cervicis Semispinalis capitis and cervicis Longissimus capitis and cervicis Trapezius and interspinales Rectus capitis posterior major and minor Obliquus capitis superior
Rotation and bend	Sternomastoid Scalenes Levator scapulae and multifidi Intercostalis and longus colli Rectus capitis lateralis

From Capen DA. Soft tissue injuries to the spine from acceleration-deceleration trauma. In: Capen DA, Haye W, editors. Comprehensive management of spine trauma. St Louis (MO): Mosby–Year Book; 1998. p. 97; with permission.

Table 6
Frequency and selected characteristics of spinal cord injuries by sport

Sport Activity	Cases No.	%	Age (y) Mean	Range	Male	White	Quadriplegia	Recreation[a]	Skilled[b]
Aquatics	97	66	21	13–47	90	91	99	100	52
Snow sports	9	6	27	17–54	89	89	33	89	50
Football	9	6	20	14–37	100	100	100	67	22
Gymnastics	8	5	18	13–21	88	100	100	88	25
Cycling	7	4	24	14–57	100	100	43	86	43
Equestrian	5	3	28	19–42	100	80	60	60	80
Hang gliding	4	3	38	21–64	75	100	25	100	75
Wrestling	3	2	20	17–22	100	100	100	100	0
Rugby	2	1	21	20–22	100	100	100	0	100
Track and field	1	1	18	—	100	100	100	0	100
Lacrosse	1	1	17	—	100	100	100	100	100
Ice skating	1	1	22	—	100	100	100	100	100
Frisbee	1	1	Unknown	—	100	100	100	100	Unknown
Total	148	100	—	—	—	—	—	—	—
Average	—	—	22	13–64	92	93	91	92	50
sans Aquatics	51	34	23	14–64	94	96	78	78	46

[a] Not a participant in an organized class or team when injured.
[b] Adept in the skills of the sport in which injured.
    From Clarke KS. Epidemiology of athletic neck injury. Clin Sports Med 1998;17:87; and *Adapted from* Clarke K. Sport-related permanent spinal cord injuries, 1980–1982. Phoenix (AZ): A report to the National Spinal Cord Injury Data Research Center; 1983.

- On-field assessment
  - Marks and colleagues[68] developed an algorithm for the initial evaluation of the injured athlete (**Fig. 29**)
  - Preparedness should include ensuring availability of proper equipment (eg, spine board, immobilization devices, airway equipment, tools to remove helmets/uniform, and stretcher), and rehearsal and review of team member roles, including assigning a captain to direct the efforts of the medical team.[70]
- Unconscious athletes
  - Should be log rolled into a supine position with someone maintaining in-line C-spine stabilization (**Fig. 30**)
  - Protective equipment (eg, helmet and shoulder pads) should be left in place until adequate immobilization of the head and neck has occurred
- Removal of protective equipment
  - Palumbo and colleagues[71] and Gastel and colleagues[72] used radiographs of cadavers to show that immobilizing neck-injured football players with only the helmet or only the shoulder pads in place causes significant cervical spine malalignment
  - Donaldson and colleagues[73] showed significant cervical spine movements during helmet and shoulder pad removal in a cadaveric model
  - Several expert recommendations describe techniques for helmet removal (See 'Techniques of Helmet Removal,' Available at: https://www.facs.org/~/media/files/quality%20programs/trauma/publications/helmet.ashx),[74] and the overall initial management of athletes with spine injuries (**Fig. 31**)

Management of specific cervical spine injuries and return-to-competition decisions following treatment of these injuries is beyond the scope of this article. However,

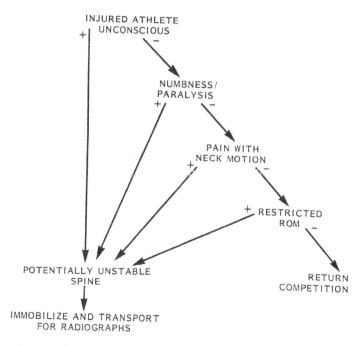

Fig. 29. Evaluation of injured athletes. (*From* Marks MR, Bell BR, Boumphrey FR. Cervical spine fractures in athletes. Clin Sports Med 1990;9:14.)

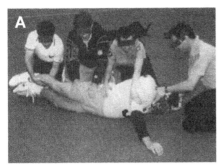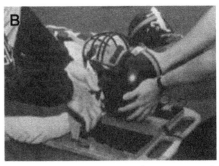

Fig. 30. Proper technique for moving an athlete thought to have a cervical spine injury. (*A*) The player is turned. One member of the medical term is responsible only for ensuring that the neck is maintained in a neutral position. The player is next placed on the long splint board, while every precaution is used to prevent secondary injury. (*B*) Proper technique for immobilizing the athlete's head and neck while another medical team member removes the face mask to gain access to the airway if necessary. (*From* Warren WL, Bailes JE. On the field evaluation of athletic neck injury. Clin Sports Med 1998;17:106.)

Fig. 32 is included for reference; Warren and Bailes[70] describe 3 types of athletic spinal injuries.

- Type I: permanent spinal cord injury
- Type II: transient neurologic deficit after trauma in persons with normal radiographic studies (SCIWORA)
  - ○ Burning hands syndrome: variant of the central cord syndrome
    - ■ Burning paresthesias and dysesthesias in both arms or hands and occasionally in the legs, accompanied by variable weakness[75]
  - ○ Cervical cord neuropraxia
    - ■ Transient quadriplegia has been estimated to occur in 7 out of 10,000 football players[76]
    - ■ Transient conduction block or a concussion of the cord
    - ■ Tingling and weakness in upper and possibly lower extremities with or without neck pain lasting from 15 minutes to 48 hours
    - ■ Recurrence rate is as high as 50% and therefore controversy exists on return to play after this injury
  - ○ Stinger injury (**Fig. 32**)
    - ■ Traction on the brachial plexus or from compression of the nerve root in the neural foramen following axial compression[77]
    - ■ Unilateral burning dysesthesias from shoulder to hand, with occasional weakness or numbness in the C5 and C6 distribution.
    - ■ Typically lasts minutes but can persist for days to weeks
    - ■ The unilaterality, brevity, and pain-free range of neck motion in the athlete can assist in discriminating between a stinger and a cord injury
      - • Some investigators suggest that symptoms that resolve in seconds to minutes may lead physicians to consider same-day return to competition
- Type III: those with radiographic findings (ie, fracture, fracture-dislocations, and ligamentous injuries) but without permanent neurologic deficits
- Continued symptoms, neck pain, incomplete range of motion, or suspicion of more serious neck injury should lead to removal from competition and further evaluation, including radiologic evaluation.[78]

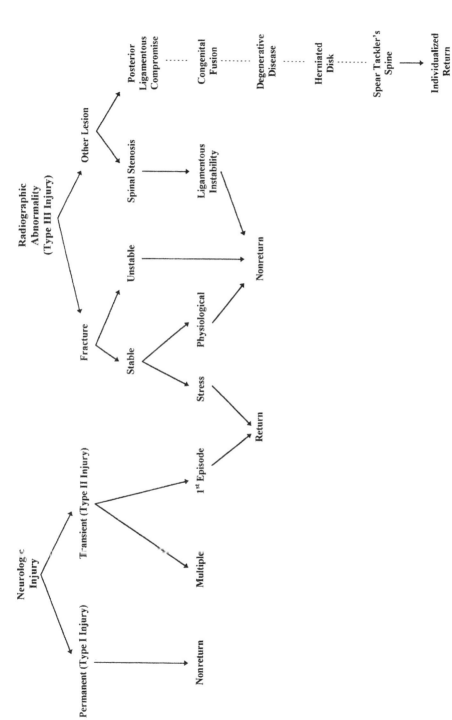

Fig. 31. Management of symptomatic athletic injuries of the cervical spine. (*From* Warren WL, Bailes JE. On the field evaluation of athletic neck injury. Clin Sports Med 1998;17:102.)

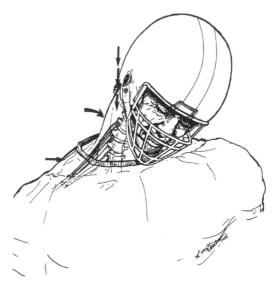

Fig. 32. Stingers or burners are thought to be caused by one of 3 mechanisms: a blow causing the neck to flex laterally away from the side of a depressed shoulder (as in tackling), stretching the upper trunk of the brachial plexus; axial loading of the head producing compression of the nerve root in the neural foramen; or, rarely, a direct blow to the trapezius or shoulder area, resulting in a contusion to the brachial plexus. (*From* Warren WL, Bailes JE. On the field evaluation of athletic neck injury. Clin Sports Med 1998;17:104.)

SUMMARY

EPs must be able to effectively and efficiently manage patients with potential cervical spine injury. The major management principle for patients with trauma with multiple injuries remains cervical spine protection during the initial evaluation and stabilization of the patient with a goal to preventing additional neurologic injury. EPs must have an understanding of the complex anatomy; types of cervical spine injury; and associated neurologic, vascular, and soft tissue injuries to manage this potentially devastating injury positively. EPs must understand the utility and limitations of different radiographic techniques for evaluating the cervical spine to manage these patients efficiently. EPs must understand the potential role of steroids and cooling, and make these decisions in conjunction with the consulting physicians. In addition, EPs who supervise prehospital providers or who function as sideline or team physicians must be aware of the specific issues related to out-of-hospital management of cervical spine injuries and return-to-competition guidelines.

REFERENCES

1. Lasfargues JE, Curtis D, Morrone F, et al. A model for estimating spinal cord injury prevalence in the United States. Paraplegia 1995;33(2):62.
2. Dryden DM, Saunders LD, Rowe BH, et al. The epidemiology of traumatic spinal cord injury in Alberta, Canada. Can J Neurol Sci 2003;30(2):113.
3. Garland DE, Lankenau JE. Epidemiology and costs of spine trauma. In: Capen DA, Haye W, editors. Comprehensive management of spine trauma. St Louis (MO): Mosby–Year Book; 1998. p. 1–5.
4. McGory BJ, Klassen RA, Chao EY, et al. Acute fractures and dislocations of the cervical spine in children and adolescents. J Bone Joint Surg Am 1993;75(7):988.

5. The National Spinal Cord Injury Statistical Center. Available at: http://www.spinalcord.uab.edu/show.asp?durki=21446. Accessed March 07, 2014.
6. Slucky AV, Eismont FJ. Treatment of acute injury of the cervical spine. Instr Course Lect 1995;44:67–80.
7. Aghababian R. Emergency medicine: the core curriculum. Philadelphia: Lippincott-Raven; 1998. p. 1210–7.
8. Hauswald M, Ong G, Tandberg D, et al. Out-of-hospital spinal immobilization: Its effect on neurologic injury. Acad Emerg Med 1998;5:214–9.
9. Orledge JD, Pepe PE. Out-of-hospital immobilization: Is it really necessary? Acad Emerg Med 1998;5:203–4.
10. Hockberger RS, Kirshenbaum KJ, Doris PE. Spinal injuries. In: Rosen P, Barkin R, Danzl D, et al, editors. Emergency medicine: concepts and clinical practice, vol. 1, 4th edition. St Louis (MO): Mosby–Year Book; 1998. p. 462–505.
11. Karasick D, Schweitzer ME, Abidi NA, et al. Fractures of the vertebrae with spinal cord injuries in patients with ankylosing spondylitis: Imaging findings. AJR Am J Roentgenol 1995;165:1205–8.
12. Olerud C, Frost A, Bring J. Spinal fractures in patients with ankylosing spondylitis. Eur Spine J 1996;5:51–5.
13. Sosner J, Avital F, Kahan BS. Odontoid fracture and C1-C2 subluxation in psoriatic cervical spondyloarthropathy: a case report. Spine 1996;21:519–21.
14. Ballard WT, Clark CR. Increased atlantoaxial instability secondary to an atraumatic fracture of the odontoid process in a patient who had rheumatoid arthritis: a case report. J Bone Joint Surg Am 1995;77:1245–8.
15. Ellis GL. Imaging of the atlas (C1) and axis (C2). Emerg Med Clin North Am 1991;9:719–32.
16. Finkelstein JA, Anderson PA. Surgical management of cervical instability. In: Capen DA, Haye W, editors. Comprehensive management of spine trauma. St Louis (MO): Mosby–Year Book; 1998. p. 144–84.
17. Walls RM. Airway management in the blunt trauma patient: how important is the cervical spine? Can J Surg 1992;35:27–30.
18. Criswell JC, Parr MJ, Nolan JP. Emergency airway management in patients with cervical spine injuries. Anaesthesia 1994;49:900–3.
19. Shatney CH, Brunner RD, Nguyen TQ. The safety of orotracheal intubation in patients with unstable cervical spine fracture or high spinal cord injury. Am J Surg 1995;170:676–80.
20. Suderman VS, Crosby ET. Occasional review: elective oral tracheal intubation in cervical spine-injured adults. Can J Anaesth 1991;38:785–9.
21. Gerling MC, Hamilton RS, Davis DP, et al. Effects of cervical spine immobilization technique and laryngoscope blade selection on unstable cervical spine injury in a cadaver model of intubation [abstract]. Ann Emerg Med 1998;32:13.
22. Robitaille A, Williams SR, Tremblay MH, et al. Cervical spine motion during tracheal intubation with manual in-line stabilization: direct laryngoscopy versus GlideScope videolaryngoscopy. Anesth Analg 2008;106(3):935–41.
23. Turkstra TP, Eng M, Eng P, et al. Cervical spine motion: a fluoroscopic comparison during intubation with lighted stylet, GlideScope, and Macintosh laryngoscope. Anesth Analg 2005;101(3):910–5.
24. Committee on Trauma. Airway and ventilator management. In: Advanced trauma life support for doctors. Chicago: American College of Surgeons; 1998. p. 72.
25. Kaji A, Hockberger RS. Evaluation and acute management of cervical spinal column injuries in adults. UpToDate. Chicago (IL): American College of Surgeons; 2014.

26. Hoffman JR, Mower WR, Wolfson AB, et al. Validity of a set of clinical criteria to rule out injury to the cervical spine in patients with blunt trauma (National Emergency X-Radiography Utilization Study Group). N Engl J Med 2000;343(2):94.

27. Hoffman JR, Wolfson AB, Todd K, et al. Selective cervical spine radiography in blunt trauma: methodology of the National Emergency X-radiography Utilization Study (NEXUS). Ann Emerg Med 1998;32(4):461.

28. Stiell IG, Wells GA, Vandemheen KL, et al. The Canadian C-spine Rule for radiography in alert and stable trauma patients. JAMA 1841;286(15):2001.

29. Steill I, Clement C, McKnight D, et al. The Canadian C-spine Rule versus the NEXUS low-risk criteria in patients with trauma. N Engl J Med 2003;349:2510–8.

30. Hunter B, Keim S, Seupaul R, et al. Are plain radiographs sufficient to exclude cervical spine injuries in low-risk adults? J Emerg Med 2014;46(2):257–63.

31. Como JJ, Diaz JJ, Dunham CM, et al. Practice management guidelines for identification of cervical spine injuries following trauma: update from the Eastern Association for the Surgery of Trauma Practice Management Guidelines Committee. J Trauma 2009;67(3):651.

32. Holmes JF, Akkinepalli R. Computed tomography versus plain radiography to screen for cervical spine injury: a meta-analysis. J Trauma 2005;58(5):902.

33. Daffner RH. Helical CT of the cervical spine for trauma patients: a time study. AJR Am J Roentgenol 2001;177(3):677.

34. Blackmore CC, Ramsey SD, Mann FA, et al. Cervical spine screening with CT in trauma patients: a cost-effectiveness analysis. Radiology 1999;212(1):117.

35. Rybicki F, Nawfel RD, Judy PF, et al. Skin and thyroid dosimetry in cervical spine screening: two methods for evaluation and a comparison between a helical CT and radiographic trauma series. AJR AM J Roentgenol 2002;179(4):933.

36. Plumb JO, Morris CG. Clinical review: spinal imaging for the adult obtunded blunt trauma patient: update from 2004. Intensive Care Med 2012;38(5):752–71.

37. Machino M, Yukawa Y, Ito K, et al. Can magnetic resonance imaging reflect the prognosis in patients of cervical spinal cord injury without radiographic abnormality? Spine 2011;36(24):1568–72.

38. Kothari P, Freeman B, Grevitt M, et al. Injury to the spinal cord without radiological abnormality (SCIWORA) in adults. J Bone Joint Surg Br 2000;82(7):1034.

39. Delinganix AV, Mann FA, Grady MS. Rapid diagnosis and treatment of a traumatic atlanto-occipital dissociation. AJR Am J Roentgenol 1998;171:986.

40. Nelson RW. Nonsurgical management of cervical spine instability. In: Capen DA, Haye W, editors. Comprehensive management of spine trauma. St Louis (MO): Mosby–Year Book; 1998. p. 134–43.

41. Henry MB, Angelastro DB, Gillen JP. Unrecognized traumatic atlanto-occipital dislocation. Am J Emerg Med 1998;16:406–8.

42. Traynalis VC, Marano GD, Dunker RO, et al. Traumatic atlanto-occipital dislocation. J Neurosurg 1986;65:863–70.

43. Ferrera PC, Bartfield JM. Traumatic atlanto-occipital dislocation: a potentially survivable injury. Am J Emerg Med 1996;14:291–6.

44. Hadley MN, Dickman CA, Browner CM, et al. Acute traumatic atlas fractures: management and long-term outcome. Neurosurgery 1988;23:31–5.

45. Rothman SL. Imaging of spinal trauma pearls and pitfalls. In: Capen DA, Haye W, editors. Comprehensive management of spine trauma. St Louis (MO): Mosby–Year Book; 1998. p. 39–95.

46. Gatrell CB. Asymptomatic cervical spine injuries: a myth? Am J Emerg Med 1985; 3:263–4.

47. Marchesi DG. Management of odontoid fractures. Orthopedics 1997;20:911–6.

48. Harris JH, Edeiken-Monroe B, Kopaniky DR. A practical classification of acute cervical spine injuries. Orthop Clin North Am 1986;17:15–30.
49. Riviello RJ, Dey CC, Townsend RN, et al. Cervical seat belt sign after motor vehicle collision [letter]. Acad Emerg Med 1997;4:335–7.
50. Andreshak JL, Dekutoski MB. Management of unilateral facet dislocations: a review of the literature. Orthopedics 1997;20:917–26.
51. Lewin MG, Pappius HM, Hansebout RR. Effects of steroids on edema associated with injury of the spinal cord. In: Reulen HJ, Schurmann K, editors. Steroids and brain edema. Berlin: Springer-Verlag; 1972. p. 101.
52. Bracken MB, Shepard MJ, Collins WF Jr, et al. Methylprednisolone or naloxone treatment after acute spinal cord injury: 1 year follow-up data (NASCIS II). J Neurosurg 1992;76(1):23.
53. Bracken MB, Shepard MJ, Holford TR, et al. Methylprednisolone or tirilazad mesylate administration after acute spinal cord injury: 1-year follow up (NASCIS III). J Neurosurg 1998;89(5):699.
54. Hulbert RJ. Strategies of medical intervention in the management of acute spinal cord injury. Spine 2006;31(Suppl 11):S16.
55. Hulbert RJ, Hadley MN, Walters BC, et al. Pharmacological therapy for acute spinal cord injury. Neurosurgery 2013;2:93–105.
56. Kao CH, Chio CC, Lin MT, et al. Body cooling ameliorating spinal cord injury may be neurogenesis-, anti-inflammation- and angiogenesis-associated in rats. J Trauma 2011;70(4):885–93.
57. Hansebout RR, Hansebout CR. Local cooling for traumatic spinal cord injury: outcomes in 20 patients and review of the literature. J Neurosurg Spine 2014;20:550–61.
58. Giacobetti FB, Vaccaro AR, Bos-Giacobetti MA, et al. Vertebral artery occlusion associated with cervical spine trauma: a prospective analysis. Spine 1997;22:188–92.
59. Prabhu V, Kizer J, Patil A, et al. Vertebrobasilar thrombosis associated with nonpenetrating cervical spine trauma. J Trauma 1996;40:130–7.
60. Schippinger C, Spork E, Obernosterer A, et al. Injury of the cervical spine associated with carotid and vertebral artery occlusion: case report and literature review. Injury 1997;28:315–8.
61. Yelon JA, Barrett L, Evans JR. Distal innominate artery transection and cervical spine injury. J Trauma 1995;39:590–2.
62. Willis BK, Greiner F, Orrison WW, et al. The incidence of vertebral artery injury after midcervical spine fracture or subluxation. Neurosurgery 1994;34:435.
63. Capen DA. Soft tissue injuries to the spine from acceleration-deceleration trauma. In: Capen DA, Haye W, editors. Comprehensive management of spine trauma. St Louis (MO): Mosby–Year Book; 1998. p. 96–104.
64. Huelke DF, Mackay GM, Morris A. Vertebral column injuries and lap-shoulder belts. J Trauma 1995;38:547–56.
65. Grauer JN, Panjabi MM, Cholewicki J, et al. Whiplash produces an S-shaped curvature of the neck with hyperextension at the lower levels. Spine 1997;22:2489–94.
66. Panjabi MM, Cholewicki J, Nibu K, et al. Simulation of whiplash trauma using whole cervical spine specimens. Spine 1998;23:17–24.
67. Borchgrevnik GE, Kaasa A, McDonagh D, et al. Acute treatment of whiplash neck sprain injuries: a randomized trial of treatment during the first 14 days after a car accident. Spine 1998;23:25–31.
68. Marks MR, Bell GR, Boumphrey FR. Cervical spine fractures in athletes. Clin Sports Med 1990;9:13–29.

69. Bailes JE, Hadley MN, Quigley MR, et al. Management of athletic injuries of the cervical spine and spinal cord. Neurosurgery 1991;29:4.
70. Warren WL, Bailes JE. On the field evaluation of athletic neck injury. Clin Sports Med 1998;17:99–110.
71. Palumbo MA, Hulstyn MJ, Fadale PD, et al. The effect of protective football equipment on alignment of the injured cervical spine—radiographic analysis in the cadaveric model. Am J Sports Med 1996;24:446–53.
72. Gastel JA, Palumbo MA, Hulstyn MJ, et al. Emergency removal of football equipment: a cadaveric cervical spine injury model. Ann Emerg Med 1998;32:411–7.
73. Donaldson WF, Lauerman WC, Heil B, et al. Helmet and shoulder pad removal from a player with suspected cervical spine injury—a cadaveric model. Spine 1998;23:1729–33.
74. McSwain NE, Camelli RL. Helmet removal from injured patients. Chicago: American College of Surgeons Committee on Trauma; 1997.
75. Wilberger JE. Athletic spinal cord injuries—guidelines for initial management. Clin Sports Med 1998;17:111–20.
76. Loftus C. Neurosurgical emergencies. 2nd edition. Rolling Meadows (IL): Thieme; 2007.
77. Cantu RC. Stingers, transient quadriplegia, and cervical spine stenosis: return to play criteria. Med Sci Sports Exerc 1997;29:S233–5.
78. Cantu RC, Bailes JE, Wilberger JE. Guidelines for return to contact or collision sport after a cervical spine injury. Clin Sports Med 1998;17:137–46.

Emergency Department Evaluation and Treatment of Wrist Injuries

 CrossMark

Alina Tsyrulnik, MD

KEYWORDS

• Wrist injury • Dislocation • Carpal bone • Scaphoid

KEY POINTS

- Correct diagnosis of wrist injuries is critical in preventing prolonged pain and dysfunction.
- Plain radiographs cannot diagnose a large percentage of injuries.
- Distal radius fractures are treated by splinting. Colles fractures are splinted in neutral or pronation; Smith's fractures are splinted in supination.
- The scaphoid is the most commonly-injured carpal bone. If fracture is suspected but not seen on radiographs, it should be treated by thumb spica splinting to prevent complications.
- Carpal dislocations are relatively rare, but can lead to significant disfunction if not emergently treated. Emergent orthopedic consultation is warranted.

The wrist, although a comparatively small part of the human body, is complex in its mechanics and function and, when injured, can lead to significant morbidity.

- Approximately 2.5% of all emergency department (ED) visits in the United States are for wrist injuries.[1]
- Approximately 1.5% of all ED visits are for hand and/or forearm fractures.[2]
- Approximately 20% of hand and wrist fractures are carpal bone fractures.[3]
- The elderly have the highest rates of carpal bone injury, with most injuries occurring as a result of accidental falls in the home.[2]
- The scaphoid is the most commonly fractured carpal bone.[3]

Correct diagnosis of wrist injuries is critical in preventing prolonged pain and dysfunction. It is complicated in that plain radiographs cannot diagnose a large percentage of injuries. Wrist sprain is considered one of the most common yet most treacherous ED diagnoses[1] because radiographs do not always rule out all acute injuries. Knowledge of the anatomy, normal physical examination findings, and

Disclosure: None.

Department of Emergency Medicine, Yale University School of Medicine, 464 Congress Ave, New Haven, CT 06519, USA

E-mail address: alina.tsyrulnik@yale.edu

Emerg Med Clin N Am 33 (2015) 283–296
http://dx.doi.org/10.1016/j.emc.2014.12.003
0733-8627/15/$ – see front matter © 2015 Elsevier Inc. All rights reserved.

physical examination abnormalities associated with different pathological conditions, is paramount in making the correct diagnosis. This article focuses on the anatomy, diagnosis, and ED management of acute wrist injuries, including fractures and dislocations.

NORMAL ANATOMY, RADIOGRAPHY, AND PHYSICAL EXAMINATION
Normal Anatomy and Radiography

The wrist, from proximal to distal, is comprised of the distal radius, ulna, and 8 carpal bones that are arranged into 2 arching rows (**Fig. 1**).

- The proximal carpal bones (from radial to ulnar direction) include: scaphoid, lunate, triquetrum, and pisiform (a sesamoid bone associated with the flexor carpi ulnaris tendon).[3]
- The distal carpal bones (from radial to ulnar direction) include trapezium, trapezoid, capitate, and hamate.

There is characteristic normal alignment of the 2 rows on posterior-anterior (PA) and lateral projections, with the "three lines of Gilula"[3] and the stacked C-shapes seen on each view, respectively.

- PA view: proximal and distal articular surfaces of the proximal row and the proximal surface of the distal row making up the "3 lines of Gilula" (**Fig. 2**).[4]
- Lateral view: the distal radius, lunate, capitate, and third metacarpal align in C-shapes (**Fig. 3**).[4]
- The radial height and palmar tilt angles are relevant in evaluating the distal radius (**Fig. 4**).[5]

Normal Physical Examination

On physical examination, the scaphoid can be palpated in the so-called snuff box, which is bordered by the tendons of the extensor pollicis longus and abductor pollicis longus.[3] Flexion of the wrist allows the palpation of the lunate just distal to the radius, ulnar to the scaphoid, and in line with the third phalanx. The triquetrum is distal to the ulna and the pisiform is palpated on the volar distal wrist in line with the fifth phalanx. The distal row of carpal bones is palpated just proximal to the metacarpals. The

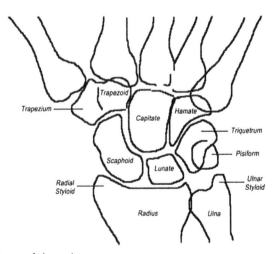

Fig. 1. Bony anatomy of the wrist.

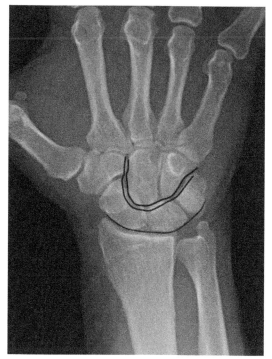

Fig. 2. The lines of Gilula: normal alignment of the carpal bones.

trapezium, trapezoid, and capitate are proximal to the first through third metacarpals (in the radial to ulnar direction) and the hamate is proximal to the fifth metacarpal. The hook of the hamate is palpated in the palm where it extends 1 to 2 cm distal and lateral to the pisiform in the hypothenar eminence.[6]

DISTAL RADIUS FRACTURES
Background

Distal radius fractures are frequently encountered in the ED. The distribution of population affected is bimodal, including children younger than 16 years and women older than 50 years of age. In the younger age group there has been a steady increase in the frequency of these injuries, which is believed to be due to increased obesity and resultant higher impact during falls.[5]

- Distal radius and/or ulna fracture account for approximately 0.66% of ED visits.[5]
- The annual incidence of distal radius fractures in the United States is 640,000.[7]
- Women older than 50 years have a 15% lifetime risk of distal radius and/or ulna fracture.[5]
- Distal radius fracture is the most common fracture in children younger than 16 years.[5]
- Fifty percent of distal radius fractures are intraarticular.[8]

Several eponyms are used to describe the various types of distal radius fractures:

- Colles fracture is a transverse fracture of distal radial metaphysis with dorsal displacement and angulation[3] often resulting from a fall onto an extended wrist.

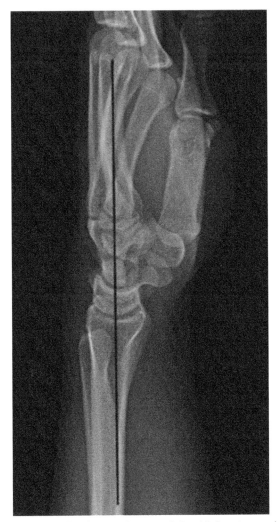

Fig. 3. Colinearity of the distal radius, capitate, and the third metacarpal.

- Smith fracture is a transverse fracture of the distal radial metaphysis with volar displacement and angulation[3] often resulting from a fall onto a flexed wrist.
- Barton fracture is a distal radius fracture with dislocation of the radiocarpal joint and either volar or dorsal angulation.[3,8]
- Hutchinson fracture is an intraarticular fracture through the radial styloid process often resulting from a direct blow or a fall onto the radial side of wrist.[3]

Diagnosis

On physical examination, Colles fractures present as the typically described silver fork or dinner fork deformity. Radiographic evidence of such fractures is accomplished with PA, anterior-posterior (AP), and lateral views, with particular attention paid to the radial height (AP and PA views) and volar tilt angle (lateral views) (see **Fig. 4**).[3,5]

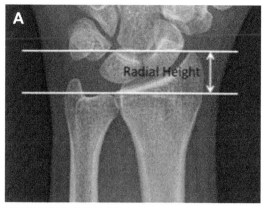

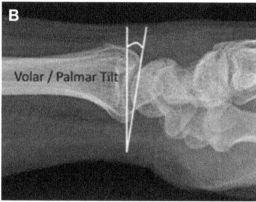

Fig. 4. (*A*) Radial height on AP view. (*B*) Palmar tilt angle on lateral view is normally 11°.

If distal radioulnar joint (DRUJ) instability is suspected, the fracture has significant intraarticular extension, or has significant comminution, a CT scan can provide additional information and aid in diagnosis and treatment (see later discussion).[8,9]

Treatment

Management of Colles and Smith fractures usually includes closed reduction. This is accomplished with regional anesthesia with a hematoma block and the use of finger traps. After reduction, a long-arm splint is applied.

- Colles fracture is splint in neutral position or pronation.[3]
- Smith fracture is splint in supination.[3]

With successful reduction of a closed Colles fracture without evidence of neurovascular compromise, the patient can wait to be seen by an orthopedist for a week to 10 days.[3] The wrist will be immobilized for 4 to 6 weeks.[5] Smith fractures have a higher incidence of instability and always require urgent specialist follow-up.[3] Barton fractures always require emergent orthopedic consultation for early surgical treatment.[3] Nondisplaced Hutchinson fractures are treated with a short arm splint and routine orthopedic follow-up. Displaced Hutchinson fractures require careful emergent reduction with complete anatomic alignment.[3] For this reason, emergent specialist consultation should be considered if alignment is not adequate.

Any open fracture requires an emergent orthopedic or hand surgery consultation, as well as administration of intravenous antibiotics and tetanus status assessment.[10]

Complications

There is a wide variance in the reported complication rate of distal radius fractures of between 6% and 80%, with an increased rate in open fractures.[10] Nerve injury occurs in up to 17% of distal radius fractures, with the median nerve being the most vulnerable, followed by the ulnar and radial nerves.[10,11] Immediate or delayed carpal tunnel syndrome (CTS) is the most common complication of distal radius fracture.[12] Transient neuropathy may also occur. The high frequency of median nerve involvement is due to its central location within the carpal tunnel as well as proximity to the distal radius.[11] Both Colles and Smith fractures can lead to median nerve injury. This complication is more likely with a higher degree of dorsal displacement of the distal fragment, more comminuted fractures, and those undergoing multiple closed reduction attempts.[3,5,10] Of note, CTS is a term used to describe the compression of the median nerve and its subsequent dysfunction that is acute and progressive. This compression is either from direct damage to the nerve or secondarily from swelling of surrounding tissues. Acute CTS develops rapidly after the injury whereas secondary CTS can happen months to years later.[12] CTS may require surgical intervention. In contrast, transient median nerve contusion, occurring in 4% of cases, resolves with conservative management.[11]

Factors that lead to instability and long-term disability after distal radius fracture include a dorsal angulation angle of more than 20° (with normal angulation being 11°) and greater than 5 mm of radial shortening.[5]

Another complication of a distal radius fracture is disruption of the DRUJ. This injury can occur in isolation (without associated fractures); however, this is less common. When isolated, it is the result of distal ulnar dislocation that can be in the volar or dorsal (more common) direction depending on the rotational component during impact. Radiographic evidence of this injury will be seen on PA radiographs as overlap of the distal radius and ulna; lateral radiographs will show ulnar displacement (dorsal or volar).[3,9]

- Dorsal dislocations are associated with pronation during impact and pain with supination on physical examination.
- Volar dislocations are associated with supination during impact and pain with pronation on physical examination.

Disruption of the supporting structures, including the triangular fibrocartilage complex (TFCC) of the DRUJ (without dislocation), is a complication of a displaced distal radius fracture. Up to 60% to 84% of distal radius fractures are associated with injury to the TFCC.[9] Signs of DRUJ instability are[3,9]

- Ulnar styloid fracture involving the base with more than 2 mm displacement
- DRUJ dislocation that can not be reduced
- Fracture of the sigmoid notch of the radius
- Wide DRUJ displacement
- Shortened radius.

DRUJ instability requires emergent orthopedic or hand surgery consultation for reduction and immobilization.[3,9]

Other common complications of distal radius fractures include arthrosis, malunion, nonunion, tendon rupture, chronic regional pain syndrome, ulnar impaction, loss of rotation, and finger stiffness.[12]

Isolated fractures of the distal ulna (within 5 mm of distal articular surface) are rare. However, they commonly occur with distal radius fractures.

- Sixty percent of distal radius fractures are associated with fractures of the ulnar styloid.[13]
- These fractures will often reduce during distal radius reduction.[13]

Many complications of distal radius fractures are iatrogenic, stemming from the treatment rather than the trauma that caused the injury.

- Splinting in extreme flexion increases carpal tunnel pressures, which causes median nerve damage.[10]
- Overlying skin of the distal radius can be very thin (especially in the elderly). Closed fractures can be converted to open fractures during reduction.[10]
- Compartment syndrome can occur acutely from the fracture itself or as a result of completely circumferential casting.[10,11]

SCAPHOID INJURIES
Background

The most commonly fractured carpal bone, the scaphoid,[3] is located at the anatomic snuff box. Fractures of the scaphoid occur as a result of a fall on an outstretched hand or during forced dorsiflexion of the wrist.[14] Initial diagnostic imaging should start with plain radiographs in 4 views: PA, lateral, radial oblique, and ulnar oblique.[15] Diagnosis of fracture is complicated by the frequency of false-negative radiographs.

- Prevalence of scaphoid fractures among patients with acute wrist injuries is 7%.[16]
- Incidence of false-negative initial radiographs for scaphoid fractures is 1% to 16%.[16,17]
- Sensitivity of initial plain radiographs for scaphoid fractures is 70% to 86%.[5]
- CT scan sensitivity is 89% to 100% and specificity is 85% to 100% for diagnosing acute scaphoid fracture.[16,18]
- MRI sensitivity is 98% to 100% and specificity of 100% for diagnosing acute scaphoid fracture.[16]

Diagnosis

Patients with tenderness on the physical examination that is suggestive of scaphoid fracture but negative radiographs deserve special consideration. Several recent studies have focused on the diagnostic value of physical examination, CT scan, and MRI in these situations. Physical examination findings most predictive of bony injury (any bone) in patients who had tenderness at the snuffbox and scaphoid tubercle after a fall on outstretched hand and negative radiographs were

- Thumb-index finger pinch with elicited pain at snuffbox: sensitivity of 73% and specificity of 75%[19]
- Pronation of the arm with elicited pain at snuffbox: sensitivity of 79% and specificity of 58%.[19]

Another study examined the sensitivity and specificity of combining the most common physical examination findings associated with scaphoid fractures[17]:

- Tenderness at the anatomic snuffbox
- Tenderness at the scaphoid tubercle

- Tenderness with longitudinal compression of thumb onto scaphoid
- Pain with active movement of the thumb.

The investigators found that

- The first 3 maneuvers had an individual sensitivity of 100%[17]
- The fourth maneuver (thumb movement) had a sensitivity of 69%[17]
- The specificities for these maneuvers were: 9%, 30%, 48%, and 66%, respectively[17]
- When the first 3 maneuvers where combined and tenderness was present on all 3, the sensitivity remained at 100% but the specificity increased to 74%.[17]

Another study compared the sensitivity of MRI and CT scan for detecting bony injuries in patients with snuffbox tenderness and negative radiographs. The investigators found that both imaging modalities had a sensitivity of 67% for detecting injury within 10 days of wrist trauma (with the gold standard being radiographs in 4 views at 6 weeks postinjury).[16]

Treatment

If a scaphoid fracture is definitively identified, the ED treatment includes application of a long-arm thumb spica splint and immediate hand surgery consultation.[3] Typically, when a scaphoid fracture is suspected without radiographic confirmation, a thumb spica splint should be applied with hand surgeon follow-up in 7 to 10 days. At that point, repeat imaging is done.[3] The argument for doing this has been that the cost of CT scan or MRI is too high to justify immediate use of these modalities. Recent studies looking at the costs incurred with prolonged immobilization (lost income, lost productivity, repeat imaging, follow-up appointments) versus immediate CT scan or MRI are showing mixed results.[14]

Complications

Avascular necrosis (AVN) and nonunion are the most common complications of scaphoid injury and the reason why even suspected fractures are treated with immobilization.

- Approximately 15% of scaphoid wrist fractures result in malunion or nonunion.[3]
- Approximately 20% of all scaphoid fractures result in AVN.[3]
- Approximately 80% of proximal scaphoid fractures result in AVN.[3]

The incidence of complications depends on the location and degree of displacement of the fracture. Nondisplaced fractures have a lower chance of poor outcomes. Furthermore, if the fracture is located in the middle or distal thirds of the scaphoid, the expected healing rate is 95% with short arm thumb spica for 10 to 12 weeks. Fractures in the proximal third of the scaphoid have a 34% chance of nonunion when treated conservatively.[5]

CARPAL FRACTURES EXCLUDING THE SCAPHOID

Compared with the incidence of scaphoid injury, other carpal bones are injured much less frequently. Nonscaphoid fractures account for 13% to 38% of carpal bone fractures.[20] See **Table 1** for a summary of carpal bone fractures, their ED treatment, and interval to specialist follow-up.[3]

Lunate

- Isolated lunate fractures are extremely rare because 70% of this bone sits on the radius and 30% articulates with the TFCC.[20]

Table 1
Carpal fracture splinting and referral recommendation

Fracture	Splint	Orthopedic Referral
Scaphoid	Thumb spica: long or short	Definite fracture: emergent Suspected fracture: nonemergent referral
Hamate Hook	Thumb spica with flexed wrist and metacarpophalangeal at 90°	Specialist referral within 1 wk
Hamate Body	Short-arm cast	Specialist referral within 1 wk
Lunate	Short-arm splint	Referral in 1–2 wk
Triquetral	Short-arm splint	Nonemergent
Pisiform	Short-arm splint	Emergent if signs of ulnar neuropathy
Capitate	Short-arm thumb spica	Emergent if associated with dislocation
Trapezium	Short-arm thumb spica	Nonemergent
Trapezoid	Short-arm spica	Emergent if displaced

- The mechanism of injury is extreme dorsiflexion with ulnar deviation.[20]
- Oblique radiographic views are necessary for the diagnosis of lunate fractures.[20]
- Emergent treatment includes immobilization with a short-arm cast for 6 weeks.[20]

Triquetrum

- Triquetrum fractures account for 4% to 20% of carpal bone fractures.[20]
- The mechanisms of injury are hyperextension with ulnar deviation or a fall on an outstretched hand.[20]
- Locations for triquetrum fractures include dorsal cortex (93%), body, or palmar cortex.[20]
- Treatment of dorsal cortical fractures is a wrist splint or short arm cast for 4 to 6 weeks.[20]
- Treatment of nondisplaced body fractures is a short arm cast for 6 weeks; displaced fractures require surgery.[20]
- Treatment of palmar cortical fractures is surgical.[20]

Pisiform

- Pisiform fractures account for 0.2% to 1% of all carpal fractures.[20,21]
- The pisiform is the last carpal bone to ossify (at age 8 to 12 years) thus making the distinction between incomplete ossification and fracture difficult in young children.[20,21]
- The mechanisms of injury are direct trauma to the hypothenar eminence, avulsion when the flexor carpi ulnaris resists forcible hyperextension (during strain to lift heavy object), or repetitive trauma associated with stick-handling sports (golf, tennis, baseball).[20,21]
- Patients may present with diminished grip strength and ulnar and/or medial nerve paresthesias.[21]
- Radiographic views, such as the reverse oblique of the wrist, clenched fist PA with ulnar deviation, wrist extension in 45° supination, and carpal tunnel view,[20,21] may aid in diagnosing pisiform fractures.
- Emergent treatment of pisiform fractures is immobilization for 4 to 6 weeks.[20,21]
- Complications include prolonged ulnar nerve palsy and diminished grip strength.[20,21]

Trapezium

- Trapezium fractures account for 3% to 5% of all carpal fractures.[20]
- The mechanisms of injury are a fall on an outstretched palm, axial loading through the first metacarpal, or hyperextension-abduction of the thumb.[20]
- An oblique radiographic view is necessary in the diagnosis of trapezium fracture (PA and lateral views fail to show the entire trapezium).[20]
- Missed diagnosis and/or inadequate treatment of this injury can result in permanent impairment of pinch and grip.[20]
- Trapezium fractures are emergently treated by short-arm thump spica cast for 4 to 6 weeks.[20]

Trapezoid

- Trapezoid fractures account for 0.2% of carpal bone fractures.[20]
- The mechanisms of injury are axial load on second metacarpal or extreme second metacarpal palmar flexion.[20]
- Plain radiography often miss the injury, CT scan may be required.[20]
- Nondisplaced fractures are treated with a short-arm thumb spica cast for 4 to 6 weeks.[20]

Capitate

- Capitate fractures account for 1.3% of carpal bone fractures.[20,22]
- Most capitate fractures are associated with scaphoid fractures.[20]
- The mechanisms of injury are a direct blow to dorsum of wrist; dorsiflexion force to wrist in neutral, ulnar, or radial deviation; force applied to second through fourth metacarpals; or a flexion force to the wrist.[22]
- Radiographic views that aid in the diagnosis of capitate fractures include PA radial and ulnar deviation views.[20]
- Clinically suspected injury that is not evident by pain radiography may warrant CT scan or MRI.[20]
- Nondisplaced fractures are treated with short-arm thumb spica cast immobilization for 6 to 8 weeks.[20]
- Displaced fractures are treated by closed or open anatomic reduction.[20]
- Complications of capitate fracture (most often resulting from delayed or missed diagnosis) include nonunion, AVN, and posttraumatic arthritis.[20]

Hamate

- Areas of fracture involve the body and hook (most common, accounting for 2% to 4% of all carpal bone fractures).[20,21]
- The mechanisms of injury are repeated microtrauma, a fall, a direct blow to hand, or stick-handling sports (golf, baseball, racquet sports).[6,20,21]
- Clinical presentation may include tenderness over the hypothenar eminence, pain with flexion of the fourth and fifth digit, pain on gripping, diminished grip strength, and ulnar and/or medial nerve paresthesias.[20,21]
- Radiographic views, such as the PA, lateral, supinated oblique, and carpal tunnel view, may aid in diagnosis.
- Plain radiography has a sensitivity of 71% (all views are combined). CT scan imaging has a sensitivity of 100%.[20,21]
- Emergent treatment of hamate fracture is an ulnar gutter short-arm cast for 3 weeks, followed by short-arm cast for 3 weeks.[20]
- Complications include ulnar and/or median nerve neuropathies and diminished grip strength.[6,21]

CARPAL DISLOCATIONS

Carpal dislocations and fracture dislocations are relatively infrequent (together they account for 7% of carpal injuries[23]). They occur as a result of carpal ligamentous injuries from hyperextension and ulnar deviation. Normally, equal spacing is seen between the carpal bones on PA imaging. There are 4 distinct stages of dislocation, each stage representing its own injury pattern[24]:

- Stage 1: scapholunate dissociation
- Stage 2: perilunate dislocation
- Stage 3: perilunate and triquetrum dislocation
- Stage 4: lunate dislocation.

Median nerve injury, acute or subacute CTS, scapholunate advanced collapse (SLAC) deformity, avascular changes, and degenerative changes are known complications of carpal dislocations.[1,23–25] A delay in treatment will increase the likelihood of a poor outcome.[26]

Scapholunate Dissociation

The normal space between the scaphoid and lunate in PA view should be 2 mm or less. Scapholunate dissociation is the widening of that gap, also known as the Terry Thomas sign, on radiographs (**Fig. 5**).[27] This widening can by accentuated by taking the radiograph while the wrist is in ulnar deviation with a clenched fist.[4] Another radiographic finding that indicates scapholunate dissociation is the signet ring sign (**Fig. 6**), which is the result of the scaphoid's rotary motion and repositioning of its distal pole in a palmar position.[4]

Lunate and Perilunate Dislocations

Injuries at and around the lunate are usually the result of hyperextension; high-energy trauma, such as fall on outstretched hand; or car or motorcycle accidents.

- Perilunate dislocation occurs when the head of the capitate dislocates from the distal surface of lunate (**Fig. 7**).

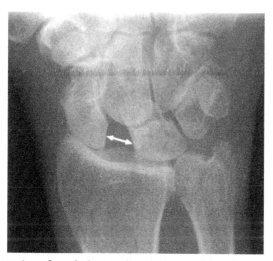

Fig. 5. Terry Thomas sign of scapholunate dissociation or dislocation.

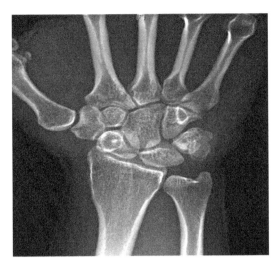

Fig. 6. Signet ring sign of scapholunate dissociation or dislocation.

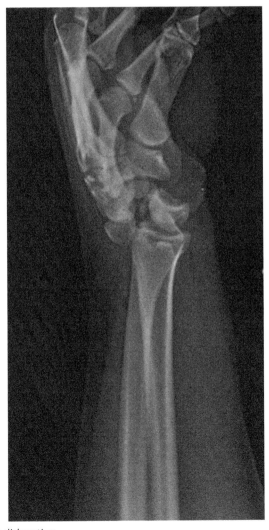

Fig. 7. Perilunate dislocation.

- Lunate dislocation occurs when the lunate no longer sits in the lunate fossa of the distal radius.

Although the more common injury is a perilunate dislocation, lunate dislocations are more severe.[1] Lunate and perilunate dislocations are often associated with other injuries:

- 61% to 65% are associated with scaphoid fractures[26]
- 26% are associated with polytrauma[26]
- 11% are associated with other upper extremity injuries.[26]

Although often accompanied by significant deformities, lunate and perilunate dislocations can be subtle and thus 16% to 25% are missed on initial presentation.[26]

Treatment of Carpal Dislocations

Carpal bone dislocations should prompt consultation of a hand specialist in the ED. For open dislocations, the patient needs operative management. Surgical intervention is also mandated if median nerve symptoms are present. For closed dislocations without median nerve damage, the dislocation can be managed by prompt closed reduction. Closed reductions are often unsuccessful, requiring open reduction with internal fixation by an orthopedic specialist.[26,28] Even if successfully reduced, early surgical correction is ideal for best outcomes because closed reduction and immobilization has been found to result in unacceptable failure rates.[25]

REFERENCES

1. Perron AD, Brady WJ. Evaluation and management of the high-risk orthopedic emergency. Emerg Med Clin North Am 2003;21:159–204.
2. Chung KC, Spilson SV. The frequency and epidemiology of hand and forearm fractures in the United States. J Hand Surg Am 2001;26(5):908–15.
3. Abraham MK, Scott S. The emergent evaluation and treatment of hand and wrist injuries. Emerg Med Clin North Am 2010;28(4):789–809.
4. Caggiano N, Matullo KS. Carpal instability of the wrist. Orthop Clin North Am 2014;45(1):129–40.
5. Bielak KM, Kafka J, Terrell T. Treatment of hand and wrist injuries. Prim Care 2013; 40(2):431–51.
6. Bishop AT, Beckenbaugh RD. Fracture of the hamate hook. J Hand Surg Am 1988;13A(1):135.
7. Diaz-Garcia RJ, Chung KC. Common myths and evidence in the management of distal radius fractures. Hand Clin 2012;28(2):127–33.
8. Wulf CA, Ackerman DB, Rizzo M. Contemporary evaluation and treatment of distal radius fractures. Hand Clin 2007;23(2):209–26, vi.
9. Carlsen BT, Dennison DG, Moran SL. Acute dislocations of the distal radioulnar joint and distal ulna fractures. Hand Clin 2010;26(4):503–16.
10. Turner RG, Faber KJ, Athwal GS. Complications of distal radius fractures. Orthop Clin North Am 2007;38(2):217–28, vi.
11. Oren TW, Wolf JM. Soft-tissue complications associated with distal radius fractures. Operat Tech Orthop 2009;19(2):100–6.
12. Niver GE, Ilyas AM. Carpal tunnel syndrome after distal radius fracture. Orthop Clin North Am 2012;43(4):521–7.
13. Dalal S, Murali SR. The distal radio-ulnar joint. Orthop Trauma 2012;26(1):44–52.
14. Adams JE, Steinmann SP. Acute scaphoid fractures. Hand Clin 2010;26(1): 97–103.

15. Farnell RD, Dickson DR. The assessment and management of acute scaphoid fractures and non-union. Orthopaedics and Trauma 2010;24(5):381–93.
16. Mallee W, Doornberg JN, Ring D, et al. Comparison of CT and MRI for diagnosis of suspected scaphoid fractures. J Bone Joint Surg Am 2011;93(1):20–8.
17. Parvizi J, Wayman J, Kelly P, et al. Combining the clinical signs improves diagnosis of scaphoid fractures. A prospective study with follow-up. J Hand Surg Br 1998;23B(3):324–7.
18. Adey L, Souer JS, Lozano-Calderon S, et al. Computed tomography of suspected scaphoid fractures. J Hand Surg Am 2007;32(1):61–6.
19. Unay K, Gokcen B, Ozkan K, et al. Examination tests predictive of bone injury in patients with clinically suspected occult scaphoid fracture. Injury 2009;40(12):1265–8.
20. Vigler M, Aviles A, Lee SK. Carpal fractures excluding the scaphoid. Hand Clin 2006;22(4):501–16 [abstract: vii].
21. O'Shea K, Weiland AJ. Fractures of the hamate and pisiform bones. Hand Clin 2012;28(3):287–300, viii.
22. Rand JA, Linscheidm RL, Dobynsm JH. Capitate fractures: a long-term follow-up. Clin Orthop Relat Res 1982;(165):209–16.
23. Sauder DJ, Athwal GS, Faber KJ, et al. Perilunate injuries. Orthop Clin North Am 2007;38(2):279–88, vii.
24. Grabow RJ, Catalano L 3rd. Carpal dislocations. Hand Clin 2006;22(4):485–500 [abstract: vi–vii].
25. Herzberg G. Perilunate and axial carpal dislocations and fracture-dislocations. J Hand Surg Am 2008;33(9):1659–68.
26. Budoff JE. Treatment of acute lunate and perilunate dislocations. J Hand Surg Am 2008;33(8):1424–32.
27. Frankel VH. The Terry-Thomas sign. Clin Orthop Relat Res 1978;(135):311–2.
28. Herzberg G, Comtet JJ, Linscheid RL, et al. Perilunate dislocations and fracture-dislocations: a multicenter study. J Hand Surg Am 1993;18(5):768–79.

Emergency Department Evaluation and Treatment of the Shoulder and Humerus

James Bonz, MD*, Bradford Tinloy, MD

KEYWORDS

- Shoulder trauma • Humerus fracture • Dislocated shoulder • Shoulder injury

KEY POINTS

- Always assess neurologic function and vascular status in the upper extremity when examining the shoulder, as many injuries have the potential to harm these systems.
- Open or displaced fractures, or compromise to either the neurologic or vascular systems, require orthopedic consult.
- Fractures to the body of the scapula necessitate a thorough evaluation for other occult injury.
- Emergency department physicians should be comfortable with several of the standard shoulder reduction techniques for optimum success.

BACKGROUND

Injuries to the shoulder are a common emergency department (ED) complaint. The intrinsic anatomy and function of the shoulder subject it to injury from repetitive stress, exertion, and trauma. Injuries range from fracture of the bones, dislocation of joints, or injury to the ligaments and tendons.

EPIDEMIOLOGY

The prevalence of chronic shoulder injury has been difficult to estimate for a variety of reasons; however, among Western populations, it appears to range from 8% to 26% and represents more than 2% of all yearly primary care visits.[1–3] Shoulder pain is the third most common musculoskeletal complaint, third only to low back and neck pain.[4] The epidemiology of specific injuries is variably understood.

Disclosures: None.
Department of Emergency Medicine, Yale School of Medicine, 464 Congress Avenue, New Haven, CT 06519, USA
* Corresponding author.
E-mail address: james.bonz@yale.edu

- The estimated incidence rate of shoulder dislocations in the United States is 23.9 per 100,000 persons; male individuals are more than 2.5 times as likely to present with dislocation than female individuals.[5]
- Clavicle fractures are common and represent 1 in 20 of all adult fractures.[6]
- Proximal humerus fractures are most common in the elderly, and among US EDs have an annual incidence of 60 per 100,000, with more than 75% of those occurring in patients older than 65 years.[7–9]
- Full-thickness rotator cuff tears are present in 5% to 30% of people older than 40.[10,11]

IMAGING

The American College of Radiology (ACR) has published guidelines on appropriate imaging for acute shoulder pain, and these recommendations set the baseline for ED imaging.[12] Three views are required for the evaluation of acute shoulder pain, 2 of which are to be orthogonal.

1. Anteroposterior (AP) projection
2. Axillary view
3. Scapular Y view

Anteroposterior Projection

In a straight AP projection, the patient is perpendicular to the beam; however, ACR recommends a "Grashey view," which is a slight variant of the AP.[12] In the Grashey view, or "true" AP, the patient is angled 45° away (obliquely) from the x-ray beam. This view allows for better visualization of the glenohumeral joint. The straight AP can be done with either internal or external rotation, allowing for either better visualization of the lesser tuberosity (internal rotation) or greater tuberosity (external rotation).

Axillary View

The axillary view is taken with the patient's arm ideally abducted to 90°. The cassette is placed superior to the shoulder and the beam projected on a plane perpendicular to the cassette through the axilla. The axillary view is often difficult to obtain secondary to patient pain with positioning. This has led to modifications of the axillary view, which are still able to pick up the injuries most commonly seen with this view, notably posterior shoulder dislocation and the Hill-Sachs deformity.[13]

Y View

The Y view is a lateral projection. The x-ray beam hits the scapula in profile, as it is "floating" on the posterior thoracic wall. The coracoid and the acromion form a "Y" with the body of the scapula. It has been noted that for diagnosis of suspected shoulder dislocation, the Y view has higher sensitivity than the axillary view and is less painful.[14]

PROXIMAL HUMERUS FRACTURES

On examination, the patient with a proximal humerus fracture will typically hold the affected arm in an adducted position. A step-off may be appreciated but is often obscured by surrounding musculature or subcutaneous tissue. A radiograph of the proximal humerus is indicated for diagnosis and classification of the fracture. An axillary view is most helpful in determining the degree of angulation and displacement of fracture parts.

Several classification systems exist to characterize proximal humerus fractures, but the Neer classification is the most frequently used.[15] This classification system divides the proximal humerus into 4 parts.

1. The humeral head
2. The humeral shaft
3. The greater tuberosity
4. The lesser tuberosity

The number of distinct parts involved then characterizes the fracture. This system divides fracture types into 1-part, 2-part, 3-part, or 4-part fractures. A fracture segment is considered a separate part if the amount of angulation is greater than 45° or if it is displaced by more than 1 cm. A 1-part fracture designates a fracture in which there is less than 45° of angulation and less than 1 cm of displacement of any of the 4 parts. Conversely, a 3-part fracture in this system is defined by having 2 individually displaced fragments from the remaining proximal humerus.

Nearly 80% of proximal humerus fractures are nondisplaced or minimally displaced and stable.[16] These are treated nonoperatively. There exists considerable controversy in the orthopedic literature regarding the treatment of 2-part fractures, with many undergoing operative treatment.[17,18] Three-part and 4-part fractures, open fractures, and fractures through the anatomic neck of the humerus require orthopedic consultation and likely operative repair, as studies have demonstrated poor outcome when treated nonoperatively.[9,19,20] Fractures through the anatomic neck raise concern for injury to the primary blood supply to the humeral head, which stems from the antero-lateral branch of the anterior humeral circumflex artery; when the blood supply is disrupted, avascular necrosis may occur.[21,22]

Management of nondisplaced and minimally displaced proximal humerus fractures consists of sling and ice application. Nonoperative 1-part fractures benefit from early immobilization and initiation of physical therapy within 3 days.[23] All proximal humeral fractures require orthopedic follow-up. Two-part, 3-part, and 4-part fractures require orthopedic consultation with regard to potential early surgical management.

HUMERAL SHAFT FRACTURES

The humeral shaft is the segment distal to the surgical neck of the humerus and proximal to the supracondylar ridge. The incidence of humeral shaft fractures increases with age after the fifth decade of life, such that these fractures are most common in elderly patients in the eighth and ninth decades of life and often result from a simple fall; high-energy trauma is more likely to be the cause of fracture in the younger male population and represents a smaller number of all humeral shaft fractures.[24]

Humeral shaft fractures are described by location and type. The shaft is divided into thirds:

- Proximal third
- Middle third
- Distal third

Fracture types are described as:

- Transverse
- Oblique
- Spiral

The radial nerve is at risk for injury in the setting of a humeral shaft fracture because of its close proximity and limited mobility at several locations along the length of the humerus. In a systemic review reflecting 4517 fractures, Shao and colleagues[25] determined the overall prevalence of radial nerve palsy after humeral shaft fracture to be 11.8%. Radial nerve injury is most likely to occur with fractures of the middle and distal thirds of the humerus.[24,26] Physical examination of the patient with a humeral shaft fracture should include a thorough neurologic examination to evaluate for radial nerve injury.

Most humeral shaft fractures can be managed with closed reduction and immobilization.[27] Functional bracing is associated with a high rate of union and acceptable angulation.[28] Most humeral shaft fractures are initially treated with a coaptation splint or hanging arm cast for the first 1 to 3 weeks, then placed in a functional brace.

Orthopedic consultation for potential operative repair is indicated for failed closed reduction with persistent excess angulation, radial nerve palsy development after reduction, open fractures, comminuted humeral fractures, and pathologic fractures.

CLAVICLE FRACTURES

Clavicle fractures occur commonly in the setting of direct blunt trauma to the shoulder. The proximal segment of the clavicle is cylindrical in shape and thus provides strength to the clavicle so as to protect vital structures that lie medially. The middle and distal segments of the clavicle are flattened, weaker, and more susceptible to injury.

A clavicle fracture may present with visible deformity and/or palpable step-off. Tenting of the skin may be present in severe fractures. Tenderness to palpation over the affected area is typically present. The proximity of the clavicle to the brachial plexus, particularly the ulnar nerve, raises concern for possible concomitant nerve injury with clavicle fracture. A thorough neurologic examination should be performed to evaluate for possible injury.

Clavicle radiographs are helpful in confirming the diagnosis and also differentiating fractures from acromioclavicular (AC) joint separations. This differentiation is of particular importance in the lateral segment of the clavicle, where the physical examination may be misleading.

Management of clavicle fractures focuses on minimization of nonunion, defined as absence of clinical or radiographic healing at 4 to 6 months after injury, and malunion, defined as angulation, shortening, or poor cosmetic appearance. Minimally or nondisplaced fractures can be managed conservatively with a sling and immobilization for 4 to 6 weeks, with studies showing nonunion rates from 0.03%–5.9%.[29,30] A figure-of-8 brace was recommended in the past, but studies comparing the figure-of-8 brace with a sling showed equivocal outcomes.[31] Additionally, the sling provides benefits in terms of comfort, ease of allowing periodic range-of-motion exercises, and less skin breakdown.[32]

Emergent orthopedic consultation should be initiated in the setting of severely displaced fractures with tenting of the skin, comminuted fracture, open fractures, and fractures associated with neurovascular compromise.[29,33] Most frequently, clavicle fractures can be managed with outpatient orthopedic follow-up.

SCAPULA FRACTURES

Scapula fractures are uncommon and can be divided by location.

- Body (spine) fractures
- Acromion fractures

- Neck fractures
- Glenoid fractures

Scapular Body Fractures

This fracture requires significant force, usually from blunt trauma. Given the amount of force required to cause a scapula fracture, patients should be evaluated for other associated injuries. In a retrospective chart review of 11,500 patients with blunt trauma with 92 identified scapular fractures, Stephens and colleagues[34] found that 76% of patients with scapular fractures had other associated injuries, and 49% had associated thoracic injuries. Scapula fractures have been to found to be associated with the following:

- Pneumothorax
- Pulmonary contusions
- Clavicle fractures
- Rib fractures
- Brachial plexus injuries

Treatment for nondisplaced (isolated) scapular body fractures requires sling or sling and swathe with orthopedic follow-up. Displaced scapular body fractures infrequently are considered for open reduction internal fixation (ORIF).[35,36]

Acromion Fractures

Fractures of the acromion are generally caused by significant blunt force to the shoulder directed inferiorly. They are often associated with other injuries, specifically AC joint dislocation and distal clavicle fractures. Nondisplaced fractures may be treated with a sling immobilizer. Displaced fractures infrequently require surgical fixation.[36,37]

Scapular Neck Fractures

Fractures of the glenoid neck often occur from falling on an outstretched arm, or blunt force, and frequently are found in conjunction with humerus fractures or shoulder dislocations. Scapular neck fractures account for one-quarter of scapular fractures.[36,38]

Nondisplaced fractures are stable for outpatient follow-up, whereas displaced fractures need early referral.

Glenoid Fractures

Glenoid fractures of the scapula often result from a direct lateral blow to the shoulder or force transmitted up the humerus (as from falling on the elbow).

- Glenoid fossa fractures make up nearly 50% of all scapular fractures.[38]
- Glenoid rim fractures account for only 7% of all scapular fractures, but are associated with up to 1 in 5 shoulder dislocations.[36,38]
- Fractures of the glenoid can directly affect joint mobility, and therefore these fractures, even if nondisplaced by radiograph, are frequently evaluated by computed tomography.
- Displaced glenoid fossa fractures are the most likely to undergo ORIF of all scapular fractures.[39,40]

Up to 90% of scapula fractures are nondisplaced.[36] Nondisplaced or minimally displaced scapula fractures tend to heal well, with good return of function without surgical fixation.[36,41,42] In general, most scapular fractures will heal within 6 weeks, but full functional recovery may not occur for several months. Open reduction is rarely indicated unless there is glenohumeral joint disruption, marked angulation or displacement of a fracture fragment, or neurovascular injury.[36–38]

ACROMIOCLAVICULAR DISLOCATIONS

AC joint separations are injuries commonly sustained by athletes and those who are otherwise active. The mechanism of injury involves a direct blow to the AC joint or a fall with an adducted arm and subsequent transmission of force from the humerus to the AC joint. A history of such injury mechanism should raise suspicion for an AC joint injury.

In the ED, initial imaging should start with plain radiographs. The typical shoulder film includes an AP, lateral, and axial view, although other specialized views have been advocated.[43] In general, however, plain film radiography for AC pathology has a sensitivity of 41% and specificity of 90%, so that physical examination contributes largely to the diagnosis of AC injury.[44]

AC dislocations are commonly classified as type I to VI separations, with types I to III being the most common subtypes.

I. A *type I separation* is an AC ligament injury, or sprain, without severe tearing of either the AC ligament or the coracoclavicular ligament. Radiographs are normal.
II. A *type II separation* involves a complete tear of the AC ligament, but an intact coracoclavicular ligament. There may be a visible and palpable protuberance on physical examination. A radiograph also may demonstrate elevation of the lateral aspect of the clavicle.
III. A *type III separation* results from complete tears of both the AC and the coracoclavicular ligaments with complete AC joint dislocation. A significant protuberance can be seen on physical examination due to a "high-riding" clavicle, which is the result of inferior displacement of the acromion and the remainder of the upper extremity.
IV. In a *type IV separation*, the distal clavicle is posteriorly dislocated through the trapezius muscle and may result in tenting of the skin.
V. A *type V separation* is a severe form of the type III separation that has a 100% to 300% increase in the AC distance on radiograph. This results from stripping of the trapezial and deltoid fascia from both the acromion and the clavicle.
VI. A *type VI separation* is a rare injury that results from severe trauma thought to involve hyperabduction and external rotation of the arm in addition to retraction of the scapula. It results in inferior dislocation of the distal clavicle into 1 of 2 positions, either subacromial or subcoracoid.

The goal of treatment is to achieve normal strength, full range of motion, pain relief, and prevent limitation of activities.

- Management of type I and II AC separations is generally nonoperative. Treatment consists of a sling, ice, appropriate analgesia, and a brief period of immobilization ranging from 3 to 7 days.
- The more severe type IV to VI separations will most often require surgical management, given the larger degree of tissue injury and joint dislocation.
- Treatment of type III separations is more controversial and must be evaluated based on the patient's occupation or sport, hand dominance, and degree of dysfunction. The current preferred approach to the type III separation is nonoperative, unless the patient has persistence of symptoms for 3 to 6 months.[45–47]

ANTERIOR GLENOHUMERAL SHOULDER DISLOCATIONS

Shoulder dislocations are one of the most common joint dislocations encountered in the ED and make up 50% of all joint dislocations.[48] They are classified as anterior, posterior, inferior, and superior, with the anterior dislocation accounting for 90% to 98% of all shoulder dislocations.[49]

On examination, patients with anterior shoulder dislocations will typically keep the affected arm at their side in an externally rotated position. The head of the humerus can usually be palpated anteriorly, and a sulcus may be seen over the lateral aspect of the shoulder.

Possible complications associated with anterior shoulder dislocations include the following:

- Bankart lesions, often difficult to diagnose initially, as high as 87% in repeat dislocations[50,51]
- Hill-Sachs lesion (54%–76%)[50–52]
- Rotator cuff tear (14%)[50]
- Axillary nerve injury (3%)[53]

A *Bankart lesion* is a deformity of the anterior glenoid rim (often separating capsule and/or labrum from the rim) that most often occurs after repeated anterior shoulder dislocations. The term often is used to refer to bony disruption of the glenoid rim. It may contribute to further joint instability and to repeated anterior dislocations, and thus may require surgical correction.

A *Hill-Sachs deformity* is a cortical depression in the posterolateral head of the humerus that occurs when force of the humeral head is directed against the anteroinferior glenoid rim during anterior shoulder dislocation. The Hill-Sachs lesion may occur concomitantly with the Bankart lesion.

The *axillary nerve* arises from the posterior cord of the brachial plexus at the axilla, crosses the inferolateral surface of the subscapularis, and proceeds along the inferior border of the shoulder capsule. It is thus susceptible to injury with anterior shoulder dislocations. To test for axillary nerve palsy, sensation over the lateral aspect of the deltoid and arm abduction should be assessed.

Prereduction Radiography

A prospective observational study conducted by Hendey[54] in 2000 demonstrated that emergency physicians were 98% to 100% accurate in their clinical diagnosis of a shoulder dislocation. The missed diagnoses in this study were in those with fractures. Although radiographs are typically taken before reduction, this study's data argue that clinical assessment may be sufficient for diagnosis in the absence of concern for concomitant fracture. Factors likely to predict fracture include traumatic mechanism, age older than 40, and first time dislocation.[54–56] In a retrospective cohort study, concomitant fractures were found in only 0.7% of individuals in their second and third decade of life, and thus this age group could be excluded from prereduction films.[57] Omission of these films would decrease cost, length of stay, and prevent additional muscle spasm that may inhibit the reduction process. Postreduction films, however, are merited to confirm reduction.

ANTERIOR SHOULDER DISLOCATION REDUCTION TECHNIQUES

Various techniques exist for anterior shoulder dislocation reduction. The success of each technique varies, and no technique is 100% successful. Technique selection most often varies based on physician comfort with a particular technique, resources available to the physician (ie, an assistant), and body habitus of the patient.

Traction-Countertraction Technique

A common reduction technique used by emergency physicians is the traction-countertraction technique, otherwise known as the modified Hippocratic technique. Its use has been advocated in dislocations that are difficult to reduce by other methods, although its success rate is between 70% and 90%.[58] Its use may be associated with higher brachial plexus nerve injuries.[50] This technique requires significant force and most often requires some form of conscious sedation. With this technique, one operator applies longitudinal traction in an inferolateral direction to the affected arm while a second operator applies countertraction, usually with the aid of a bed sheet wrapped around the patient's thorax.

Scapular Manipulation

The scapular manipulation method may be performed in either the seated or prone position. This method focuses on repositioning the glenoid fossa so that the humeral head may be placed back into its appropriate position. In the prone position, the affected arm is held at a 90° angle, downward traction is applied by either an assistant or weights, and the inferior tip of the scapula is adducted by applying pressure with the operator's thumbs. In the seated position, an assistant applies downward traction to the affected arm while the operator applies pressure to the inferior tip of the scapula. This is a preferred method of the authors, and has high first-attempt success (90%–92%) with 100% overall success reported.[59,60]

Stimson Technique

The Stimson technique is performed by placing the patient in the prone position on a stretcher, with the affected extremity hanging downward toward the ground. Reduction can be accomplished with gentle downward traction by the physician or with the use of weights that can be attached to the arm. This technique can be advantageous in a busy ED, as the patient can be monitored by an assistant while gravitational pull aids in reduction. The overall success rate is between 70% and 90%.[58]

External Rotation

The external rotation technique has reported first-attempt success between 78% and 81%.[61,62] With the external rotation technique, the physician holds the patient's affected arm in the adducted position with the elbow flexed to 90°. The operator supports the elbow with one hand while at the same time gently externally rotating the affected arm. Successful reduction typically occurs at 70 to 110° of external rotation.

Milch Technique

Milch[63,64] first reported his technique in 1938 and advocated its use as a highly successful single-operator reduction technique not requiring anesthesia. The Milch technique is performed by gradually abducting the patient's affected arm to an overhead position while the operator's other hand places pressure on the dislocated humeral head, not allowing it to slip more inferiorly. When the arm is fully abducted at the shoulder, gentle longitudinal traction and external rotation are performed. The operator then gently applies pressure to the humeral head to ease it over the glenoid and complete reduction. First-attempt success is reported to be as high as 89% to 100%.[65,66]

Spaso Technique

The Spaso technique is another technique that can be performed by a single operator. With the patient in a supine position, the affected arm is held upright toward the ceiling. The operator grasps the patient's wrist and applies upward traction while gently externally rotating the arm. It has been advocated as a highly effective reduction technique, even for inexperienced operators, not requiring sedation or an assistant, with first-attempt success of 87.5%.[67]

After successful reduction of an anterior shoulder dislocation, the affected arm should be placed in a sling. Careful examination of neurovascular status is imperative. Ice is given and outpatient orthopedic referral is appropriate. In 5% to 10% of cases, an anteriorly dislocated shoulder is unable to be reduced in the ED.[58] These cases need emergent orthopedic consultation.

POSTERIOR DISLOCATION

Posterior shoulder dislocations are rare and are usually related to seizures or an electrical shock, such as a lightning strike. A patient with a posterior dislocation will typically present with the affected arm in a flexed, adducted, and internally rotated position. Radiographs can be helpful in the diagnosis and may reveal a complication known as the reverse Hill-Sachs lesion, which is a cortical depression of the anteromedial segment of the humeral head. Closed reduction can be performed with the patient in the supine position. Lateral traction is applied to the affected arm as it is externally rotated. Posterior pressure may be applied to the humeral head to complete the reduction.

INFERIOR DISLOCATION (LUXATIO ERECTA)

Inferior glenohumeral dislocations are rare, accounting for less than 1% of all dislocations.[68] They are referred to as luxatio erecta ("to place upward") because of the appearance of the patient with the affected arm positioned above the head with elbow in flexion. In this type of dislocation, the humeral head lies inferior to the glenoid fossa. Soft tissue injuries including avulsion of the supraspinatus, pectoralis major, and teres minor muscles may occur. Brachial plexus injury is also common. Radiographs are helpful in aiding the diagnosis of the inferior glenohumeral dislocation. Reduction of this dislocation requires a traction-countertraction technique in which longitudinal traction is placed on the affected arm while it is slowly and gently adducted. Closed reduction is frequently successful, although treating physicians have reported using fluoroscopy given the rare nature of this injury.[00] Operative management may be necessary in the setting of associated displaced humeral head fracture or instability in patients with recurrent dislocations.[69]

SUPERIOR DISLOCATION

Superior glenohumeral dislocations are very uncommon. They are caused by severe anterior and upward force imparted on the adducted arm. Patients will often present with their arm in adduction with significantly restricted range of motion. In the setting of a superior dislocation, an AP view of the shoulder will demonstrate the humeral head overlying the acromion or the lateral aspect of the clavicle. An axillary view of the shoulder may show displacement of the humeral head anterior to the acromion and coracoid. Complications of superior glenohumeral dislocations include fractures of the clavicle, acromion, coracoid, AC separation, and neurovascular compromise.[70]

ROTATOR CUFF INJURIES

The rotator cuff is the sum of 4 individual muscles and their tendinous attachments: the supraspinatus, infraspinatus, teres minor, and subscapularis. These muscles, in concert, help maintain the position of the head of the humerus in the glenoid cavity during movement of the shoulder. Rotator cuff injuries are felt to be due to prolonged microtrauma, often resulting in partial or complete tendon rupture. Impingement syndromes and tendonitis therefore play a direct role in tendon injury.

Neer[71] characterized the degradation of tendons into 3 phases:

1. Edema and microhemorrhage
2. Tendonitis and fibrosis
3. Tearing of the tendon

According to Neer,[71] this degradation was due to anatomic impingement in 95% of patients. Microtrauma from impingement is most frequently due to the hood over the glenoid capsule, specifically the physical proximity of the acromion and the coracoacromial ligament to the collective bundle of tendons making up the rotator cuff. The supraspinatus tendon is affected by physical impingement most commonly. Chronic impingement is a degenerative condition that over time leads to weakening of the tendon. This will, with or without an acute traumatic stress, eventually cause partial or complete rupture.

Impingement and its downstream physiologic effects are thought to interact with other factors to varying degrees. Several investigators have noted the relative avascularity[72,73] of the supraspinatus portion of the rotator cuff and believe that frequent microtrauma and subsequent inflammation coupled with poor blood supply promotes fibrosis and eventual rupture.[74] Poor vascularity in this region appears to worsen with age.[75] In addition, there appears to be a higher incidence of rotator cuff tendon injury in people with a "hooking" of the acromion, a physical morphology in which the acromion curves abruptly downward.[76] It is important to note that impingement and rotator cuff tears also occur in individuals without this anatomic morphology.

Tendonitis

Tendonitis may occur in any of the rotator cuff tendons, but most frequently is seen in the supraspinatus tendon and long head of the biceps (bicipital tendonitis). It is the inflammation in the tendon that occurs in a continuum, as noted previously. The inflammation can result in calcium deposition, which further decreases the subacromial space and causes pain with movement, most often elicited with abduction or external rotation. Tendonitis is managed conservatively with orthopedic follow-up.

Impingement Syndrome

Impingement syndrome refers to the mechanical compression of the rotator cuff between the humeral head and the overlying ligaments, which leads to a syndrome of pain most frequently felt in the lateral shoulder. Impingement syndrome is often found in athletes with overhead arm motion (pitchers, swimmers, tennis players) and the elderly. Initial treatment consists of analgesic and steroid injection with physical therapy.

Rotator Cuff Tears

In patients older than 50 years, rotator cuff tears may occur with little or no trauma. In younger patients, acute trauma frequently precipitates tearing. Most often, patients have pain or weakness with abduction, and internal or external rotation. Physical examination has poor sensitivity in diagnosing even moderate tears.[77] Rotator cuff tears are frequently missed in the ED and require clinical suspicion. Rotator cuff tears are at the end of a spectrum of pathology that often includes impingement and tendonitis, and the symptoms and examination are often the same as for these precipitating conditions. Acute intervention is conservative, but outpatient orthopedic referral is important, as missed lesions may influence ultimate prognosis due to delayed surgical repair.[78] Younger and more active patients, as well as those whose occupations involve lifting or overhead movement, are likely to benefit from surgical repair.

REFERENCES

1. Linsell L, Dawson J, Zondervan K, et al. Prevalence and incidence of adults consulting for shoulder conditions in UK primary care; patterns of diagnosis and referral. Rheumatology (Oxford) 2006;45(2):215–21.
2. Luime JJ, Koes BW, Hendriksen IJ, et al. Prevalence and incidence of shoulder pain in the general population; a systematic review. Scand J Rheumatol 2004; 33(2):73–81.
3. McBeth J, Jones K. Epidemiology of chronic musculoskeletal pain. Best Pract Res Clin Rheumatol 2007;21(3):403–25.
4. Parsons S, Breen A, Foster NE, et al. Prevalence and comparative troublesomeness by age of musculoskeletal pain in different body locations. Fam Pract 2007; 24(4):308–16.
5. Zacchilli MA, Owens BD. Epidemiology of shoulder dislocations presenting to emergency departments in the United States. J Bone Joint Surg Am 2010; 92(3):542–9.
6. Allman FL Jr. Fractures and ligamentous injuries of the clavicle and its articulation. J Bone Joint Surg Am 1967;49(4):774–84.
7. Lind T, Kroner K, Jensen J. The epidemiology of fractures of the proximal humerus. Arch Orthop Trauma Surg 1989;108(5):285–7.
8. Kim SH, Szabo RM, Marder RA. Epidemiology of humerus fractures in the United States: nationwide emergency department sample, 2008. Arthritis Care Res (Hoboken) 2012;64(3):407–14.
9. Lanting B, MacDermid J, Drosdowech D, et al. Proximal humeral fractures: a systematic review of treatment modalities. J Shoulder Elbow Surg 2008;17(1): 42–54.
10. Bokor DJ, Hawkins RJ, Huckell GH, et al. Results of nonoperative management of full-thickness tears of the rotator cuff. Clin Orthop Relat Res 1993,(294).103–10.
11. Clark J, Sidles JA, Matsen FA. The relationship of the glenohumeral joint capsule to the rotator cuff. Clin Orthop Relat Res 1990;(254):29–34.
12. Wise JN, Daffner RH, Weissman BN, et al. ACR Appropriateness Criteria(R) on acute shoulder pain. J Am Coll Radiol 2011;8(9):602–9.
13. Geusens E, Pans S, Verhulst D, et al. The modified axillary view of the shoulder, a painless alternative. Emerg Radiol 2006;12(5):227–30.
14. Silfverskiold JP, Straehley DJ, Jones WW. Roentgenographic evaluation of suspected shoulder dislocation: a prospective study comparing the axillary view and the scapular 'Y' view. Orthopedics 1990;13(1):63–9.
15. Neer CS 2nd. Displaced proximal humeral fractures. I. Classification and evaluation. J Bone Joint Surg Am 1970;52(6):1077–89.
16. Helmy N, Hintermann B. New trends in the treatment of proximal humerus fractures. Clin Orthop Relat Res 2006;442:100–8.

17. Handoll HH, Ollivere BJ. Interventions for treating proximal humeral fractures in adults. Cochrane Database Syst Rev 2010;(12):CD000434.
18. Vallier HA. Treatment of proximal humerus fractures. J Orthop Trauma 2007;21(7): 469–76.
19. Olerud P, Ahrengart L, Ponzer S, et al. Internal fixation versus nonoperative treatment of displaced 3-part proximal humeral fractures in elderly patients: a randomized controlled trial. J Shoulder Elbow Surg 2011;20(5):747–55.
20. Olerud P, Ahrengart L, Ponzer S, et al. Hemiarthroplasty versus nonoperative treatment of displaced 4-part proximal humeral fractures in elderly patients: a randomized controlled trial. J Shoulder Elbow Surg 2011;20(7):1025–33.
21. Jakob RP, Miniaci A, Anson PS, et al. Four-part valgus impacted fractures of the proximal humerus. J Bone Joint Surg Br 1991;73(2):295–8.
22. Lee CK, Hansen HR. Post-traumatic avascular necrosis of the humeral head in displaced proximal humeral fractures. J Trauma 1981;21(9):788–91.
23. Lefevre-Colau MM, Babinet A, Fayad F, et al. Immediate mobilization compared with conventional immobilization for the impacted nonoperatively treated proximal humeral fracture. A randomized controlled trial. J Bone Joint Surg Am 2007;89(12):2582–90.
24. Ekholm R, Adami J, Tidermark J, et al. Fractures of the shaft of the humerus. An epidemiological study of 401 fractures. J Bone Joint Surg Br 2006;88(11): 1469–73.
25. Shao YC, Harwood P, Grotz MR, et al. Radial nerve palsy associated with fractures of the shaft of the humerus: a systematic review. J Bone Joint Surg Br 2005;87(12):1647–52.
26. Klenerman L. Fractures of the shaft of the humerus. J Bone Joint Surg Br 1966; 48(1):105–11.
27. Ekholm R, Tidermark J, Tornkvist H, et al. Outcome after closed functional treatment of humeral shaft fractures. J Orthop Trauma 2006;20(9):591–6.
28. Sarmiento A, Zagorski JB, Zych GA, et al. Functional bracing for the treatment of fractures of the humeral diaphysis. J Bone Joint Surg Am 2000;82(4):478–86.
29. Robinson CM, Court-Brown CM, McQueen MM, et al. Estimating the risk of nonunion following nonoperative treatment of a clavicular fracture. J Bone Joint Surg Am 2004;86A(7):1359–65.
30. Zlowodzki M, Zelle BA, Cole PA, et al, Evidence-Based Orthopaedic Trauma Working Group. Treatment of acute midshaft clavicle fractures: systematic review of 2144 fractures: on behalf of the Evidence-Based Orthopaedic Trauma Working Group. J Orthop Trauma 2005;19(7):504–7.
31. Andersen K, Jensen PO, Lauritzen J. Treatment of clavicular fractures. Figure-of-eight bandage versus a simple sling. Acta Orthop Scand 1987;58(1):71–4.
32. Balcik BJ, Monseau AJ, Krantz W. Evaluation and treatment of sternoclavicular, clavicular, and acromioclavicular injuries. Prim Care 2013;40(4):911–23, viii–ix.
33. Paladini P, Pellegrini A, Merolla G, et al. Treatment of clavicle fractures. Transl Med UniSa 2012;2:47–58.
34. Stephens NG, Morgan AS, Corvo P, et al. Significance of scapular fracture in the blunt-trauma patient. Ann Emerg Med 1995;26(4):439–42.
35. Gosens T, Speigner B, Minekus J. Fracture of the scapular body: functional outcome after conservative treatment. J Shoulder Elbow Surg 2009;18(3): 443–8.
36. Goss TP. Scapular fractures and dislocations: diagnosis and treatment. J Am Acad Orthop Surg 1995;3(1):22–33.
37. Cole PA. Scapula fractures. Orthop Clin North Am 2002;33(1):1–18, vii.

38. Lantry JM, Roberts CS, Giannoudis PV. Operative treatment of scapular fractures: a systematic review. Injury 2008;39(3):271–83.
39. Kavanagh BF, Bradway JK, Cofield RH. Open reduction and internal fixation of displaced intra-articular fractures of the glenoid fossa. J Bone Joint Surg Am 1993;75(4):479–84.
40. Mayo KA, Benirschke SK, Mast JW. Displaced fractures of the glenoid fossa. Results of open reduction and internal fixation. Clin Orthop Relat Res 1998;(347):122–30.
41. Armstrong CP, Van der Spuy J. The fractured scapula: importance and management based on a series of 62 patients. Injury 1984;15(5):324–9.
42. McGinnis M, Denton JR. Fractures of the scapula: a retrospective study of 40 fractured scapulae. J Trauma 1989;29(11):1488–93.
43. Mazzocca AD, Arciero RA, Bicos J. Evaluation and treatment of acromioclavicular joint injuries. Am J Sports Med 2007;35(2):316–29.
44. Walton J, Mahajan S, Paxinos A, et al. Diagnostic values of tests for acromioclavicular joint pain. J Bone Joint Surg Am 2004;86A(4):807–12.
45. McFarland EG, Blivin SJ, Doehring CB, et al. Treatment of grade III acromioclavicular separations in professional throwing athletes: results of a survey. Am J Orthop (Belle Mead NJ) 1997;26(11):771–4.
46. Phillips AM, Smart C, Groom AF. Acromioclavicular dislocation. Conservative or surgical therapy. Clin Orthop Relat Res 1998;(353):10–7.
47. Schlegel TF, Burks RT, Marcus RL, et al. A prospective evaluation of untreated acute grade III acromioclavicular separations. Am J Sports Med 2001;29(6):699–703.
48. Blake R, Hoffman J. Emergency department evaluation and treatment of the shoulder and humerus. Emerg Med Clin North Am 1999;17(4):859.
49. Westin CD, Gill EA, Noyes ME, et al. Anterior shoulder dislocation. A simple and rapid method for reduction. Am J Sports Med 1995;23(3):369–71.
50. Beeson MS. Complications of shoulder dislocation. Am J Emerg Med 1999;17(3):288–95.
51. Perron AD, Ingerski MS, Brady WJ, et al. Acute complications associated with shoulder dislocation at an academic Emergency Department. J Emerg Med 2003;24(2):141–5.
52. Hovelius L, Augustini BG, Fredin H, et al. Primary anterior dislocation of the shoulder in young patients. A ten-year prospective study. J Bone Joint Surg Am 1996;78(11):1677–84.
53. Weaver JK. Skiing-related injuries to the shoulder. Clin Orthop Relat Res 1987;(216):24–8.
54. Hendey GW. Necessity of radiographs in the emergency department management of shoulder dislocations. Ann Emerg Med 2000;36(2):108–13.
55. Emond M, Le Sage N, Lavoie A, et al. Clinical factors predicting fractures associated with an anterior shoulder dislocation. Acad Emerg Med 2004;11(8):853–8.
56. Shuster M, Abu-Laban RB, Boyd J. Prereduction radiographs in clinically evident anterior shoulder dislocation. Am J Emerg Med 1999;17(7):653–8.
57. Orloski J, Eskin B, Allegra PC, et al. Do all patients with shoulder dislocations need prereduction x-rays? Am J Emerg Med 2011;29(6):609–12.
58. Riebel GD, McCabe JB. Anterior shoulder dislocation: a review of reduction techniques. Am J Emerg Med 1991;9(2):180–8.
59. Anderson D, Zvirbulis R, Ciullo J. Scapular manipulation for reduction of anterior shoulder dislocations. Clin Orthop Relat Res 1982;(164):181–3.

60. Baykal B, Sener S, Turkan H. Scapular manipulation technique for reduction of traumatic anterior shoulder dislocations: experiences of an academic emergency department. Emerg Med J 2005;22(5):336–8.

61. Danzl DF, Vicario SJ, Gleis GL, et al. Closed reduction of anterior subcoracoid shoulder dislocation. Evaluation of an external rotation method. Orthop Rev 1986;15(5):311–5.

62. Mirick MJ, Clinton JE, Ruiz E. External rotation method of shoulder dislocation reduction. JACEP 1979;8(12):528–31.

63. Milch H. Treatment of dislocation of the shoulder. Surgery 1938;3:732–40.

64. Milch H. Pulsion-traction in the reduction of dislocations or fracture dislocations of the humerus. Bull Hosp Joint Dis 1963;24:147–52.

65. Janecki CJ, Shahcheragh GH. The forward elevation maneuver for reduction of anterior dislocations of the shoulder. Clin Orthop Relat Res 1982;(164):177–80.

66. Russell JA, Holmes EM 3rd, Keller DJ, et al. Reduction of acute anterior shoulder dislocations using the Milch technique: a study of ski injuries. J Trauma 1981; 21(9):802–4.

67. Yuen MC, Yap PG, Chan YT, et al. An easy method to reduce anterior shoulder dislocation: the Spaso technique. Emerg Med J 2001;18(5):370–2.

68. Mallon WJ, Bassett FH 3rd, Goldner RD. Luxatio erecta: the inferior glenohumeral dislocation. J Orthop Trauma 1990;4(1):19–24.

69. Groh GI, Wirth MA, Rockwood CA Jr. Results of treatment of luxatio erecta (inferior shoulder dislocation). J Shoulder Elbow Surg 2010;19(3):423–6.

70. Downey EF Jr, Curtis DJ, Brower AC. Unusual dislocations of the shoulder. AJR Am J Roentgenol 1983;140(6):1207–10.

71. Neer CS 2nd. Impingement lesions. Clin Orthop Relat Res 1983;(173):70–7.

72. Clark JM, Harryman DT 2nd. Tendons, ligaments, and capsule of the rotator cuff. Gross and microscopic anatomy. J Bone Joint Surg Am 1992;74(5):713–25.

73. Rathbun JB, Macnab I. The microvascular pattern of the rotator cuff. J Bone Joint Surg Br 1970;52(3):540–53.

74. SooHoo NF, Rosen P. Diagnosis and treatment of rotator cuff tears in the emergency department. J Emerg Med 1996;14(3):309–17.

75. Lohr JF, Uhthoff HK. The microvascular pattern of the supraspinatus tendon. Clin Orthop Relat Res 1990;(254):35–8.

76. Balke M, Schmidt C, Dedy N, et al. Correlation of acromial morphology with impingement syndrome and rotator cuff tears. Acta Orthop 2013;84(2):178–83.

77. Hughes PC, Taylor NF, Green RA. Most clinical tests cannot accurately diagnose rotator cuff pathology: a systematic review. Aust J Physiother 2008;54(3):159–70.

78. Sorensen AK, Bak K, Krarup AL, et al. Acute rotator cuff tear: do we miss the early diagnosis? A prospective study showing a high incidence of rotator cuff tears after shoulder trauma. J Shoulder Elbow Surg 2007;16(2):174–80.

Evaluation and Treatment of Acute Back Pain in the Emergency Department

David Della-Giustina, MD

KEYWORDS

- Back pain • Epidural compression • Epidural abscess • Herniated disc
- Vertebral osteomyelitis

KEY POINTS

- Back pain is a common presenting complaint in the emergency department (ED).
- Most patients have a benign etiology for their symptoms, requiring only a red flag focused history and physical examination without any diagnostic testing or imaging.
- Most patients with a herniated disc do not require emergent imaging in the ED.
- Suspected spinal infection and epidural compression syndromes are emergent conditions that require imaging with MRI in the ED.

INTRODUCTION: NATURE OF THE PROBLEM

Low back pain is a significant problem that has an annual incidence of 5% and affects up to 90% of the population at some point in their lives. It is the fifth most common cause for physician visits and accounts for approximately 3% of emergency department (ED) visits in the United States.[1–4] Approximately 30% of patients who present to the ED with back pain undergo diagnostic imaging with plain radiography; 10% undergo CT (Computed Tomography) or MRI.[5] Low back pain is the most common cause of work-related disability in persons younger than 45 years and the second most common cause of temporary disability for all ages. Approximately 2% of the US work force is compensated for back pain annually.

Most studies show that up to 85% to 90% of patients with acute low back pain resolve their symptoms in 4 to 6 weeks without any clear cause determined for their symptoms.[1–3,6] Because it is such a common complaint with a benign outcome for most, the provider can be lulled into a false sense of security and potentially miss clues to more serious disease that can have significant morbidity and mortality. To help

Disclosure: None.
Emergency Medicine, Yale School of Medicine, 464 Congress Avenue, Suite 260, New Haven, CT 06519-1315, USA
E-mail address: david.della-giustina@yale.edu

Emerg Med Clin N Am 33 (2015) 311–326
http://dx.doi.org/10.1016/j.emc.2014.12.005
0733-8627/15/$ – see front matter © 2015 Elsevier Inc. All rights reserved.

prevent this, the provider should approach every patient with a complaint of back pain systematically, with a focus on "red flags" in the history and physical examination that are markers for more serious disease, and use the presence or absence of these to drive the diagnostic and treatment plan.

The "red flags" of back pain are important historical and physical features that point to potentially dangerous conditions. Identification of a red flag warrants close attention and potentially further evaluation with diagnostic testing. These red flags were defined in a set of guidelines on acute low back pain published by the Agency for Health Care Policy and Research.[6]

PATIENT HISTORY

A focused history is the most critical tool for identifying risk factors for serious disease in a patient who presents with low back pain. Directing the history toward the red flags allows for an efficient, cost-effective assessment (**Table 1**).

Duration of Symptoms

- Low back pain falls into 3 categories based on duration:
  - *Acute pain* lasts less than 6 weeks;
  - *Subacute pain* continues for 6 to 12 weeks; and
  - *Chronic pain* persists for longer than 12 weeks.
- Pain lasting longer than 6 weeks is a red flag because 80% to 90% of episodes have resolved by that time.

Table 1
Clues in the history that raise a "red flag" in the evaluation of low back pain

Red Flags	Possible Cause
Duration >6 wk	Tumor, infection, rheumatologic
Age <18 y	Congenital defect, tumor, infection, spondylolysis, spondylolisthesis
Age >50 y	Tumor, infection, intra-abdominal process (abdominal aortic aneurysm, pancreatitis, kidney stone)
Major trauma, or minor trauma in elderly	Fracture
Cancer	Tumor
Fever, chills, night sweats	Tumor, infection
Weight loss	Tumor, infection
Injection drug use	Infection
Immunocompromised status	Infection
Recent genitourinary or gastrointestinal procedure	Infection
Night pain	Tumor, infection
Unremitting pain	Tumor, infection
Pain worsened by coughing, sitting, or Valsalva maneuver	Herniated disc
Pain radiating below knee	Herniated disc or nerve root compression below the L3 nerve root
Incontinence	Epidural compression syndrome
Saddle anesthesia	Epidural compression syndrome
Severe or rapidly progressive neurologic deficit	Epidural compression syndrome

- A common ED presentation is the patient who has had pain for 4 to 6 weeks without any medical evaluation or treatment regimen. In these cases, it is reasonable to delay the workup and to have them followed closely by their primary care provider, as long as there are no other red flags.
- Another common, yet higher risk, presentation is the patient who has chronic back symptoms but has acute worsening of the pain. In these patients, review the previous evaluation to ensure it has been thorough and that important findings have not been overlooked.

Age

- Back pain in patients younger than 18 or older than 50 years is a red flag.
- In both of these age groups, a serious etiology, such as tumor or infection, should be considered.
- Patients under age 18 have also have an higher incidence of congenital and bony abnormalities, such as spondylolisthesis or spondylolysis.
- Patients older than 50 years are more likely to have nonmechanical causes, such as a rupturing abdominal aortic aneurysm or other intra-abdominal processes.
- Spinal stenosis is more common in persons older than 65 years.

Location and Radiation of the Pain

- Pain that originates from muscular or ligamentous strain, or from degenerative disc disease without nerve involvement, is located primarily in the back, although it may radiate into the buttocks or thighs.
- Pain that radiates below the knee is a red flag for a herniated disc or nerve root compression below the L3 nerve root.
  - This is based on the dermatomal distribution of the nerve roots and the fact that the pain associated with compression or inflammation is referred along the entire pathway of the nerve.
  - More than 90% of herniated discs occur at the L4-5 or the L5-S1 disc space. This means that they impinge on the L5 or S1 nerve roots respectively, and produce a radiculopathy that extends into the lower leg and foot along the pathway of that nerve root.[1,7]
- The location of the pain helps to distinguish mechanical low back pain from sciatica.
  - Sciatica is a radicular pain that travels into the legs in the distribution of a lumbar or sacral nerve root and is accompanied often by sensory and motor deficits.[1,7]
  - Sciatica may be associated with low back pain, but patients with sciatica typically complain primarily about the leg symptoms more so than the back pain.
  - Only 1% to 3% of patients with low back pain have associated sciatic symptoms.[1,7,8]

History of Trauma

- Major trauma is a red flag for the possibility of fracture and should prompt the physician to order plain radiographs of the involved spine.
- Minor trauma in the elderly, such as falling from a standing or seated position, should also raise concern for fracture owing to osteoporosis.

Systemic Complaints

- Constitutional symptoms, such as fever, chills, night sweats, malaise, or unintended weight loss, suggest infection or malignancy.

- Constitutional symptoms are especially worrisome if the patient is immunocompromised, including diabetes, or has other risk factors for infection, such as a recent bacterial infection or injection drug use.
  - Back pain in an injection drug user is generally assumed to be a spinal infection until ruled out with imaging studies.
  - A recent pneumonia, urinary tract infection, or genitourinary or gastrointestinal procedure may predispose the patient to infection secondary to bacteremia.

Atypical Pain Features

- Benign low back pain is typically described as a dull, aching pain that generally worsens with movement and improves with lying still.
- Red flags for tumor and infection include pain that is much worse at night or is unrelenting, despite appropriate analgesia and rest.
- Pain from a herniated disc may be worsened by coughing, sitting, or the Valsalva maneuver and is relieved by lying supine.[7–9]
- Spinal stenosis is a bilateral sciatic pain worsened by activities such as walking, prolonged standing, and back extension, and is relieved by rest and forward flexion.
- In the author's experience, night pain and unrelenting pain are the most worrisome symptoms that are commonly overlooked in the evaluation of patients with back pain.

Associated Neurologic Deficits

- Most patients with a benign etiology for low back pain will have no neurologic deficits.
- Any severe or rapidly progressive neurologic deficit is a red flag.
  - Consider an epidural compression syndrome, such as spinal cord compression, cauda equina syndrome, or conus medullaris syndrome, in a patient who reports bowel or bladder incontinence with low back pain.
  - Patients with a history of urinary incontinence (whether just 1 episode or many) may be evaluated by measuring a postvoid residual volume.
    - A large postvoid residual indicates overflow incontinence. In the setting of low back pain, this suggests significant neurologic compromise and mandates an immediate evaluation for an epidural compression syndrome.
    - A negative postvoid residual rules out significant neurologic compromise.[1,10]
  - Other neurologic complaints, such as paresthesias, numbness, weakness, and gait disturbances, need to be further evaluated during the history and physical examination to determine whether the symptoms involve single or multiple nerve roots.

History of Cancer

- Patients with a history of cancer are at risk of spinal metastases. The more common malignancies that involve the spine are breast, lung, thyroid, kidney, and prostate cancers, and myeloma, lymphoma, and sarcoma.
- In more than 90% of these patients, back pain is the initial symptom of spinal metastases.[1,11–13]

Urinary, Abdominal, or Chest Complaints

- Review these areas to avoid overlooking disease processes referring to the back.
- The most serious of these is a ruptured abdominal aortic aneurysm. Other potential causes of pain referred to the back include pancreatitis, a posterior lower lobe pneumonia, nephrolithiasis, and renal infarct.

PHYSICAL EXAMINATION

The examination is neither complicated nor prolonged. It is directed toward ruling out red flags and identifying specific neurologic deficits (**Table 2**).

Vital Signs

- Fever strongly suggests infection.
  - The sensitivity of fever is low: 27% for tuberculous osteomyelitis, 50% for pyogenic osteomyelitis, 60% to 70% for pyogenic discitis, and 66% to 83% for spinal epidural abscess.[10,14–16]
  - Approximately 2% of patients with nonspecific back pain present with a fever that is not owing to a spinal infection. In these cases, it is usually attributed to a concomitant viral illness.[10] Noting this, the principal concern should still be for spinal infection until further history, examination, and possibly diagnostic testing rule it out.

General Appearance

- The patient with benign back pain is most comfortable when lying still.
- In the patient who is writhing and cannot get comfortable, consider spinal infection, abdominal aortic aneurysm or dissection, and nephrolithiasis.

Abdomen

- All patients require an abdominal examination evaluating for masses, tenderness, or evidence of an aortic aneurysm.

Back

- Examine for any signs of underlying disease.
- Erythema, warmth, and purulent drainage are signs of infection.
- Contusion or swelling raises a red flag for trauma.
- Point tenderness to percussion is found with fractures and bacterial infection, with a sensitivity of 86% and specificity of 60% for infection.[10]

Perform a Straight Leg Raise Test

- With the patient lying supine, passively lift each leg individually to approximately 70° in an attempt to produce pain.
- A positive result consists of the reproduction of the patient's radicular pain that travels below the knee of the affected leg.
  - This radicular pain is worsened by ankle dorsiflexion and improved with ankle plantar flexion or decreased elevation.

Table 2	
Red flags in the physical examination	
Red Flags	**Possible Cause**
Fever	Infection
Unexpected anal sphincter laxity	Epidural compression syndrome
Perianal/perineal sensory loss	Epidural compression syndrome
Major motor weakness	Nerve root compression
Point tenderness to percussion	Fracture or infection
Positive straight leg raise test result	L5 or S1 herniated disc

- ○ Reproduction of the patient's back pain or pain in the hamstring area does not constitute a positive result.
- A positive straight leg raise is about 80% sensitive for an L4-5 or L5-S1 herniated disc.
- Radicular pain in the affected leg when the asymptomatic leg is lifted (positive crossed straight leg raise) is highly specific but not sensitive for a herniated disc.[1,2,7,8]

Neurologic Examination

- This is the most important portion of the examination.
- Test sensation using light touch initially, followed by a pinprick, temperature, proprioception, and vibration if there are abnormalities on the initial examination.
- Test strength and reflexes by focusing on each muscle group and reflex innervated by a specific nerve root.
- Spinal nerve root examination:
  - ○ The L1 through L3 nerve roots supply sensation over the anterior thigh and provide strength to the hip flexors. There is no well-defined reflex for these nerve roots.
  - ○ The L4 nerve root provides sensation over the medial surface of the leg and foot, including the medial surface of the great toe, but not the first dorsal web space. The motor component of L4 involves leg extension (L2–L4) and ankle dorsiflexion and inversion. The patellar reflex is innervated predominantly by the L4 nerve root, with some contribution from L2 and L3.
  - ○ The L5 nerve root provides sensation over the lateral leg and the dorsum of the foot, including the first dorsal web space. The muscular innervation from L5 is the extensor hallucis longus (great toe dorsiflexion) and dorsiflexors of the foot. There is no well-defined reflex for L5.
  - ○ The S1 nerve root provides sensation over the plantar and lateral surface of the foot. It innervates the peroneal muscles, which evert the foot and, along with the S2 nerve root, is responsible for the muscles that plantarflex the foot and allow toe walking. The S1 nerve root innervates the Achilles' reflex.
  - ○ The S2 through S4 nerve roots supply sensation to the perineum, forming concentric rings surrounding the rectum. They are responsible for innervating the bladder and intrinsic muscle of the foot. They innervate the anal wink reflex.

Rectal Examination

- A rectal examination is not mandated for all patients with low back pain. It is indicated in those patients with red flags, especially those with neurologic complaints or severe pain.
- Evaluate rectal tone and sensation, for prostatic and rectal masses, and for abscess.
- Poor rectal tone in association with back pain and saddle anesthesia indicates an epidural compression syndrome.

IMAGING AND ADDITIONAL TESTING

In the majority of patients, no testing is required. However, diagnostic testing is indicated in the ED if the physician has a concern for fracture, infection, epidural compression, spinal metastases, or rheumatologic causes of the back pain.

Laboratory Tests

- Order a complete blood count, erythrocyte sedimentation rate (ESR), and urinalysis when considering spinal infection, neoplastic disease, or rheumatologic disease.
- With infection, the white blood cell count may be normal or elevated, but one cannot rely on a normal white blood cell count to rule out infection.
- With infection, the ESR is typically elevated (>20 mm/h), even in those with immunocompromise, with a sensitivity of 90% to 98% for an infectious etiology of spine pain.[14–18] The ESR is also elevated in patients with a rheumatologic etiology of their symptoms, as well as in the majority of patients with neoplastic disease of the spine.[1,19]
- C-reactive protein is a commonly ordered test and it is increased with acute spinal infection.[1,14,20]
- Urinalysis is obtained to rule out urinary tract infection as an infectious source.
- Blood cultures should be drawn if there is a concern for spinal infection because they are frequently positive and help with long-term management.

DIAGNOSTIC IMAGING
Plain Radiographs

- Obtain plain radiographs if there is suspicion of a fracture.
- Only anteroposterior and lateral films of the lumbar spine are necessary; oblique projections add little information and more than double gonadal radiation exposure and cost.[8]

MRI

- MRI is the preferred imaging modality for most patients with low back pain.
- MRI offers the best resolution of lesions in the vertebral bodies, soft tissue, spinal canal, and spinal cord, and provides excellent visualization of disc disease.
- Emergent MRI is the gold standard study for the evaluation of suspected spinal infection and epidural compression syndrome.
- MRI is indicated for routine or urgent use in the evaluation of neoplastic processes of the spine and of disc disease or when the patient's symptoms fail to resolve after 6 to 8 weeks.

Computed Tomography

- CT is most useful in evaluating vertebral fractures, the facet joints, and the posterior elements of the spine.
- Its widespread availability makes it useful in emergencies when MRI is either unavailable or unsuitable.
- CT myelography is the best alternative when lesions involving the spinal canal are suspected and MRI is unavailable or if the patient is unable to undergo MRI.

DIFFERENTIAL DIAGNOSIS
Nonspecific Back Pain

Most patients with acute low back pain have conditions that may be generally classified as having nonspecific back pain; a more precise diagnosis is never made in up to 85% of these patients.[1,2] The patient typically complains of a mild to moderate low back pain that is aggravated with movement and relieved with rest. There is usually no significant identifiable cause of the pain, nor are there any remarkable findings on the physical examination. The evaluation of any red flags noted in the history or on physical examination reveals no significant underlying condition.

Treatment options

- These patients can be treated conservatively and monitored for 4 to 6 weeks to see if symptoms improve before requiring diagnostic evaluation. This is because 85% to 90% of these patients will recover spontaneously during this period.[1,6]
- If any red flags appear or if the patient fails to improve, then diagnostic testing is indicated.[1,6]
- Relapses of nonspecific low back pain occur in approximately 40% of patients within the first 6 months.[21] A recurrence unaccompanied by red flags may not require immediate referral or further diagnostic evaluation.

PHARMACOLOGIC TREATMENT OPTIONS
Nonsteroidal Anti-inflammatory Drugs

- Nonsteroidal anti-inflammatory drugs (NSAIDs), which are all equally efficacious, are considered as first-line therapy for acute low back pain.[1,22–24]
- However, 1 meta-analysis showed that NSAIDs vary in their side effect profiles and toxicity.[25] Ibuprofen was the least toxic, particularly with regard to upper gastrointestinal tract bleeding. The concomitant use of misoprostol or omeprazole reduces the risk of clinically important gastrointestinal tract bleeding during NSAID therapy.[25]

Acetaminophen

- There is no definitive evidence that NSAIDs are more effective than acetaminophen for symptomatic relief of low back pain.[1,25]
- The author recommends using acetaminophen in combination with NSAIDs or as the sole initial agent when treating patients at risk for adverse effects of NSAIDs.

Opiate Analgesics

- Opiate analgesics may be prescribed for patients with moderate to severe pain. It is best not to prescribe more than 1 to 2 weeks of medication.
- When prescribing combination opiate–acetaminophen analgesics, warn patients not to combine them with other acetaminophen products.

Muscle Relaxants

- Muscle relaxants are as effective as NSAIDs, but they do not have a synergistic benefit when used in combination with NSAIDs.[1,22]

Steroids

- Systemic steroids are not recommended, because their benefit has not been demonstrated.[1,22,26]

NONPHARMACOLOGIC TREATMENT OPTIONS
Activity Modification

- Patients who resume their normal activities to the extent tolerable recover faster than those who stay in bed or perform back mobilizing exercises.[1,27,28]
- Counsel patients to continue their routine activities, using their pain as the limiting factor.

Spinal Manipulation

- Spinal manipulation is among the more controversial treatments of acute low back pain.
- Research has shown that manipulation administered acutely was no better than physical therapy and only slightly better, in terms of patient satisfaction with care at 1 and 4 weeks, than an inexpensive educational booklet.[29]
- A second study demonstrated that clinical outcomes with manipulation were no better than with standard medical therapy.[30]
- A Cochrane review concluded that spinal manipulative therapy was no better than standard interventions for acute low back pain.[31]

Other Physical Modalities

- None of the following have been proven effective for acute low back symptoms: traction, diathermy, cutaneous laser treatment, exercise, ultrasound treatment, and transcutaneous electrical nerve stimulation.[1,2]
- Heat or ice may provide temporary symptomatic relief in some patients.

HERNIATED DISC

Patients with a herniated disc typically present with back pain and radicular symptoms, commonly called sciatica. Sciatica affects only 1% to 3% of all patients with low back pain, but is present in 95% of patients with a symptomatic herniated disc.[1,2,7,8] A herniated disc is the most common cause of sciatica; others include foraminal stenosis, intraspinal tumor or infection, extraspinal plexus compression, piriformis syndrome, and lumbar canal stenosis (spinal stenosis).

Patients who present with low back pain owing to a herniated disc complain more frequently about the radicular symptoms than the back pain. Because more than 95% of disc herniations occur at the L4-5 or L5-S1 level, the radicular pain typically extends below the knee in the dermatomal distribution of that specific nerve root.[1,2,7,8] This radicular component is useful in differentiating true sciatica from nonsciatic conditions, such as trochanteric bursitis, hip osteoarthritis and meralgia paresthetica.[9] The approximately 5% of patients who have disc herniation above the L4-5 level are older persons. In this group, there is a relatively increased risk of disc herniation at the L2-3 and L3-4 levels. These herniations cause pain in the anterior thigh, weakness of the quadriceps, and a diminished patellar reflex on the affected side.[7,8] An additional distinguishing feature of sciatica caused by a herniated disc is that the pain is aggravated by sitting, coughing, or Valsalva maneuver and is relieved by lying supine.[2,7–9] The physical examination generally demonstrates localization of pain and a neurologic deficit in a unilateral single nerve root, and usually a positive result on the straight leg raise test.

Treatment Options

- If the patient has no other red flags, treat him or her conservatively and do not perform any diagnostic tests for the first 4 to 6 weeks of symptoms.[1,2,7–9] In the ED, the physician should explain to the patient why radiographs are not being ordered, because this is a common patient expectation.
- If the patient has a demonstrable neurologic deficit, the physician may consider obtaining plain radiographs. These will not diagnose the herniated disc, but are used to rule out other possible causes of the patient's symptoms, such as tumor, fracture, spondylolisthesis, and infection.

- If the patient's condition worsens or the sciatica fails to improve, order an imaging study, preferably an MRI.[32]

PHARMACOLOGIC TREATMENT OPTIONS
Nonsteroidal Anti-inflammatory Drugs, Acetaminophen, and Muscle Relaxants
- The use of analgesics and muscle relaxants is the same as that described for nonspecific back pain.
- Interestingly, NSAIDs are less effective for herniated disc than they are for nonspecific back pain.[1,7,22,24]

Steroids
- Systemic steroids are no better than placebo and not recommended.[8,33]
- Although not an ED procedure, epidural steroid injection is a treatment that may be offered to a patient with a herniated disc as a follow-up option.
- Epidural steroid injection may provide a short-term improvement in leg pain and sensory symptoms. However, no long-term benefit has been demonstrated.[22,33,34]

NONPHARMACOLOGIC TREATMENT OPTIONS
Activity Modification
- The treatment mirrors that of patients with nonspecific back pain.
- In 1 study, 2 weeks of bed rest was no more effective than watchful waiting when factors such as intensity of pain, bothersomeness of symptoms, and functional status were assessed. If a patient's symptoms are severe enough to warrant bed rest, the shortest possible period is recommended, in most instances no longer than 2 to 3 days.[1,27,35]

Manipulation and Other Physical Modalities
- The use of manipulation as treatment for sciatica is more controversial than its use in nonspecific back pain.
- Manipulation is generally not recommended for the routine management of symptoms from a herniated disc.[6,8,36]
- Forceful manipulation may cause or aggravate neurologic deficits.[8]
- Other physical modalities have not been shown to be useful in managing sciatica, although, as in the case of nonspecific back pain, heat or ice may provide temporary relief.

Surgical Treatment Options
- It is important to understand the surgical considerations for patients who present with a herniated disc so that the physician may appropriately educate them about their options.
- Most patients with a herniated disc can be treated and monitored without specialist referral; more than 50% recover in 6 weeks and approximately 80% of patients improve with nonsurgical therapy.[1,2,7,8,37]
- Most spine surgeons agree that surgery is appropriate only when all of the following criteria are met[7,37]:
  ○ Definitive evidence of herniation on an imaging study.
  ○ A corresponding clinical picture and neurologic deficit.
  ○ Failure of conservative treatment to produce improvement in 4 to 6 weeks.
- Emergency decompressive surgery is required only in patients with acute epidural compression syndromes.[8,37]

- Conservative nonsurgical treatment has been compared with surgery for herniated discs in several studies. The results showed that patients who underwent surgery had improved function and fewer symptoms at 1 and 2 years postoperatively, compared with those treated conservatively; however, by 4 and 10 years postoperatively, the results in both groups were comparable.[2,8,37,38]

SPINAL INFECTION

Spinal infections (vertebral osteomyelitis, discitis, and spinal epidural abscess) are uncommon but serious causes of back pain. Although these are different entities, they may all be part of the continuum of spinal infection. The most important issue is that, when the emergency physician considers spinal infection, those patients should be evaluated thoroughly owing to the potential morbidity and mortality from a delay in diagnosis. Unfortunately, these infections are missed commonly on initial assessments; some patients with vertebral osteomyelitis have symptoms for longer than 3 months.[14,17,39]

A concerning history is that of unremitting back pain and night pain in association with fever or other constitutional symptoms in a patient who is at risk for infection. Risk factors for infection include immunocompromised states (diabetes, human immunodeficiency virus infection, and organ transplant recipients), alcoholism, recent invasive procedures, spinal implants and devices, injection drug use, and skin abscesses.[14,15,17,20] On physical examination, approximately one-half of patients have a fever.[14,39] The white blood cell count may be normal but the ESR and C-reactive protein are almost always elevated, although this is nonspecific.[14,15,20,39–41] Blood cultures are positive in approximately 40% to 60% of cases and should be obtained routinely when spinal infection is considered. For all spinal infections, MRI is the gold standard imaging study that should be obtained to rule out infection. CT detects osteomyelitis and discitis; however, it does not visualize inside the spinal canal very well and as such may miss an epidural abscess.

Treatment Options

- Spinal infection requires emergent evaluation and management by a spine surgeon.
- In most cases of epidural abscess, the patient will undergo surgery, but there are situations beyond the scope of this review wherein the patient may not be taken to the operating room and will only be treated with intravenous (IV) antibiotics.
- Most cases of vertebral osteomyelitis and discitis are treated with IV antibiotics alone; however, the spine surgeon should directs the definitive treatment.
- All spinal infections require IV antibiotics. For vertebral osteomyelitis and discitis, consult with a spine surgeon before antibiotic administration, because antibiotics may result in negative culture results from a bone biopsy. However, do not withhold antibiotics unless specifically directed by the spine surgeon.
- Empiric antibiotic therapy should be directed against Staphylococcus aureus. Parenteral piperacillin–tazobactam and vancomycin, or similar agents with broad-spectrum coverage, can be given until culture results are available.[14,40–42]

EPIDURAL COMPRESSION SYNDROME

Epidural compression syndrome is a general term that encompasses spinal cord compression, cauda equina syndrome, and conus medullaris syndrome. Although the diagnosis of a complete epidural compression is obvious, evaluating patients with early signs and symptoms is more difficult because the initial differential diagnosis is broad and includes most conditions that cause weakness, sensory changes, or autonomic dysfunction. The history and physical examination enables the physician to narrow the differential to a potentially compressive lesion of the spinal cord or cauda equina. When the emergency physician has a suspicion of epidural compression, this clinical suspicion should be confirmed with an MRI.

The history of patients with epidural compression usually includes back pain with associated neurologic deficits, incontinence, and sciatica in 1 or both legs. The duration of symptoms does not help to differentiate these syndromes from benign causes of back pain. Important features are a history of malignancy and rapid progression of neurologic symptoms, especially bilateral symptoms.

The physical examination findings depend on the level of compression and the extent to which the spinal cord or cauda equina is compressed. The most common finding in cauda equina syndrome is urinary retention with overflow incontinence; it has a sensitivity of 90% and a specificity of about 95%.[1,10] This measure proves useful in patients who present with back pain and an ambiguous history of urinary incontinence. Evaluate these patients by checking urinary postvoid residual volume. The absence of a postvoid residual volume has a negative predictive value for cauda equina syndrome that approaches 99.9%.[10] However, this test alone should not constitute the entire evaluation of a patient who presents with other major neurologic deficits. Other common findings in patients with epidural compression include weakness or stiffness in the lower extremities, paresthesias or sensory deficits, gait difficulty, and abnormal results on straight leg raising.[10] The most common sensory deficit is "saddle anesthesia," which is diminished to absent sensation over the buttocks, posterosuperior thighs, and perineal regions. Anal sphincter tone is decreased in 60% to 80% of patients.[10]

The differential diagnosis for a patient who presents with an epidural compression includes spinal canal hemorrhage, spinal canal infections, massive midline disc herniation, and spinal tumor. Although less common, clinicians should have concern for spinal canal hemorrhage in the patient who is on anticoagulants and presents with a sudden onset of back pain and a neurologic deficit. Transverse myelitis is a noncompressive condition that may present exactly like a compressive lesion of the spinal cord.

Treatment Options

- When epidural compression is suspected clinically, especially when it may be associated with a tumor, administer corticosteroids before ordering tests or attempting to make a definitive diagnosis.
- The acute use of steroids in the patient with epidural compression from disc herniation, epidural abscess, and hematoma is controversial and there is no definitive recommendation.
- For the patient with potentially metastatic disease, the current recommended approach is to administer 10 to 16 mg of dexamethasone IV to the patient with known cancer and signs of epidural compression.[11,12,43,44]
- After administering the dexamethasone, the patient requires emergent imaging with MRI. In the past, the recommendation was to obtain plain radiographs initially and then to use those to help determine whether further imaging was necessary. This is no longer recommended because plain films add time and expense, but not much important information to the initial evaluation.[12,43]
- If epidural compression resulting from cancer is suspected, an MRI of the entire spine is recommended. This is because 10% of patients with vertebral metastases have additional silent epidural metastases that would be missed by a localized imaging study.[12,43,44] The presence of these tumors remote from the symptomatic site may change the management strategy.

- If cauda equina syndrome resulting from a massive central disc herniation is suspected, it is reasonable to obtain a localized MRI.
- Consult a spine surgeon to direct the management once the etiology for the symptoms is diagnosed.
- For patients who have epidural compression attributable to tumors, the outcome depends on presenting symptoms.
  - Patients who cannot walk before treatment rarely walk again.
  - Those who are too weak to walk without assistance but who are not paraplegic have a 50% chance of walking again.
  - Those who are able to walk when treatment begins are likely to remain ambulatory.[12,43–45]
  - Of patients who require a catheter for urinary retention before treatment, most continue to require the catheter afterward.[12,43,45]

BACK PAIN IN THE PATIENT WITH A HISTORY OF CANCER

The best approach is to divide patients into 3 groups based on symptoms.

1. Group I: Patients with New or Progressive Symptoms
   a. This group includes patients with new or progressing signs or symptoms of epidural compression that have developed over several hours to days.
   b. Treat this group with immediate corticosteroid therapy and obtain an emergent MRI.[11,12,44,46]
2. Group II: Patients with Stable Symptoms
   a. This group includes patients with symptoms that are not progressive and have been present for several days to weeks.
   b. Stable signs include an isolated Babinski sign or radiculopathy without other neurologic deficits or evidence of cord compression.
   c. Radiculopathy is characterized by radicular pain, weakness, sensory changes, or reflex changes involving only one nerve root. Involvement of more than 1 nerve root places them in group I.
   d. Evaluation and treatment are similar to those for group I, although MRI can be obtained within 24 hours if not available emergently.
   e. If MRI cannot be performed within 24 hours, then obtain a CT of the involved area to look for evidence of metastatic disease.[11,12,46]
      i. If there is evidence of metastatic disease, obtain an emergent MRI in the ED or transfer the patient to a facility that has MRI available.
      ii. If CT shows no evidence of metastatic disease, it is reassuring, but the patient should still undergo imaging with MRI in the future to better evaluate for disease in the spinal canal or spinal cord.
   h. One should administer 10 mg of oral dexamethasone while awaiting definitive diagnostic evaluation.[44]
3 Group III: Patients without Neurologic Signs or Symptoms
   a. Group III includes those patients with back pain only without any neurologic signs or symptoms.
   b. In the ED, obtain anteroposterior and lateral radiographs of the involved spine.
      i. If any focal bony lesions are discovered, obtain an MRI of the entire spine.
      ii. Normal findings on plain radiographs do not exclude the presence of epidural metastases. In fact, more than 60% of patients with lymphoma and epidural metastases have normal plain radiographs.[44]
      iii. If plain films are negative, refer the patient for follow-up by their primary physician within 5 to 7 days.

SUMMARY

Low back pain is a common presenting complaint to the ED that usually has a benign etiology and improves in most patients in 4 to 6 weeks. A red flag–focused history and physical examination will drive the diagnostic evaluation, if one is even necessary. For those benign etiologies for the low back pain, conservative management with NSAIDs, acetaminophen, limited opiates, and activity modification is the primary treatment regimen. When considering serious etiologies for the symptoms, laboratory testing is helpful, but MRI is the gold standard study that should be obtained. Consider treatment with steroids early before embarking on a prolonged diagnostic evaluation in those patients whose symptoms may be owing to neoplastic disease of the spine.

REFERENCES

1. Chou R, Qaseem A, Snow V, et al. Diagnosis and treatment of low back pain: a joint clinical practice guideline from the American College of Physicians and the American Pain Society. Ann Intern Med 2007;147(7):478–91.
2. Deyo RA, Weinstein JN. Low back pain. N Engl J Med 2001;344(5):363–70.
3. Andersson GB. Epidemiological features of chronic low-back pain. Lancet 1999; 354(9178):581–5.
4. Waterman BR, Belmont PJ Jr, Schoenfeld AJ. Low back pain in the United States: incidence and risk factors for presentation in the emergency setting. Spine J 2012;12(1):63–70.
5. Friedman BW, Chilstrom M, Bijur PE, et al. Diagnostic testing and treatment of low back pain in United States emergency departments: a national perspective. Spine (Phila Pa 1976) 2010;35(24):E1406–11.
6. Bigos SJ, United States Agency for Health Care Policy and Research. Acute low back problems in adults. Clinical practice guideline. Rockville (MD): U.S. Department of Health and Human Services, Public Health Service, Agency for Health Care Policy and Research; 1994. viii.
7. Deyo RA, Loeser JD, Bigos SJ. Herniated lumbar intervertebral disk. Ann Intern Med 1990;112(8):598–603.
8. Frymoyer JW. Back pain and sciatica. N Engl J Med 1988;318(5):291–300.
9. Mazanec DJ. Back pain: medical evaluation and therapy. Cleve Clin J Med 1995; 62(3):163–8.
10. Deyo RA, Rainville J, Kent DL. What can the history and physical examination tell us about low back pain? JAMA 1992;268(6):760–5.
11. Chamberlain MC. Neoplastic meningitis and metastatic epidural spinal cord compression. Hematol Oncol Clin North Am 2012;26(4):917–31.
12. Penas-Prado M, Loghin ME. Spinal cord compression in cancer patients: review of diagnosis and treatment. Curr Oncol Rep 2008;10(1):78–85.
13. McCurdy MT, Shanholtz CB. Oncologic emergencies. Crit Care Med 2012;40(7): 2212–22.
14. Cottle L, Riordan T. Infectious spondylodiscitis. J Infect 2008;56(6):401–12.
15. Darouiche RO. Spinal epidural abscess. N Engl J Med 2006;355(19):2012–20.
16. Reihsaus E, Waldbaur H, Seeling W. Spinal epidural abscess: a meta-analysis of 915 patients. Neurosurg Rev 2000;23(4):175–204 [discussion: 205].
17. Davis DP, Wold RM, Patel RJ, et al. The clinical presentation and impact of diagnostic delays on emergency department patients with spinal epidural abscess. J Emerg Med 2004;26(3):285–91.
18. Wisneski RJ. Infectious disease of the spine. Diagnostic and treatment considerations. Orthop Clin North Am 1991;22(3):491–501.

19. Deyo RA, Diehl AK. Cancer as a cause of back pain: frequency, clinical presentation, and diagnostic strategies. J Gen Intern Med 1988;3(3):230–8.
20. Sendi P, Bregenzer T, Zimmerli W. Spinal epidural abscess in clinical practice. QJM 2008;101(1):1–12.
21. Carey TS, Garrett JM, Jackman A, et al. Recurrence and care seeking after acute back pain: results of a long-term follow-up study. North Carolina Back Pain Project. Med Care 1999;37(2):157–64.
22. Deyo RA. Drug therapy for back pain. Which drugs help which patients? Spine (Phila Pa 1976) 1996;21(24):2840–9 [discussion: 2849–50].
23. Malanga GA, Dennis RL. Use of medications in the treatment of acute low back pain. Clin Occup Environ Med 2006;5(3):643–53, vii.
24. van Tulder MW, Deyo RA, Koes BW, et al. Non-steroidal anti-inflammatory drugs for low back pain. Cochrane Database Syst Rev 2000;(2):CD000396.
25. Gotzsche PC. Non-steroidal anti-inflammatory drugs. BMJ 2000;320(7241): 1058–61.
26. Friedman BW, Holden L, Esses D, et al. Parenteral corticosteroids for Emergency Department patients with non-radicular low back pain. J Emerg Med 2006;31(4): 365–70.
27. Dahm KT, Brurberg KG, Jamtvedt G, et al. Advice to rest in bed versus advice to stay active for acute low-back pain and sciatica. Cochrane Database Syst Rev 2010;(6):CD007612.
28. Malmivaara A, Häkkinen U, Aro T, et al. The treatment of acute low back pain–bed rest, exercises, or ordinary activity? N Engl J Med 1995;332(6):351–5.
29. Cherkin DC, Deyo RA, Battié M, et al. A comparison of physical therapy, chiropractic manipulation, and provision of an educational booklet for the treatment of patients with low back pain. N Engl J Med 1998;339(15):1021–9.
30. Andersson GB, Lucente T, Davis AM, et al. A comparison of osteopathic spinal manipulation with standard care for patients with low back pain. N Engl J Med 1999;341(19):1426–31.
31. Rubinstein SM, Terwee CB, Assendelft WJ, et al. Spinal manipulative therapy for acute low-back pain. Cochrane Database Syst Rev 2012;(9):CD008880.
32. Deen HG Jr. Diagnosis and management of lumbar disk disease. Mayo Clin Proc 1996;71(3):283–7.
33. Gregory DS, Seto CK, Wortley GC, et al. Acute lumbar disk pain: navigating evaluation and treatment choices. Am Fam Physician 2008;78(7):835–42.
34. Carette S, Leclaire R, Marcoux S, et al. Epidural corticosteroid injections for sciatica due to herniated nucleus pulposus. N Engl J Med 1997;336(23):1634–40.
35. Vroomen PC, de Krom MC, Wilmink JT, et al. Lack of effectiveness of bed rest for sciatica. N Engl J Med 1999;340(6):418–23.
36. Rubinstein SM, Terwee CB, Assendelft WJ, et al. Spinal manipulative therapy for acute low back pain: an update of the Cochrane review. Spine (Phila Pa 1976) 2013;38(3):E158–77.
37. Awad JN, Moskovich R. Lumbar disc herniations: surgical versus nonsurgical treatment. Clin Orthop Relat Res 2006;443:183–97.
38. Hahne AJ, Ford JJ, McMeeken JM. Conservative management of lumbar disc herniation with associated radiculopathy: a systematic review. Spine (Phila Pa 1976) 2010;35(11):E488–504.
39. Murillo O, Roset A, Sobrino B, et al. Streptococcal vertebral osteomyelitis: multiple faces of the same disease. Clin Microbiol Infect 2014;20(1):O33–8.
40. Pradilla G, Ardila GP, Hsu W, et al. Epidural abscesses of the CNS. Lancet Neurol 2009;8(3):292–300.

41. Jaramillo-de la Torre JJ, Bohinski RJ, Kuntz CT. Vertebral osteomyelitis. Neurosurg Clin N Am 2006;17(3):339–51, vii.
42. Tompkins M, Panuncialman I, Lucas P, et al. Spinal epidural abscess. J Emerg Med 2010;39(3):384–90.
43. Cole JS, Patchell RA. Metastatic epidural spinal cord compression. Lancet Neurol 2008;7(5):459–66.
44. Portenoy RK, Lipton RB, Foley KM. Back pain in the cancer patient: an algorithm for evaluation and management. Neurology 1987;37(1):134–8.
45. Helweg-Larsen S. Clinical outcome in metastatic spinal cord compression. A prospective study of 153 patients. Acta Neurol Scand 1996;94(4):269–75.
46. Kwok Y, Tibbs PA, Patchell RA. Clinical approach to metastatic epidural spinal cord compression. Hematol Oncol Clin North Am 2006;20(6):1297–305.

Emergency Department Evaluation and Treatment of Acute Hip and Thigh Pain

Matthew Jamieson Stein, MD*, Christopher Kang, MD,
Vincent Ball, MD*

KEYWORDS

- Hip pain • Hip fracture • Hip dislocation • Emergency medicine • Ultrasound
- Avascular necrosis • Tourniquet

KEY POINTS

- Ultrasound guidance for hip aspirations and femoral nerve blocks is safe and efficient for emergency department use.
- High index of suspicion is necessary for often missed diagnoses such as occult femoral neck fracture and those diagnoses associated with high morbidity such as compartment syndrome of the thigh.
- Application of tourniquets for massive extremity hemorrhage is safe and life saving.

INTRODUCTION

Hip and thigh pain are common presentations to the emergency department (ED). Etiologies range from benign to life threatening, and disposition varies from outpatient follow-up to emergent operative management. Hip fractures resulted in 306,000 hospital visits in 2010. Although the incidence of hip fractures is decreasing, the overall prevalence continues to increase because of an aging population. People older than 65 suffer fractures at a rate of 0.6% per year, a rate that increases to 2% per year for persons older than 85.[1–3] One in 5 patients suffering a hip fracture will die within a year.[4] Additionally, the emergency physician (EP) must consider entities such as avascular necrosis (AVN), compartment syndrome, and muscular disruption. This article reviews patterns and complications of acute hip and thigh injuries and clinically relevant diagnostic, anesthetic, and treatment options that facilitate timely, appropriate, and effective ED management.

Disclosures: None.
Department of Emergency Medicine, Madigan Army Medical Center, 9040 Jackson Avenue, Tacoma, WA 94804, USA
* Corresponding authors.
E-mail addresses: mstein1985@gmail.com; docball40@gmail.com

APPROACH

The differential diagnosis for hip pain is broad, and suspicion for specific disease is critical. History should include past surgeries, typical function and activity, recent lifestyle changes, and mechanism of injury. Physical examination should be diligent with specific muscle group and sensory testing. For atraumatic pain, the differential diagnosis includes degenerative and chronic mechanical, autoimmune, infectious, anatomic, and vascular etiologies; neoplastic etiologies; overuse; and occult trauma. Special attention should be paid to often missed entities such as stress and occult fractures, Lyme arthritis, AVN, prostatitis, and psoas abscess and "can't miss" diagnoses such as septic arthritis. Imaging will typically identify the cause after a traumatic event, but elderly and vulnerable populations may report or exhibit vague complaints.

The diagnosis may not involve the hip itself. Pain may refer to the hip from pelvic sources such as prostatitis or prostate cancer, urinary tract infections, pelvic inflammatory disease, or a psoas abscess.[5,6] Knee pain also frequently refers to the hip, particularly in children and the elderly, and conversely traumatic knee pain necessitates a close evaluation for hip pathology.[7,8]

TRAUMA
Epidemiology and Mechanism

Hip fractures and dislocations are common entities in the ED. The presence of one injury should raise suspicion for the other. Fractures of the femur may include the femoral head, neck, trochanters, or shaft. Timely identification is important, as delayed diagnosis is associated with increased mortality, surgical intervention, duration of hospitalization, or nursing home residency and dramatically decreased functionality. A delay in treatment of just 2 days doubles the mortality rate, and a missed occult fracture can convert necessary treatment from percutaneous fixation to open hemiarthroplasty. As always, the most commonly missed fracture in the ED is "the second one," and the EP should not cease investigation at the obvious injury.[9–11]

Leading mechanisms of injury vary by age. A younger patient requires a significant mechanism such as a fall from height or motor vehicle collision. Elderly or chronically ill patients may present after a more subtle insult. Vulnerable populations such as those suffering from deconditioning, osteoporosis, poor nutrition, vision impairment, or decreased balance all are more likely to sustain an injury and with it the increased risk of morbidity and complications.[12] Patient vulnerability or a suspicious mechanism should prompt advanced imaging, as up to 11% of patients with suspected fractures and negative radiographs will have delayed diagnosis of an injury.[13,14] A low threshold for the use of computed tomography (CT) or MRI is therefore warranted.

Relevant Anatomy

The femoral neck and head articulate the axial force of weight from the shaft of the femur into the axis of the pelvis. With its angle and compression, the femoral neck is a uniquely vulnerable point focusing at Ward's triangle, where femoral neck fractures most commonly occur. It is formed by a paucity of strain-bearing trabeculations. The medial and lateral circumflex arteries arise from the profunda femoris artery and anastomose around the femoral neck. They are particularly vulnerable to disruption, which causes an AVN. The femoral head runs anteromedially to the femoral nerve and the sciatic nerve runs posterior to it. Posterior dislocations may be complicated by sciatic nerve injury. Femoral nerve injury will present with quadriceps weakness and diminished sensation to the anterior thigh and medial shin.

Imaging Choices

Plain films are first-line studies and will frequently suffice to identify a fracture or dislocation. However, these studies miss 3% to 4% of occult fractures. CT is widely available but misses 2% of fractures, most often nondisplaced fractures, and is associated with higher levels of radiation exposure. Bone scanning is another alternative in patients who may have a contraindication to MRI but requires good follow-up, availability of the isotope, and willingness to accept a 1- to 3-day delay to complete the evaluation.[15,16]

MRI is the imaging modality of choice for hip fracture. Its use is limited by access, time, and expense. Similar to a stroke series, a limited study with the focal aim of diagnosing occult fracture has been proposed. In one study, abbreviated MRI using coronal T1-weighted or STIR (short T1 inversion recovery) was as sensitive as a full-series MRI with a sensitivity of 99.4% for fractures. It was also sensitive for AVN and muscular or ligamentous injury, while taking 10 to 12 minutes rather than the 30 to 45 minutes for a regular complete MRI study.[17]

Ultrasound scan is an evolving modality for the identification of fractures. Although CT and MRI are often considered for adults, the need for sedation and exposure to radiation limits their use for pediatric patients. Ultrasound scan has been used to screen for hip fractures in the setting of nonaccidental trauma. In a meta-analysis, sensitivity for fracture in adults was reported at 85% to 100%, rivaling or surpassing that of plain radiographs. Specificity varied from 75% to 100%. However, results vary and may be operator dependent.[18,19]

Femur Fracture

ED identification of fractures is critical, as up to 25% of affected patients will require full-time nursing home care, and half of all patients will require long-term assistance with ambulation.[20] The EP must be especially cautious in the elderly person. Fractures are managed based on their location and pattern.

Recent solidification of evidence has led to changes in the standard management of hip fractures. The traditional use of preoperative traction for fractures is not substantiated by the literature and should be abandoned except for select patients. The importance of timely surgical intervention has been reinforced. Although low-molecular-weight heparin is generally used postoperatively, pressure gradient stockings should be applied preoperatively. Adequate analgesia is absolutely essential and may even mitigate chronic pain. Femoral nerve blocks are increasingly used and gaining acceptance because of the excellent analgesia they provide.[21–24]

Femoral Head Fractures

Femoral head fracture typically occurs with anterior dislocation. Worse prognosis occurs with progressive dislocation. Multiple classification systems are in use and include the Epstein, Thompson-Epstein, and Stewart-Milson systems. Femoral head fractures are associated with posttraumatic arthritis and AVN. Increased severity may require surgical intervention after, or instead of, closed ED reduction.

Femoral Neck Fractures

Femoral neck, or subcapital, fractures are common and dangerous. They result from substantial force and are associated with 10% incidence of femoral shaft fracture.[25,26] The patient may present with shortening, external rotation, and pain with abduction with any range of motion of the affected leg. The prognostic Garden classification is the most referenced system (**Box 1**). Complications include AVN and nonunion caused

> **Box 1**
> **Garden classification of femoral neck fractures**
>
> Type I: valgus impaction only, incomplete fracture
>
> Type II: complete fracture without displacement
>
> Type III: displaced less than 50%
>
> Type IV: displaced greater than 50%

by weight-bearing stress on the curvature of the femoral neck. Paradoxically, younger patients have far worse outcomes, likely because of higher functional demands, with AVN and nonunion rates reported as high as 85% and 60%, respectively, and especially poor prognosis with posterior comminution.[27,28]

ED management includes identification through a high index of suspicion, advanced imaging, analgesia, positioning, and early surgical intervention. Patients will be more comfortable with a pillow under the knee of the affected side. Femoral nerve block should be strongly considered. If available, MRI is the preferred study. If not readily available, CT or bone scan is appropriate.[29]

These fractures are considered surgical emergencies because treatment within 8 hours is associated with lower incidence of AVN. Although under debate, treatment may include arthroplasty or closed versus open reduction and internal fixation (ORIF). Traditional treatment was based on the degree of displacement. Nondisplaced fractures are now typically treated with closed reduction and internal fixation. For displaced fractures, the trend has been ORIF for younger and arthroplasty for older patients. Better outcomes have been observed for total hip arthroplasty in the functional elderly versus hemiarthroplasty for the cognitively impaired elderly.[30,31]

Intertrochanteric and Subtrochanteric Fractures

These fractures are typically similar to femoral neck fractures, and similarly dangerous, with a 6-month mortality rate of 10% to 30%. The intertrochanteric region includes from below the femoral neck to above the lesser trochanter. The subtrochanteric region spans from the lesser trochanter extending 5 cm distally. Unlike femoral neck fractures, these types are associated with greater blood loss caused by the vascularity of the involved bone. Theses fractures also hold far less risk of AVN, at 0.5% to 1%.[32] Management is similar, typically either open or closed reduction with intermedullary nails or dynamic screws for intertrochantric fractures and various fixation implants for subtrochanteric fractures.[33–36]

It is critical to identify and treat hemorrhage from these injuries, as they can ultimately lead to hypovolemic shock. Preoperative anemia can predict perioperative mortality.[37] The EP should be vigilant for identifying blood loss into the thigh and initiating appropriate resuscitation. Blood loss averages 25% of body volume and is typically greater than estimated by both EPs and surgeons.[38] Application of a traction splint may reduce hemorrhage and pain. The EP may consider the use of tranexamic acid. Although thrombotic events are increased 4 to 6 weeks postoperatively in patients who received tranexamic acid at time of surgery, the CRASH-2 (Clinical Randomization of an Antifibrinolytic in Significant Hemorrhage) trial speaks in its favor if given within 3 hours.[39–41]

Trochanteric Fractures

Greater and lesser trochanter fractures are rare and have good prognosis. In young patients, they are typically an avulsion fracture caused by forceful contraction of the gluteus medius and minimus in the case of the greater trochanter and the iliopsoas in the case of the lesser. In adults, they usually result from trauma. Both types may be components of an intertrochanteric fracture. Patients bear weight with a limp, report groin or lateral hip pain, and have resisted range of motion. Greater trochanteric fractures displaced less than 1 cm may be treated with 3 days of bed rest and a month of crutch use with gradual return to activity. If further displaced, they are treated with ORIF. Lesser trochanteric fractures are managed with early mobilization rather than crutches.[33,42]

Femoral Shaft Fractures

The femoral shaft is exceedingly difficult to fracture. Shaft fractures indicate a high-energy mechanism and should trigger a search for intra-abdominal, thoracic, and retroperitoneal injuries. These fractures result from fall from height, gunshot wound, motor vehicle collision, or nonaccidental trauma. The thigh can conceal significant blood loss, and resuscitation should be initiated aggressively. A low-energy fracture may indicate underlying bone pathology, such as malignancy or metastasis, and should prompt further investigation. Special considerations include the risk of fat embolism and injury to the femoral artery and sciatic nerve. Femoral shaft fractures are graded by the Winquist classification system (**Box 2**). Despite its dramatic presentation, prognosis is good, although rates of amputation and malunion increase in trauma and complicity of neurovascular injury.[43,44]

ED management should focus on resuscitation, pain management, diagnosis of associated hemorrhage, nerve and vascular injury, and early orthopedic consultation. Patients with open fractures should receive broad-spectrum antibiotics and irrigation.[45] Because the femur derives its innervation from both the femoral and sciatic nerves, blocks of both nerves should be considered. Traction splinting should be applied, except in cases of sciatic nerve injury, for open fractures in which a bone fragment may be seeded with bacteria or when traction may exacerbate other nerve injuries.

Fat embolism is a potentially deadly complication commonly recognized by the classic triad of acute respiratory distress, petechial rash, and altered mental status. The patient displays hypoxemia, hypocapnia, and an increased A-a gradient. Unfortunately, CT scan may be normal. Treatment is supportive, focusing on respiratory status and volume resuscitation. Early surgery significantly decreases the incidence of fat embolism from 22% to 1%, although multiple injuries may force delayed reduction after traction or external fixation.[46–48]

Shaft fracture may cause vascular injury. Arteriography is indicated in the presence of bruit, obvious arterial bleeding and when distal ischemia is suggested by symptoms such as pain, paresthesias, pulselessness, poikilothermia, pallor, and paralysis. Prioritization of vascular repair versus orthopedic stabilization is still contentious. Anticoagulation reduces amputation rates in the absence of active hemorrhage.[49–54]

Box 2
Winquist classification of femoral neck fractures

Type I: minimal to no comminution, less than 25% of cortical circumference involvement

Type II: comminuted fragments involve 25% to 50% circumference of bone

Type III: comminuted fragments involve more than 50% circumference, minimal contact

Type IV: comminution involves entire bony circumference without cortical contact

Stress Fractures

These fractures are typically repetitive stress injuries in the young and those serving in the military. Although they only represent 2% to 5% of all fractures, stress fractures are associated with an insidious onset, are difficult to diagnose, and exert disproportionate morbidity.[55] Delayed diagnosis may lead to displacement. Nondisplaced fractures are treated with rest, protected range of motion, and gradual return to activity. Displaced fractures may require ORIF. Associated factors include distance running, female gender, eating disorders, amenorrhea, osteoporosis, and pain in the groin region that worsens with use and resolves with rest. The patient may report pain on internal rotation or hip flexion. MRI and radionuclide scanning may be required.

HIP DISLOCATION

The femoral head is a ball held deep in its acetabular socket by strong stabilizers, reinforced by a sturdy capsule and labrum. Dislocations imply high-energy insults but may result from less significant forces in the elderly, infants, or artificial hips. Direction of dislocation and presence of fracture determines treatment. The femur most commonly dislocates posteriorly but may dislocate anteriorly or centrally. The EP must resuscitate appropriately, appreciating the energy involved and search for distal injury or underlying cause. If there is no associated fracture, reduction should be accomplished as soon as possible to reduce the incidence of AVN and arthritis. Postreduction stability should be assessed. If instability is discovered, operative management may be required.[56] Prereduction CT or MRI is recommended, as reducing a fractured hip can cause displacement or other secondary injuries, necessitating surgical intervention.

Posterior dislocations result from a cephalad force to a flexed knee and hip, classically from a dashboard. They typically present with leg shortening, flexion, internal rotation, and adduction. The affected femoral head, closer to the film cassette, will cast a smaller x-ray shadow than the unaffected head and may obscure the lesser trochanter. Sciatic nerve injury is common, causing weakness and sensory deficit to the lower leg and posterior thigh. The peroneal portion of the nerve is most commonly injured, either by direct stretching or trauma from fragments of the posterior acetabular wall.

Roughly 10% of dislocations are anterior.[57] History is typically a fall from height, a dashboard injury to an abducted hip, or a posterior blow to a flexed hip. The leg may be externally rotated. The affected femoral head casts a larger shadow on plain film than the unaffected head, with a visible lesser trochanter. Anterosuperior dislocations may cause injury to the femoral neurovascular bundle with ischemia, pulse deficit, compartment syndrome, or motor deficit to the quadriceps and sensory deficit to the anterolateral thigh. An associated femoral head fracture portends a worse functional outcome, and the EP should investigate the presence of a femoral head fracture before attempting reduction.[58]

Central dislocations are rare, occurring from lateral strikes to the hip with intrusion of the head through the acetabulum. The patient typically experiences extreme pain with any hip range of motion. The fractured pelvis may result in exsanguination, necessitating aggressive resuscitation. Most patients require open reduction and internal fixation. A small study suggests that nonoperative management in patients with high operative risk or stable hip joints may have some potential.[59]

Dislocation of hip arthroses is increasingly prevalent, complicating 1% to 3% of arthroplasties in the first 6 postoperative weeks. Risk factors include age, laxity, female gender, comorbidity, and reoperation. The first postoperative dislocation is typically treated with closed reduction and a knee immobilizer. Repetitive dislocation typically requires operative management.[60–62]

Treatment of Uncomplicated Dislocations

Unless a fracture is identified, anterior and posterior dislocations should be reduced in the ED. Indications for surgery include an associated femoral neck or shaft fracture, an irreducible head, and a nonconcentric reduction.[56,63,64] An irreducible dislocation (10%–15%) constitutes a surgical emergency.[65] Loose fragments around the femoral head may require arthroscopy or open management. Management of dislocations with femoral head fractures should take place in consultation with an orthopedist.

In the Allis technique, the patient is placed supine. The provider applies in-line traction and flexes the hip to 90° with pelvic stabilization by an assistant. Slight adduction and "wiggling" internal and external rotation may help. Although the provider classically stands on the bed while performing this procedure, another variation, the "Captain Morgan technique", may also be used in which the provider places his or her knee on the bed underneath the patient's knee and cantilevers the patient's leg over his or her own while applying downward pressure on the patient's ankle (**Fig. 1**).

In the Stimson method, the patient is placed prone. The affected leg is placed off the edge of the stretcher to 90° of hip and knee flexion. With pelvic stabilization by an assistant, the provider holds the ankle and applies downward and anterior traction to the back of the knee. Hip dislocations reduced in the ED require procedural sedation, and appropriate pain control is critical. An opiate-benzodiazepine combination is common for use in sedation, but ketamine, propofol, and etomidate are frequently used as alternatives and are increasingly well described.[66–68] Ketamine may be administered intranasally early on.[69] Ketofol, a 1:1 mix of ketamine and propofol, may cause less hypotension than propofol alone with a shorter duration than ketamine alone.[70–73]

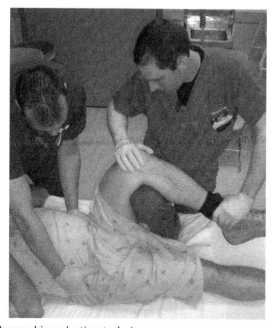

Fig. 1. Captain Morgan hip reduction technique.

The incidence of AVN increases from 5% to more than 50% if reduction is not accomplished within 6 hours from injury.[74] Heavy physical activity appears to accelerate posttraumatic arthritis, which complicates 24% of all reductions and 37% of those pursuing heavy physical activity.[75] After an uncomplicated reduction, early immobilization is recommended to avoid arthritis and intra-articular adhesions. Patients should avoid significant hip flexion for 4 weeks. Early weight-bearing status is debated because of a possible contribution to AVN. Strengthening exercises are mandatory. Sciatic nerve injuries are generally self-limited but may persist in delayed reduction.[76]

AVASCULAR NECROSIS

The femoral head features a unique vascular supply predisposing it to ischemic insult. The femoral head derives its major blood supply from a ring of the medial and lateral circumflex arteries. The head derives some blood supply from its foveal artery at the articular apex and from metaphyseal arteries, but AVN most frequently results from insult to the circumflex arteries.[77,78] Although most commonly caused by direct stretching from a displaced femoral neck fracture or hemorrhagic tamponade, AVN can follow dislocation, slipped capital femoral syndrome, or occlusion in sickle cell disease and decompression sickness. AVN may also complicate systemic conditions such as vasculitis, autoimmunity, alcoholism, radiation, and steroid use.[79–82] Delayed diagnosis can result in need for additional or more invasive surgery and increased morbidity. AVN complicates up to 40% of displaced femoral neck fractures, 10% of nondisplaced neck fractures, 3% of anterior dislocations, and 12% of posterior dislocations.[83,84] Idiopathic AVN may be bilateral in up to 60% of cases.[85] In the United States, up to 18% of total hip arthroplasties are performed because of AVN.[86,87]

Presentation is typically delayed by days to months after the initial insult. Patients may limp and feature a gradually worsening dull or boring groin pain or have pain radiating to the buttock or lateral hip, exacerbated by weight bearing or passive range of motion. Physical examination may be difficult because of pain. Internal rotation and adduction are particularly painful. Resistive muscle action may provoke pain from tensile stresses across the trabeculations of the femoral head. Advanced disease may result in joint deformity.

The EP should have a low threshold for advanced imaging for suspected AVN. The classic finding is the crescent subchondral collapse. Although radiographic evidence may be absent in the first stages, abnormal lucencies may become evident and increasingly severe with later stages. If plain radiographs are nondiagnostic, MRI is the imaging study of choice.[88] CT scan may show lucencies or deformity but is less sensitive than MRI. Angiography may also be considered but is associated with risks of arterial dissection and hematoma and requires interventional radiology consultation. Bone scans may show increased reactivity of the infarcted border with a cold center, but this modality is often impractical in the ED.[89]

Treatment of AVN depends on the underlying cause. An orthopedist should be involved early in traumatic cases. The traditional and definitive late treatment remains total hip arthroplasty, although procedures including resurfacing are showing promise for younger patients. Risk factor modification such as smoking cessation, statins, and hyperbaric oxygen may palliate the early underlying process. Core decompression of necrotic material may stimulate repair of salvageable bone if undertaken before subchondral collapse occurs, highlighting the importance of early diagnosis. Grafts may palliate or prevent collapse and preserve structural function but reoperation and completion arthroplasty are common.[89,90]

TOURNIQUETS

Devices to arrest bleeding date to antiquity.[91] Tourniquets fell out of favor for decades because of concerns of pain, compartment syndrome, rhabdomyolysis, reperfusion injury, and efficacy.[92] Recent wartime injury patterns resulting in uncommonly massive hemorrhage required immediate, easily accessible, and effective prehospital management.[93] The efficacy of tourniquets to reduce mortality from traumatic extremity injury is now well documented and has eliminated extremity hemorrhage as the leading cause of battlefield death.[94–97] The morbidity of tourniquets has been debated, but recent experience weighs favorably.[98] Use should not be delayed in the face of life-threatening hemorrhage.

The classic windlass tourniquet is the easiest to improvise and apply. It may also be self-applied. Pneumatic and locking screw tourniquets are alternative options.[99] Truncal tourniquets may be applied to the femoral artery for proximal bleeding or disarticulation. Further proximally, abdominal aortic tourniquets are also available.[100,101]

A tourniquet should be applied when direct pressure, elevation, and packing fail to adequately control bleeding, regardless of when an operating room will be available. Tourniquets lend themselves to use in wilderness or rural settings, prolonged extrication or inaccessible extremity scenarios, or in mass casualty incidents in which static providers are scarce.[102]

Occlusion of arterial flow is critical, requiring a surprising amount of force. Venous occlusion may cause backflow to the wound, increasing blood loss. Active hemorrhage control should be the primary metric of success. Resuscitation may increase systolic blood pressure and surpass tourniquet pressure, requiring frequent reassessment and adjustment. Tourniquet failure should lead to application of a second proximally adjacent "kissing" tourniquet sparing intervening skin. When removed, reperfusion injury should be anticipated, and the EP should prepare for hyperkalemia and renal injury. Severe ischemic pain can evolve in as few as 10 minutes. Nerve blocks and ketamine are attractive alternatives to opiates to control pain.

MUSCULOTENDINOUS INJURIES OF THE HIP AND THIGH

Although less common than with the knee or ankle, acute musculotendinous injuries involving the hip and thigh are increasing in prevalence, in large part because of the increase in athletic activities. Of particular interest are strains of the hip adductors and hamstrings.

Hip adductor strain, or pulled groin, is seen in high-energy or contact athletic activities such as football, soccer, basketball, baseball, and hockey.[103] The hip adductors comprise the adductor magnus, minimus, brevis, and longus as well as the gracilis and pectineus. This muscle group inserts focally at the pubic ramus, richly innervated with modest vascularity.[104] The most common mechanisms involve sudden acceleration, twisting, and abrupt changes in direction. Diagnosis can be made with localized swelling and tenderness in the proximal medial thigh and pain with resisted adduction of the leg with extended hip and knee. Ultrasound scan, CT, and MRI are often unnecessary, as complete ruptures requiring surgery are rare. Plain radiographs have limited utility but may show avulsion fractures. Initial treatment includes ice and avoidance of painful activities with possible crutches and physical therapy.

Hamstring injuries are common with sprinting during track and field, football, soccer, tennis, and waterskiing.[105,106] The hamstrings comprise the semimembranosus, semitendinosus, and biceps femoris. Strains most commonly occur with high tension during eccentric contraction of the long head of the proximal biceps femoris.

Waterskiing injuries may involve proximal avulsions after forceful hip extension while falling forward on an extended knee.[107] Diagnosis can be made with abrupt pain in the posterior thigh with resisted knee flexion. Complete rupture may cause a palpable defect and pronounced weakness. As with adductor strain, imaging is often unnecessary. Initial treatment includes rest, ice, compression, elevation, and avoidance of painful activities. Crutches, immobilization in knee extension, and physical therapy may be warranted for more serious injuries. In complete rupture, orthopedic consultation or referral is recommended.

Compartment Syndrome of the Thigh

Compartment syndrome of the thigh is uncommon with high resultant morbidity and mortality. It is traditionally associated with trauma such as femur fracture or crush injuries.[108] Other reported causes include seemingly mild contusions, muscle tears, drug abuse and strenuous exercise.[109–115] Cases have also been associated with anticoagulation.[116–118] Osteofascial pressures may exceed perfusion pressure in one or more of the anterior, medial, posterior, and psoas compartments.[119,120] Clinical diagnosis begins with the identification of a tense and edematous thigh with pain out of proportion to the injury and exacerbated by passive stretching.[121] Distal paresthesias and diminished pulses are possible but unreliable early findings, with reports of delayed presentation days to 2 weeks after injury.[122] If not clinically evident, diagnosis may be confirmed by measurement of compartment pressure within 30 mm Hg of diastolic blood pressure. ED management consists of elevation to heart level, analgesia, treatment of contributing factors such as fracture reduction and reversal of coagulopathy, and expeditious surgical consultation.[116,121,123]

PERIPHERAL NERVE BLOCKADE

An alternative or adjunct to opiates for hip and proximal thigh injuries is the femoral nerve block (FNB). The femoral nerve courses under the inguinal ligament and splits into the lateral cutaneous nerve of the thigh supplying sensation to the anterior thigh and the more posterior obturator nerve supplying the quadriceps muscles and the medial knee and medial calf. This ultrasound-guided block is a safe and simple technique for anesthesia in femur fractures and soft tissue injuries of the anterior thigh.[124–133] The 3-in-1 FNB is a variation of the fascia iliaca and FNB, targeting the lateral cutaneous nerve of the thigh and obturator nerve. It requires more local anesthetic and direct pressure 2–4 cm distal to the injection site to allow anesthesia of both branches of the femoral nerve.[125–127] An EP can perform the 3-in-1 block in an average of 8 minutes with minimal training.[125,127,132,134–136]

The EP should be aware that any nerve block may mask compartment syndrome by compromising the limb's neurologic examination. The authors advise consulting the admitting team before performing FNB. Complications are rare but include infection, hematoma, accidental injection of local anesthetic into the circulation, and transient neurologic deficit. The largest review to date showed a rate of procedural paresthesia in 2.0% and transient neurologic deficit lasting 5 days to 6 months in 1.9% of patients.[137]

The ultrasound machine is positioned opposite the provider with the patient supine and the leg slightly abducted. Using a linear probe, the landmarks of femoral nerve, femoral artery, vein, and fascia lata and iliaca should be identified. The authors recommend using sterile technique. Constant visualization of the needle tip helps avoid femoral nerve injury. The needle is directed anterior or lateral to the femoral nerve, avoiding the femoral artery. A pop should be palpable as the needle pierces the fascia lata and iliaca. Ten to 20 mL of 1% local anesthetic under the fascia iliaca is standard, but up to 30 mL may be necessary for a 3-in-1 block. After injection, pressure should be held 2 to 4 cm distal to the site for 3 minutes to achieve a 3-in-1 block.

SUMMARY

Hip injury is a common and challenging complaint in the ED and exists in a changing context of practice. Significant injuries to the bony architecture require timely and aggressive intervention and resuscitation and should initiate a search for additional distant injuries. The differential diagnosis frequently includes subtle entities such as occult or stress fracture and osteonecrosis. The EP is equipped with powerful imaging and diagnostic capability including ultrasound scan, MRI, and advancing therapeutic options such as tourniquets and nerve blocks. Emergency medicine must continue to develop its stewardship of these assets through evidence-based clinical decision making.

REFERENCES

1. Centers for Disease Control and Prevention (CDC). Fatalities and injuries from falls among older adults — United States, 1993-2003 and 2001-2005. MMWR Morb Mortal Wkly Rep 2006;55(45):1221–4.
2. Centers for Disease Control and Prevention. National Center for Health Statistics. Health Data Interactive. Available at: www.cdc.gov/nchs/hdi.htm. Accessed March 15, 2014.
3. Stevens JA, Rudd RA. The impact of decreasing US hip fracture rates on future hip fracture estimates. Osteoporos Int 2013;24(10):2725–8.
4. Farahmand BY, Michaëlsson K, Ahlbom A, et al. Survival after hip fracture. Osteoporos Int 2005;16(12):1583–90.
5. DeAngelis NA, Busconi B. Assessment and differential diagnosis of the painful hip. Clin Orthop Relat Res 2003;406:11–8.
6. Lishchnya N, Henderson S. Acute onset-low back pain and hip pain: a case report. J Can Chiropr Assoc 2004;48(1):5–11.
7. Chern CH, Hu SC, Kao WF. Psoas abscess: making an early diagnosis in the ED. J Emerg Med 1997;15(1):83–8.
8. Emms NW, O'Connor M, Montogmery SC. Hip pathology can masquerade as knee pain in adults. Age Ageing 2002;31(1):67–9.
9. Rashid A, Brooks TB, Bessman E, et al. Factors associated with emergency department length of stay for patients with hip fracture. Geriatr Orthop Surg Rehabil 2013;4(3):78–83.
10. Belmont PJ, Garcia EJ, Romano D, et al. Risk factors for complications and in-hospital mortality following hip fractures: a study using the National Trauma Data Bank. Arch Orthop Trauma Surg 2014;134(5):597–604.
11. Harty JA, McKenna P, Moloney D, et al. Anti-platelet agents and surgical delay in elderly patients with hip fractures. J Orthop Surg (Hong Kong) 2007;15(3):270–2.
12. Cummings SR, Nevitt MC. A hypothesis: the causes of hip fractures. J Gerontol Jul 1989;44(4):M107–11.
13. Parker MJ. Missed hip fractures. Arch Emerg Med 1992;9(1):23–7.
14. Dominguez S, Liu P, Roberts C, et al. Prevalence of traumatic hip and pelvic fractures in patients with suspected hip fracture and negative initial standard radiographs—a study of emergency department patients. Acad Emerg Med 2005;12(4):366–9.

15. Cannon J, Silvestri S, Munro M. Imaging choices in occult hip fracture. J Emerg Med 2009;37(2):144–52.
16. Hakkarinen DK, Banh KV, Hendey GW. Magnetic resonance imaging identifies occult hip fractures missed by 64-slice computed tomography. J Emerg Med 2012;42(2):303–7.
17. Khurana B, Okanobo H, Ossiani M, et al. Abbreviated MRI for patients presenting to the emergency department. Am J Roentgenol 2012;198(6):W581–8.
18. Joshi N, Lira A, Mehta N, et al. Diagnostic accuracy of history, physical examination, and bedside ultrasound for diagnosis of extremity fracturesin the emergency department: a systematic review. Acad Emerg Med 2013;20(1):1–15.
19. Warkentine FH, Horowitz R, Pierce MC. The use of ultrasound to detect occult or unsuspected fractures in child abuse. Pediatr Emerg Care 2014;30(1):43–6.
20. Pasco JA, Sanders KM, Hoekstra FM, et al. The human cost of fracture. Osteoporos Int 2005;16(12):2046–52.
21. Mak JC, Cameron ID, March LM, et al. Evidence-based guidelines for the management of hip fractures in older persons: an update. Med J Aust 2010;192(1):37–41.
22. Moja L, Piatti A, Pecoraro V, et al. Timing matters in hip fracture surgery: patients operated within 48 hours have better outcomes. A meta-analysisand meta-regression of over 190,000 patients. PLoS One 2012;7(10):e46175.
23. Handoll HH, Qually JM, Parker MJ. Pre-operative traction for hip fracture in adults. Cochrane Database Syst Rev 2011;(12):CD000168.
24. Sachdeva A, Dalton M, Amargiri SV, et al. Elastic compression stockings for prevention of deep vein thrombosis. Cochrane Database Syst Rev 2010;(7):CD001484.
25. Swiontkowski MF, Hansen ST Jr, Kellam J. Ipsilateral fractures of the femoral neck and shaft. A treatment protocol. J Bone Joint Surg Am 1984;66(2):260–8.
26. O'Toole RV, Dancy L, Dietz AR, et al. Diagnosis of femoral neck fracture associated with femoral shaft fracture: blinded comparison of computedtomography and plain radiography. J Orthop Trauma 2013;27(6):325–30.
27. Polacek M, Smabrekke A. Displaced stress fracture of the femoral neck in young active adults. BMJ Case Rep 2010: bcr0220102749.
28. Protzman RR, Burkhalter WE. Femoral-neck fractures in young adults. J Bone Joint Surg Am 1976;58(5):689–95.
29. Swiontkowski MF, Winquist RA, Hansen ST Jr. Fractures of the femoral neck between the ages of twelve and forty-nine years. J Bone Joint Surg Am 1984;66(6):837–46.
30. Forsch DA, Ferguson TA. Contemporary management of femoral neck fractures: the young and the old. Curr Rev Musculoskelet Med 2012;5(3):214–21.
31. Lowe JA, Crist BD, Bhandari M, et al. Optimal treatment of femoral neck fractures according to the patient's physiologic age: an evidence-based review. Orthop Clin North Am 2010;41(2):157–66.
32. Mallina R, Dinah F. Avascular necrosis of the femoral head: a rare complication of a common fracture in an octogenarian. Geriatr Orthop Surg Rehabil 2013;4(3):74–7.
33. Kyle RF, Cabanela ME, Russell TA, et al. Fractures of the proximal part of the femur. Instr Course Lect 1995;44:227–53.
34. Baixauli EJ, Baixauli F Jr, Baixauli F, et al. Avascular necrosis of the femoral head after intertrochanteric fractures. J Orthop Trauma 1999;13(2):134–7.
35. Bartonicek J, Fric V, Skala-Rosenbaum J, et al. Avascular necrosis of the femoral head in pertrochanteric fractures: a report of 8 cases and a review of the literature. J Orthop Trauma 2007;21(4):229–36.

36. Baumgaertner MR, Oetgen ME. Intertrochanteric hip fractures. In: Browner BD, editor. Skeletal trauma. Philadelphia: Saunders; 2009. p. 1913–52.
37. Smith GH, Tsang J, Molyneux SG, et al. The hidden blood loss after hip fracture. Injury 2011;42(2):133–5.
38. Gardner RC. Blood loss after fractures of the hip. Results of ten high femoral osteotomies using a radioactive tracer and an electronic blood volume computer. JAMA 1969;208(6):1005–7.
39. Roberts I, Shakur H, Coats T, et al. The CRASH-2 trial: a randomised controlled trial and economic evaluation of the effects of tranexamic acid ondeath, vascular occlusive events and transfusion requirement in bleeding trauma patients. Health Technol Assess 2013;17(10):1–79.
40. Zuffery PJ, Miquet M, Quenet S, et al. Tranexamic acid in hip fracture surgery: a randomized controlled trial. Br J Anesth 2010;104(1):23–30.
41. Ker K, Edwards P, Perel P, et al. Effect of tranexamic acid on surgical bleeding: a systematic review and cumulative meta-analysis. BMJ 2012;344:e3054.
42. Steele MT, Stubbs AM. Hip and femur fractures. In: Tintinalli J, editor. Tintinalli's emergency medicine: a comprehensive study guide. 7th edition. New York: McGraw Hill; 2011. p. 1930.
43. Bucholz R, Brumback R. Fractures of the shaft of the femur. In: Rockwood C, Green D, Bucholz R, et al, editors. Rockwood and green's fractures in adults. 4th edition. Philadelphia: Lippincott-Raven; 1996.
44. Gruber JE. Injuries to the proximal femur. In: Rosen P, Barkin R, editors. Emergency medicine: concepts and clinical practice. 4th edition. St Louis (MO): CV Mosby; 1998.
45. Zalvaras CG, Marcus RE, Levin LS, et al. Management of open fractures and subsequent complications. Instr Course Lect 2008;57:51–63.
46. Bone LB, Giannoudis P. Femoral shaft fracture fixation and chest injury after polytrauma. J Bone Joint Surg Am 2011;93(3):311–7.
47. Parisi DM, Koval K, Egol K. Fat embolism syndrome. Am J Orthop 2002;31(9):507–12.
48. Shaikh N. Emergency management of fat embolism syndrome. J Emerg Trauma Shock 2009;2(1):29–33.
49. Cakir O, Subasi M, Erdem K, et al. Treatment of vascular injuries with limb fractures. Ann R Coll Surg Engl 2005;87(5):348–52.
50. Starr AJ, Hunt JL, Reinert CM. Treatment of femur fracture with associated vascular injury. J Trauma 1996;40(1):17–21.
51. Fowler J, Macintyre N, Rehman S, et al. The importance of surgical sequence in the treatment of lower extremity trauma with concomitant vascular injury: a meta-analysis. Injury 2009;40(1):72–6.
52. Halvorson JJ, Anz A, Langfitt M, et al. Vascular injury associated with extremity trauma: initial diagnosis and management. J Am Acad Orthop Surg 2011;19(8):495–504.
53. Seligson D, Ostermann PA, Henry SL, et al. The management of open fractures associated with arterial injury requiring vascular repair. J Trauma 1994;36(6):938–40.
54. Guerrero A, Gibson K, Kralovich KA, et al. Limb loss following lower extremity arterial trauma: what can be done proactively? Injury 2002;33(9):765–9.
55. Kupferer KR, Bush DM, Cornell JE, et al. Femoral neck stress fractures in Air Force basic trainees. Mil Med 2014;179(1):56–61.
56. Sanders S, Tejwani N, Egol KA. Traumatic hip dislocation—a review. Bull NYU Hosp Jt Dis 2010;68(2):91–6.

57. DeLee JC. Fractures and dislocations of the hip. In: Rockwood CA Jr, Green DP, Bucholz R, editors. Fractures in adults, vol. 2, 4th edition. Philadelphia: Lippincott-Raven; 1996. p. 1756–803.

58. Stewart MJ, Milford MW. Fracture-dislocation of the hip; an end-result study. J Bone Joint Surg Am 1954;36(A:2):315–42.

59. Nandi SN, Manda P, Bhakta A. Result of conservative management in central fracture dislocation of the hip. J Indian Med Assoc 2012;110(7):481–4.

60. Brooks PJ. Dislocation following total hip arthroplasty: causes and cures. Bone Joint J 2013;95-B(11 Suppl A):67–9.

61. Patel PD, Potts A, Froimson MI. The dislocating hip arthroplasty: prevention and treatment. J Arthroplasty 2007;22(4 Suppl 1):86–90.

62. Bourne RB, Mehin R. The dislocating hip: what to do, what to do. J Arthroplasty 2004;19(4 Suppl 1):111–4.

63. Karthik K, Sundararajan SR, Dheenadhayalan J, et al. Incongruent reduction following post-traumatic hip dislocations is an indicator of intra-articular loose bodies: a prospective review of 117 patients. Indian J Orthop 2011;45(1):33–8.

64. Canale ST, Maniugian AH. Irreducible traumatic dislocations of the hip. J Bone Joint Surg Am 1979;61(1):7–14.

65. Tornetta P, Mostafavi H. Hip dislocation: current treatment regimens. J Am Acad Orthop Surg 1997;5(1):27–36.

66. Jewett J, Phillips WJ. Dexmedetomidine for procedural sedation in the emergency department. Eur J Emerg Med 2010;17(1):60.

67. Dela Cruz JE, Sullivan DN, Varboncouer E, et al. Comparison of procedural sedation for the reduction of dislocated total hip arthroplasty. West J Emerg Med 2014;15(1):76–80.

68. Miner JR, Martel ML, Meyer R, et al. Procedural sedation of critically ill patients in the emergency department. Acad Emerg Med 2005;12(2):124–8.

69. Andolfatto G, Willman E, Joo D, et al. Intranasal ketamine for analgesia in the emergency department: a prospective observational series. Acad Emerg Med 2013;20(10):1050–4.

70. Jamal SM, Fathil SM, Nidzwani MM, et al. Intravenous ketamine is as effective as midazolam/fentanyl for procedural sedation and analgesia in theemergency department. Med J Malaysia 2011;66(3):231–3.

71. David H, Shipp J. A randomized controlled trial of ketamine/propofol versus propofol alone for emergency department procedural sedation. Ann Emerg Med 2011;57(5):435–41.

72. Sener S, Eken C, Schultz CH, et al. Ketamine with and without midazolam for emergency department sedation in adults: a randomized controlled trial. Ann Emerg Med 2011;57(2):109–14.

73. Strayer RJ, Nelson LS. Adverse events associated with ketamine for procedural sedation in adults. Am J Emerg Med 2008;26(9):985–1028.

74. Hougaard K, Thomsen PB. Traumatic posterior dislocation of the hip–prognostic factors influencing the incidence of avascular necrosis of the femoral head. Arch Orthop Trauma Surg 1986;106(1):32–5.

75. Upadhyay SS, Moulton A, Srikrishnamurthy K. An analysis of the late effects of traumatic posterior dislocation of the hip without fractures. J Bone Joint Surg Br 1983;65(2):150–2.

76. Dwyer AJ, John B, Singh SA, et al. Complications after posterior dislocations of the hip. Int Orthop 2006;30(4):224–7.

77. Sevitt S, Thompson RG. The distribution and anastomoses of the arteries supplying the head and neck of the femur. J Bone Joint Surg Br 1965;47:560–73.

78. Nixon J. Avascular necrosis of bone: a review. J R Soc Med 1983;76:681–91.
79. Mont MA, Hungerford DS. Non-traumatic avascular necrosis of the femoral head. J Bone Joint Surg Am 1995;77(3):459–74.
80. Kaushik AP, Das A, Cui Q. Osteonecrosis of the femoral head: an update in year 2012. World J Orthop 2012;3(5):49–57.
81. Larson AN, McIntosh AL, Trousdale RT, et al. Avascular necrosis most common indication for hip arthroplasty in patients with slipped capital femoral epiphysis. J Pediatr Orthop 2010;30(8):767–73.
82. Koo KH. Risk period for developing osteonecrosis of the femoral head in patients on steroid treatment. Clin Rheumatol 2002;2(4):299–303.
83. Barnes R, Brown JT, Garden RS, et al. Subcapital fractures of the femur: a prospective review. J Bone Joint Surg Br 1976;58(1):2–24.
84. Epstein HC. Traumatic dislocation of the hip. Clin Orthop Relat Res 1973;92:116–42.
85. Mankin HJ, Brower TD. Bilateral idiopathic aseptic necrosis of the femur in adults: "Chandler's disease". Bull Hosp Joint Dis 1962;23:42–57.
86. Vail TP, Covington DB. The incidence of osteonecrosis. In: Urbaniak JR, Jones JR, editors. Osteonecrosis: etiology, diagnosis, treatment. Rosemont (IL): American Academy of Orthopedic Surgeons; 1997. p. 43–9.
87. Prokopetz JJ, Losina E, Bliss RL, et al. Risk factors for revision of primary total hip arthroplasty: a systematic review. BMC Musculoskelet Disord 2012;13:251.
88. Malizos KN, Karantanas AH, Varitimidis SE, et al. Osteonecrosis of the femoral head: etiology, imaging and treatment. Eur J Radiol 2007;63(1):16–28.
89. McGrory BJ, York SC, Iorio R, et al. Current practices of AAHKS members in the treatment of adult osteonecrosis of the femoral head. J Bone Joint Surg Am 2007;89(6):1194–204.
90. Castro FP, Barrack PL. Core decompression and conservative treatment for avascular necrosis of the femoral head: a meta-analysis. Am J Orthop 2000;29(3):187–94.
91. Mabry RL. Tourniquet use on the battlefield. Mil Med 2006;171:352–6.
92. Navein J, Coupland R, Dunn R. The tourniquet controversy. J Trauma 2003;54:219–20.
93. Jacobs N, Rourke K, Rutherford J, et al. Lower limb injuries caused by improvised explosive devices: proposed "Bastion classification" and prospective validation. Injury 2012;45(9):1422–8.
94. Lee C, Porter KM, Hodgetts TJ. Tourniquet use in the civilian prehospital setting. Emerg Med J 2007;24(8):584–7.
95. Rush RM, Arrington ED, Hou JR. Management of complex extremity injuries: tourniquets, compartment syndrome detection, fasciotomy, and amputation care. Surg Clin North Am 2012;92(4):987–1004.
96. Risk GC, Augustine J. Extreme bleeds: recommendations for tourniquets in civilian EMS. JEMS 2012;37(3):76–81.
97. Kragh JF, Wallum TE, Aden JK. Emergency tourniquet effectiveness in four positions on the thigh. J Spec Oper Med 2014;14(1):26–9.
98. Kragh JF, Walters TJ, Baer DG, et al. Practical use of emergency tourniquets to stop bleeding in major limb trauma. J Trauma 2008;64(Suppl 2):S38–49 [discussion: S49–50].
99. Taylor DM, Vater GM, Parker PJ. An evaluation of two tourniquet systems for the control of prehospital lower limb hemorrhage. J Trauma 2011;71(3):591–5.
100. Kragh JF, Murphy C, Dubick MA, et al. New tourniquet device concepts for battlefield hemorrhage control. US Army Med Dep J 2011;38–48.

101. Croushorn J, Thomas G, McCord SR. Abdominal aortic tourniquet controls junctional hemorrhage from a gunshot wound of the axilla. J Spec Oper Med 2013; 13(3):1–4.
102. Doyle GS, Taillac PP. Tourniquets: a review of current use with proposals for expanded prehospital use. Prehosp Emerg Care 2008;12(2):241–56.
103. Feeley BT, Powell JW, Muller MS, et al. Hip injuries and labral tears in the national football league. Am J Sports Med 2008;36(11):2187–95.
104. Davis JA, Stringer MD, Woodley SJ. New insights into the proximal tendons of adductor longus, adductor brevis and gracilis. Br J Sports Med 2012;46(12): 871–6.
105. Garrett WE, Speer KP, Kirkendall DT. Principles and practice of orthopaedic sports medicine. Philadelphia: Lippincott Williams & Wilkins; 2000. p. 805–17.
106. Sallay PI, Friedman RL, Coogan PG, et al. Hamstring muscle injuries among water skiers. Functional outcome and prevention. Am J Sports Med 1996;24(2):130–6.
107. Drezner JA. Practical management: hamstring muscle injuries. Clin J Sport Med 2003;13(1):48–52.
108. Ojike NI, Craig RS, Giannoudis PV. Compartment syndrome of the thigh: a systematic review. Injury 2010;41(2):133–6.
109. Uzel A, Bulla A, Henri S. Compartment syndrome of the thigh after blunt trauma: a complication to be ignored. Musculoskelet Surg 2013;97(1):81–3.
110. Burns BJ, Sproule J, Smyth H. Acute compartment syndrome of the anterior thigh following quadriceps strain in a footballer. Br J Sports Med 2004;38: 218–20.
111. Kurill JA, DeFelice GS. Acute compartment syndrome of the thigh following rupture of the quadriceps tendon: a case report. J Bone Joint Surg Am 2006; 88(2):418–20.
112. Levine M, Levitan R, Skolnik A. Compartment syndrome after "bath salts" use: a case series. Ann Emerg Med 2013;61(4):480–3.
113. DeFilippis EM, Kleiman DA, Derman PB, et al. Spinning-induced rhabdomyolysis and the risk of compartment syndrome and acute kidney injury: two cases and a review of the literature. Sports Health 2014;6(4):333–5.
114. King TW, Lerman OZ, Carter JJ, et al. Exertional compartment syndrome of the thigh: a rare diagnosis and literature review. J Emerg Med 2010;39(2):e93–9.
115. Khan SK, Thati S, Gozzard C. Spontaneous thigh compartment syndrome. West J Emerg Med 2011;12(1):134–8.
116. Olson SA, Glasgow RR. Acute compartment syndrome in lower extremity musculoskeletal trauma. J Am Acad Orthop Surg 2005;13(7):436–44.
117. Calabro LJ, Dick CG, Lutz MJ. Acute compartment syndrome of the thigh following minor trauma in a patient on dual anti-platelet therapy. Emerg Med Australas 2011;23:95–7.
118. Limberg RM, Dougherty C, Mallon WK. Enoxaparin-induced bleeding resulting in compartment syndrome of the thigh: a case report. J Emerg Med 2011;41(1): e1–4.
119. Compartment syndrome of the thigh. Lancet 1989;334(8861):485–6.
120. Mallo GS, Stanat SJ, Al-Humadi M, et al. Posterior thigh compartment syndrome as a result of a basketball injury. Orthopedics 2009;32(12):923.
121. Kanlic EM, Pinski SE, Verwiebe EG, et al. Acute morbidity and complications of thigh compartment syndrome: A report of 26 cases. Patient Saf Surg 2010; 4(13):1–9.
122. Mithöfer K, Lhowe DW, Altman GT. Delayed presentation of acute compartment syndrome after contusion of the thigh. J Orthop Trauma 2002;16(6):436–8.

123. Shadgan B, Wustrack R, Kandemir U. Diagnostic techniques in acute compartment syndrome of the leg. J Orthop Trauma 2008;22(8):581–7.
124. Beaudoin FL, Haran JP, Liebmann O. A comparison of ultrasound-guided three-in-one femoral nerve block versus parenteral opiods alone for analgresia in emergency department patients with hip fractures: a randomized controlled trial. Acad Emerg Med 2013;20(6):584–91.
125. Antonis MS, Chandwani D, McQuillen K. Ultrasound-guided placement of femoral 3-in-1 anesthetic nerve block for hip fractures. Acad Emerg Med 2006;13:S122–3.
126. O'Donnell BD, Mannion S. Ultrasound-guided femoral nerve block, the safest way to proceed? Reg Anesth Pain Med 2006;31:387–8.
127. Marhofer P, Schrogendorfer K, Koinig H, et al. Ultrasoundographic guidance improves sensory block and onset time of three-in-one blocks. Anesth Analg 1997;85:854–7.
128. Snoeck MM, Vree TB, Gielen MJ, et al. Steady state bupivacaine plasma concentrations and safety of a femoral "3-in-1" nerve block with bupivacaine in patients over 80 years of age. Int J Clin Pharmacol Ther 2003;41:107–13.
129. Fletcher AK, Rigby AS, Hayes FL. Three-in-one femoral nerve block as analgesia for fractured neck of femur in the emergency department: a randomized, controlled trial. Ann Emerg Med 2003;41:227–33.
130. Tan TT, Coleman MM. Femoral blockade for fractured neck of femur in the emergency department. Ann Emerg Med 2003;42:596–7.
131. McGlone R, Sadhra K, Hamer DW, et al. Femoral nerve block in the initial management of femoral shaft fractures. Arch Emerg Med 1987;4:163–8.
132. Williams R, Saha B. Best evidence topic report. Ultrasound placement of needle in three-in-one nerve block. Emerg Med J 2006;23(5):401–3.
133. Marhofer P, Greher M, Kapral S. Ultrasonographic guidance in regional anesthesia. Br J Anesth 2005;94:7–17.
134. Casati A, Baciarello M, Di Cianni S, et al. Effects of ultrasound guidance on the minimum effective anaesthetic volume required to block the femoral nerve. Br J Anaesth 2007;98:823–7.
135. Oberndorfer U, Marhofer P, Bosenberg A, et al. Ultrasonographic guidance for sciatic and femoral nerve blocks in children. Br J Anaesth 2007;98:797–801.
136. Marhofer P, Schrogendorfer K, Wallner T, et al. Ultrasonographic guidance reduces the amount of local anesthetic for 3-in-1 blocks. Reg Anesth Pain Med 1998;23:584–8.
137. Sites BD, Taenzer AH, Herrick MD, et al. Incidence of local anesthetic systemic toxicity and postoperative neurologic symptoms associated with 12,000 ultrasound-guided nerve blocks: an analysis from a prospective clinical registry. Reg Anesth Pain Med 2012;37(5):478–82.

Evaluation and Management of Traumatic Knee Injuries in the Emergency Department

CrossMark

Tristan Knutson, MD*, Jason Bothwell, MD, Ricky Durbin, MD

KEYWORDS

• Knee • Fracture • Dislocation • Neurovascular damage

KEY POINTS

- Utilization of clinical decision rules can reliably rule out fractures of the knee and reduce the utilization of radiography.
- If ligamentous or meniscal injury is suspected, the physician should arrange for expedited follow-up with the primary care physician or an orthopedic specialist for an MRI and further management.
- Knee dislocations are associated with popliteal artery injury. The ankle–brachial index should be measured in cases of known or suspected evaluation to assess for vascular damage.
- Tibial plateau fractures can be difficult to identify on plain radiographs. When suspected by injury mechanism or examination, CT should be performed to better evaluate for this injury.

KNEE ANATOMY AND FUNCTION

The knee is a complex joint composed of a synovial capsule, bony articular surfaces, menisci, ligaments, tendons, and muscles. An understanding of the relevant anatomy and how these components secure the stability and function of the knee allows the emergency physician to rapidly assess and recognize potential injuries.

Disclosures: The authors have no conflicts of interest or funding sources to disclose. The opinions or assertions contained herein are the private views of the authors and are not to be construed as official or reflecting the views of the Department of the Army or the Department of Defense.

Department of Emergency Medicine, Madigan Army Medical Center, 9040 Fitzsimmons Drive, Tacoma, WA 98431, USA

* Corresponding author.

E-mail address: Tristan.l.knutson.mil@mail.mil

Osseous and Meniscal Structures

The femoral and tibial condyles articulate so as to allow smooth flexion and extension. The patella articulates with the femur and serves as a platform for attachment of the quadriceps tendon and patellar tendon. The medial and lateral menisci are C-shaped, cartilaginous structures. They provide padding for the knee joint by reducing friction and preventing bone-on-bone contact during knee movement.[1,2]

Ligaments

The medial and lateral collateral ligaments (MCL and LCL) are extrinsic ligaments that provide the knee with primary resistance to valgus and varus stress, respectively. The anterior cruciate ligament (ACL) is the primary stabilizing ligament of the knee, preventing anterior displacement and internal rotation of the tibia on the femur.[3,4] The posterior cruciate ligament (PCL) primarily prevents posterior translation of the tibia on the femur and acts secondarily to prevent external rotation and varus movement of the knee.[1,2]

Neurovascular Structures

The popliteal artery and vein and the tibial and common peroneal nerves course through the popliteal fossa. Neurovascular function distal to the knee must be assessed and documented as these structures are commonly injured during high-energy injuries.[5]

HISTORY AND EXAMINATION OF THE UNDIFFERENTIATED KNEE INJURY
History

The mechanism of injury is an important factor in guiding evaluation of a knee injury in the emergency department (ED) and in predicting the ultimate diagnosis. Consider the direction of the force applied to the knee and the position of the knee at the time the force was applied. Inquire about the ability to bear weight immediately after the injury, the development of restrictions of range of motion, the location of pain, loss of sensation, any new swelling and the period of time over which it occurred, and whether a "pop" was felt or heard by the injured patient.

Physical Examination

Examination begins with a gross inspection of the knee. Compare the affected knee with the contralateral side for reference and symmetry. Skin injury, position of the patella, and the presence of any obvious deformity should be noted. If the patient is able to bear weight, gait should be assessed. Active and passive ranges of motion should be examined. Distal pulses and capillary refill distal to the site of injury as well sensory and motor testing of the affected extremity should be assessed and documented. Palpate all bony structures of the knee and note localized tenderness. The patellar tap and ballottement tests can identify knee joint effusions.[6] Maneuvers used to diagnose specific injuries are discussed subsequently.

EMERGENCY DEPARTMENT IMAGING OF THE UNDIFFERENTIATED KNEE INJURY
Clinical Decision Rules

Plain radiographs are the most common imaging modality used in the ED evaluation of knee injuries. These studies are almost always nondiagnostic.[7] In an effort to reduce the practice of ordering unnecessary radiographs, clinical decision rules have been developed and validated. The 2 widely used and cited of these are the Ottawa and Pittsburg Knee Rules.

The Ottawa Knee Rule was originally described by Stiell and colleagues[7] in 1995. They identified 5 clinical variables that, when absent, effectively ruled out a fracture

(**Box 1**), and thus obviated the need for obtaining plain radiographs in the ED. In the original study, application of the rule was 100% sensitive in ruling out a fracture, and resulted in a relative reduction in plain film use by 28%. The Ottawa Knee Rule has since been validated prospectively and can also be applied to children.[8] The Pittsburgh Decision Rule was described by Seaberg and Jackson[9] in 1994 (**Box 2**). Prospective validation of the rule by the original authors revealed a sensitivity of 100% and a specificity of 79% for diagnosing a knee fracture.

In a multicenter comparison study between the Pittsburgh and Ottawa Knee Rules, the Pittsburgh Rule resulted in greater sensitivity and specificity than the Ottawa Rule (99% and 60% vs 97% and 27%, respectively).[10] Exclusion factors for this study included patients with an altered level of consciousness, polytrauma, sensory changes, prosthetic hardware, and penetrating injuries.[7,9]

Although these rules have been validated and shown in subsequent studies to reduce the number of radiographs ordered, decreased costs, and shorten ED wait times, their application in actual ED practice is variable. A study examining barriers to implementation and noncompliance revealed that most physicians are aware of the rules, but do not follow them because of their perception of patient expectations, malpractice concerns, and the thought that a specialist may want them for later diagnosis and treatment for nonfracture, soft tissue injuries.[11]

Plain Radiography

Plain radiographs are typically the first-line study when evaluating for traumatic knee injury. Frontal and lateral plain films are generally the standard. Other views may be ordered to assess for specific injuries in the appropriate clinical setting and are discussed elsewhere in this article.

Ultrasonography

Ultrasonography is an appealing image modality owing to the dynamic nature of the test, the lack of associated radiation, and its relatively low cost.[12,13] The applications are extensive, and ultrasonography has been described as being useful in evaluating for tendon rupture, joint effusions, meniscal injury, and occult fractures. Specific indications are discussed in detail.

Computed Tomography

CT should be reserved for situations where an occult fracture (not seen on plain radiographs) is suspected based on the reported mechanism of injury or the presence of an effusion. CT may also be requested by the orthopedic surgeon when plain films

---

Box 1
Ottawa Knee Rule

The 5 variables evaluated by Stiell and colleagues that would become known as the Ottawa Knee Rule; according to Stiell, if the patient did not meet any of the below criteria then a fracture was ruled out with 100% sensitivity:

1. Age 55 years or older;

2. Tenderness at the head of the fibula;

3. Isolated tenderness of the patella;

4. Inability to flex knee to 90°; and

5. Inability to bear weight both immediately and in the emergency department (4 steps)

> **Box 2**
> **The Pittsburg Decision Rule as described by Seaberg and Jackson.**
>
> 1. Fall or blunt trauma mechanism.
> 2. Age less than 12 or greater than 50 years.
> 3. Inability to ambulate (unable to take 4 full weight-bearing steps).

demonstrate complex knee injuries, because CT often provides better characterization of exact fracture anatomy and optimizes operative planning.[14]

MRI

Most knee injuries seen in the ED are soft tissue rather than osseous.[7] MRI is an excellent test for diagnosing ligamentous and meniscal injuries and for determining whether surgery is required or if conservative management will suffice.[15] MRI has supplanted diagnostic arthroscopy as the study of choice for diagnosing internal derangement of the knee and has proven to be cost effective.[16]

However, MRI has a very limited use in the ED owing to its cost, time requirement, and limited availability. Injuries requiring MRI diagnosis are rarely emergent and can be done in the outpatient setting. Unfortunately, literature and guidelines on the subject are lacking, leaving the emergency physician in the unfortunate position of explaining why an MRI does not need to be obtained emergently.

DISPOSITION OF A PATIENT WITH AN UNDIFFERENTIATED KNEE INJURY

After obtaining a thorough history and physical examination, the need for plain radiographs should be determined using either the Ottawa or Pittsburgh Rule. If negative and there is a low suspicion for an occult fracture, the patient most likely has a soft tissue injury.

Initial ED management of undifferentiated soft tissue injuries consists of ice, compression, elevation, and crutches with partial weight bearing as tolerated. A knee immobilizer may provide comfort in the initial days following injury, particularly in an unstable knee, but range of motion exercises are crucial to prevent loss of mobility and contracture.[17] There is no universally accepted approach, but having the patient perform 10 to 20 knee flexion and extension movements 3 or 4 times a day is a reasonable approach.[1] Nonsteroidal anti-inflammatory drugs are the first-line therapy for analgesics. Urgent referral to the patient's primary care provider or directly to an orthopedic surgeon is indicated for follow-up further and evaluation.

ANTERIOR CRUCIATE LIGAMENT INJURIES
History

About two-thirds of ACL injuries are noncontact injuries, resulting from rapid deceleration, cutting, pivoting, or landing in near extension after jumping. Contact injuries represent about one-third of injuries, and result from a valgus or anteriorly directed force applied to a fixed lower leg. In either instance, the patient frequently reports hearing or feeling a "pop" and the event is associated with severe and immediate pain.[3,18] If the patient is able to ambulate at all, he or she may complain of a sensation of the knee "giving way."[19]

Physical Examination

Inspection of the knee frequently reveals an effusion, particularly if several hours have passed from the time of injury. Aspiration of a hemarthrosis is not indicated routinely, but has a few potential benefits worth mentioning. Diagnostically, the presence of a hemarthrosis suggests an ACL injury 72% of the time.[20] Additionally, the patient may experience symptomatic relief, potentially allowing the examiner to perform a more accurate physical examination.

A properly performed composite ACL examination is highly accurate for injury, with up to 82% sensitivity and 94% specificity.[19] The 3 most widely used tests for assessing ACL integrity are the Lachman test, the anterior drawer test, and the pivot-shift test. Of these, the Lachman test is the most sensitive (**Box 3**). With the knee flexed under normal conditions, the medial tibial tuberosity lies 1 cm anterior to the medial condyle. Failure to recognize this relationship could result in a false-positive Lachman or anterior drawer test.[21,22]

POSTERIOR CRUCIATE LIGAMENT INJURIES
History

Patients with PCL injuries frequently describe a direct blow to the tibia with a posteriorly directed force, as in the case of a "dashboard" injury from a motor vehicle crash, or a direct blow to the anterior tibia while playing sports. Forced hyperflexion of the knee, with a plantar flexed foot, has been cited as a common cause of noncontact isolated PCL injuries. Hyperextension can also cause PCL injuries, particularly with an associated varus or valgus force.[4]

Unlike ACL injuries, PCL injuries may occur after minor trauma, and usually without a distinct "pop." The patient may complain of posterior knee pain, pain with kneeling or deceleration, or on ascending or descending stairs. There may be a feeling of fullness from an effusion, but often without the sensation of knee instability. Sometimes the patient may say that the knee "just does not feel right."[19,22]

Physical Examination

The physical examination is highly accurate for PCL injuries. Solomon and colleagues[23] found an overall sensitivity of 91% and specificity of 98% of the composite physical examination in their review of the literature. The PCL is initially assessed via inspection, with the hip flexed to 45° and the knee flexed to 90°, with the foot flat on the examination table. PCL injury is detected by the presence of sag—visible posterior displacement of the tibia on the femur caused by gravity. The posterior drawer test is the most accurate test for the detection of PCL injuries, with sensitivity of up to

---

Box 3
ACL examination maneuvers

Lachman test: Flex knee to 30°. Stabilize femur with 1 hand. Apply anterior force with opposite hand.

Positive test: Anterior translation of tibia or no abrupt stop of tibia.

Anterior drawer test: Flex hip to 45° and knee to 90°. Foot is flat on bed. Stabilize femur with one hand. Apply anterior force with opposite hand.

Positive test: Anterior translation of tibia or no abrupt stop of tibia.

Pivot shift test: Patient lies supine with the knee slightly flexed. Place 1 hand on the fibular head and apply a valgus force to the knee. Internally rotate tibia with opposite hand.

Positive test: Anterior subluxation of the tibia at about 20° of flexion. Upon flexion to 40°, the tibia will reduce owing to contraction of the iliotibial band.

Data from Refs.[1,4,21–23]

90% and specificity of up to 99%.[19] In the same position as the sag assessment, the examiner immobilizes the patient's foot on the table, grips the tibia, and applies a rapid posterior force. Posterior displacement of the tibia, or the absence of an appreciable end point, suggest a positive test and thus a PCL injury.[3] As always, performing the initial test on the uninjured leg yields invaluable information about the patient's baseline anatomy.

COLLATERAL LIGAMENT INJURIES
History

Historical features of the injury are helpful in determining the likelihood of collateral ligament damage. The MCL is most commonly injured by a direct blow to the lateral thigh or lower leg. Other noncontact valgus stressors may also damage the MCL, such as an athlete changing direction quickly or a ski catching its medial edge, forcing abduction of the lower leg.[24] LCL injuries occur frequently with hyperextension of knee, often with rotation, and from blows to the medial side of the leg.[3] Noncontact injuries to the PCL can occur with rapid twisting on a planted foot. Patients typically complain of pain on the lateral knee joint, and the leg may feel unstable when in full extension.[25] With either injury, patients may have difficulty twisting or pivoting.

Physical Examination

Inspection may reveal relatively minor swelling, even with complete collateral ligament ruptures. Upon standing, patients with lateral collateral injuries may exhibit genu varum. Palpation of the medial and lateral joint surfaces may reveal point tenderness at the location of the ligamentous injury. To evaluate the integrity of the collateral ligaments, the knee should be flexed to 30°, with valgus and varus stress applied to the knee to investigate the MCL and LCL, respectively. The knee should then be fully extended to recruit the remaining stabilizing structures and the stress applied again. Medial opening in full extension suggests complete rupture of the MCL as well as injury to the cruciate ligaments. Lateral opening in full extension suggests rupture of the LCL as well as injury to the posterolateral corner or anterior or posterior cruciate ligaments.

RADIOGRAPHIC EVALUATION OF LIGAMENTOUS INJURIES

The majority of ligamentous injuries can be diagnosed by history and physical examination and clinical decision rules should guide the use of radiographs as discussed previously.[23,26,27] Radiographs do not reveal direct injury to the ligaments, but can show surrogate markers. In the case of ACL injury, these findings may include tibial avulsion (Segond) fractures or other bony derangements. Posterior sagging of the tibia on the lateral view, and avulsion fracture of the PCL insertion site should raise the index of suspicion for PCL injury.[4]

Ultrasonography does not readily visualize the ACL, but can aid in recognition of hematoma at the origin of the ACL in the femoral notch. This finding has demonstrated 88% sensitivity and 98% specificity for ACL tear.[28] The superficial location of the collateral ligaments make them suitable for ultrasound examination, and indeed ultrasonography has been described in the detection of collateral ligamentous injuries but with varying results.[13]

MRI remains the best diagnostic test for the evaluation of the ACL, with sensitivity between 92% and 94% and specificity between 95% and 100%.[4] It is highly sensitive and specific for complete PCL tears, and is the most accurate imaging modality for the diagnosis of collateral ligament injuries.

MANAGEMENT OF LIGAMENTOUS INJURIES

The initial ED management of suspected ligamentous injuries is the same as discussed previously in the undifferentiated knee injury section. The definitive management of most partial ligamentous injuries is nonoperative, with physical therapy and strengthening exercises. Management of complete ACL injuries depends on many factors, but surgery is generally indicated for patients who wish to continue in athletics that require rapid direction changing, and those with chronic knee instability.[29]

Management of complete PCL injuries is somewhat controversial, because many patients do well with conservative measures and physical therapy. Operative repair may be considered for patients who fail to recover with physical therapy or develop significant pain or instability.[19,22] If there is any associated avulsion fracture, however, operative repair is typically indicated.[3]

The MCL has the greatest propensity to heal of any of the 4 major ligaments in the knee, and injuries are often managed conservatively, even in cases of a complete tear. In contrast, complete LCL injuries do not heal well on their own, and are often best managed surgically.[25]

MENISCAL INJURIES
History

In younger patients, meniscal injuries are usually caused by twisting on a fixed foot, often with rapid acceleration or deceleration. Contact injuries also cause meniscal damage, often in conjunction with injuries to the MCL or ACL. In older patients, degenerative tears predominate, often with minimal or no significant trauma.[19]

The nerve and blood supply to the menisci are denser peripherally than centrally, and thus peripheral injuries produce more pain and bleeding. Patients with acute injuries typically complain of pain, swelling, or both of the involved knee.[19] With less severe injuries, the patient may be able to complete his or her activity, but with gradually increasing discomfort. Unlike effusions from ACL injuries, which often develop in just a few hours, effusions from meniscus injuries tend to develop more slowly, often over 24 hours. Patients may also experience a clicking sensation while walking, a sensation of the knee giving way, or even a "locked" flexed knee, depending on the location and mobility of the torn fragment.[23]

Physical Examination

The composite physical examination is relatively accurate in the detection of meniscal injuries, with a sensitivity of 77% and specificity of 91%.[23] Inspection and general palpation may demonstrate the presence of an effusion. Direct palpation of the medial and lateral joint lines has demonstrated good sensitivity (79%) but poor specificity (15%) for detection of meniscal injuries.[23] The Thessaly test is the most sensitive test (60%–90%), with a specificity of 96%. It is performed by having the patient stand on the affected leg, flexing the knee to 20°, and then internally and externally rotating (twisting) at the knee. A positive test is concluded when the patient experiences pain, clicking, locking, or inability to twist.[19] It is best to perform this test on the unaffected knee first to establish a baseline, and to ensure the patient has something to hold onto for balance.

The McMurray test is performed by having the patient lie supine with the thigh flexed and the knee hyperflexed. The examiner grips the knee with 1 hand, externally rotates the ankle with the other, and valgus stress is applied to the knee as it is repeatedly extended and flexed. A positive test is identified by reproduction of pain or a palpable clunk, and indicates injury to the medial meniscus. To test the lateral meniscus, the knee is gripped, the ankle internally rotated, and a varus stress applied during flexion and extension of the knee.[30] The Apley test is performed by having the patient lie prone on a low examining table. The affected knee is flexed to 90°, and the examiner places his or her thigh on the patient's posterior thigh. Axial pressure is applied to the bottom of the foot as the ankle is rotated internally and externally. Again, a positive test is concluded with reproduction of pain or clicking or clunking.[23] The composite evaluation may be more accurate than any of these maneuvers alone, so it is important to develop proficiency with each of them.

Imaging

Radiographs are not useful in directly demonstrating isolated meniscal injuries. If indicated for other reasons, radiographs often show degenerative changes, which may predispose a patient to a meniscal injury, and may be useful in detecting concomitant injuries. MRI is the most common imaging modality used to detect meniscal injuries, but is not indicated routinely from the ED. The accuracy of MRI varies greatly, with a sensitivity of 47% to 100% and a specificity of 81% to 95%, depending on the meniscus involved and the location of the injury.[19] Ultrasonography has also shown substantial variation in its accuracy for meniscal evaluation, with sensitivity from 60% to 93% and specificity from 21% to 95%. The use of ultrasonography is evolving but not routinely recommended in the ED.[13]

Management

The initial ED management of suspected meniscal injuries is the same as discussed in the undifferentiated knee injury section.

QUADRICEPS AND PATELLAR TENDON INJURIES

Rupture of the extensor mechanisms of the knee are relatively uncommon injuries, and include injuries of either the quadriceps or patellar tendon. Injury to the patella itself can also disrupt the extensor function, and is discussed separately in this article. Although there may be considerable overlap, quadriceps injuries are more common in patients over the age of 40, with some underlying degenerative disease. Patellar tendon ruptures are more common in younger patients. Knee extensor injuries require a high index of suspicion, as the initial miss rate has been reported as high as 10% to 50%.[31]

History

Knee extensor injury may result from a sudden, violent contraction of the knee extensor, usually with the foot planted and the knee partially flexed. The patient may report stumbling or sudden pain when trying to prevent an unexpected fall, often missing a step or stepping into an unseen hole.[32,33] In the case of patellar tendon rupture, a direct blow to the tendon may be the precipitating event. Patients typically report an abrupt onset of pain that is tearing in nature, followed by an inability to ambulate or extend the knee.[31] They may experience a popping sound or sensation as well. Many patients have some form of underlying disease or injury, so obtaining the patient's past medical history is often contributory. Risk factors include diabetes mellitus, chronic renal failure, chronic steroid use or steroid injection, flouroquinolone use, and connective tissue disorders.

Physical Examination

On physical examination, tenderness and swelling are expected at the site of injury. A palpable tendon defect is often felt, particularly immediately after the injury.[33] Over hours to days, swelling and hematoma may make this finding less reliable, and aspiration of hematoma may aid in the physical examination. The inability to raise the straightened leg while fully supine, complete inability to extend the knee, or to maintain position after passive extension, suggests rupture of the patellar or quadriceps tendon. The presence of weak knee extension or extension lag may indicate intact patellar retinaculum despite complete tendon rupture.[31]

Imaging

The initial evaluation of the extensor mechanism begins with plain radiographs of the knee. Complete rupture of the quadriceps tendon may result in a low-riding patella (patella baja), whereas rupture of the patellar tendon may result in a high-riding patella (patella alta; **Fig. 1**). The Insall–Savati ratio, which is defined as the patellar tendon length divided by the greatest patellar diagonal length, can be useful in making this determination. Classically, patella baja is defined as a ratio of less than 0.8, and patella alta as greater than 1.2. However, there is considerable variance in normal values, and interobserver reliability is considered poor.[31] Radiographs of the contralateral knee may be helpful in unclear cases. Ultrasonography has been shown to be useful in the diagnosis of quadriceps and patellar tendon ruptures and has the advantage of being available for bedside use in many EDs. However, its utility is operator dependent.[34,35] MRI, although often not readily available, is useful when the diagnosis remains suspected but unconfirmed.[32]

Management

If complete rupture of either tendon is suspected, the knee should be immobilized in full extension and the patient placed immediately in non–weight-bearing status. ED orthopedic evaluation is recommended in the case of a complete rupture. In either injury, early surgical repair is considered definitive treatment. Delay in diagnosis or repair may result in retraction of the extensor muscles, the need for a more complicated operation, and worse clinical outcomes for the patient. For suspected partial injuries, the knee should be immobilized and weight bearing should be avoided to prevent complete disruption while the patient awaits urgent orthopedic follow-up.[31,33] Partial tears may be managed nonoperatively, but this decision is best made by an orthopedic surgeon.

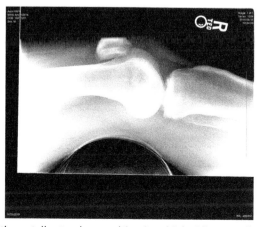

Fig. 1. Rupture of the patellar tendon resulting in a high-riding patella (patella alta).

PATELLAR SLEEVE FRACTURE

Children may present after knee injury with a high-riding patella that is initially concerning for a rupture of the patellar tendon. Patellar tendon ruptures, however, are extremely rare in children, and in these cases patellar sleeve fracture is the more likely diagnosis.[36]

Patellar sleeve fractures typically occur when a load comes in contact with a contracted quadriceps while the knee is in flexion. This results in a degloving of the protective cartilage that surrounds the patella, pulling it inferiorly. A small avulsion from the inferior pole of the patella may be seen on plain film, but this finding can be subtle (**Fig. 2**). If there is clinical suspicion for a patellar sleeve fracture despite an apparently normal plain film, an MRI should be obtained.[37] Identifying sleeve fractures is critical because prompt operative correction is required for recovery of function.[38] Delay may result in complications such as reduced knee flexion, ectopic bone formation, or avascular necrosis.[38,39]

PATELLAR DISLOCATION

History

Patella dislocations are relatively common injuries, particularly among young athletes.[40] They usually occur when a rotational force is applied to a contracted quadriceps, such as when a basketball player externally pivots on a planted leg. This strains the medial patellar retinaculum, which is much weaker than the lateral retinaculum, and allows the patella to dislocate laterally. A direct blow to the medial or anterior patella may also result in a patella dislocation.[1]

After a patellar dislocation, patients may report that their knee "gave out" and that they are unable to bear weight on the extremity. The patient is typically unable to fully flex or extend the affected knee. Spontaneous reductions are common, particularly among patients who have had patellar dislocations in the past.

Physical Examination

Patients usually present with tenderness along the medial aspect of the patella. An effusion is often present, and the knee is held in partial flexion. Often, the patella is easily seen in a lateral, unnatural position. Patients who have spontaneously reduced,

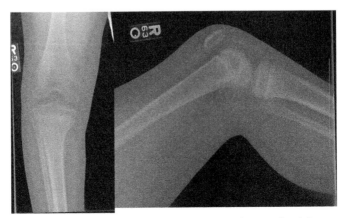

Fig. 2. Patellar sleeve fracture. A small avulsion from the inferior pole of the patella may be seen on plain film, but this finding can be subtle.

or those who frequently dislocate, may have a positive apprehension sign. In this test, the patient experiences pain or anxiety and contracts the quadriceps when the examiner attempts to displace the patella laterally.[41]

Imaging

Radiography is typically unnecessary to confirm the diagnosis, but some recommend obtaining anteroposterior and lateral views to evaluate for concomitant avulsion fractures.[1]

Management

After providing adequate analgesia, closed reduction should be performed by gently extending the knee and guiding the patella medially. If this action does not succeed in reduction, then the hip should be flexed in addition to the knee extension. Reduction is confirmed with a palpable clunk as the patella resumes its normal position. Postreduction radiographs may be obtained to evaluate for avulsion fractures. After successful reduction, the knee should be immobilized in full extension and referred for orthopedic follow-up. Approximately 15% of patients experience recurrent dislocations. Operative intervention may be effective in preventing further episodes.[42]

PATELLAR FRACTURES

History

Patellar fractures typically occur as a result of a direct trauma to the knee, such as a fall or blow from an external source such as a vehicle or a bat.[1,43] Patients who have sustained this injury experience pain and swelling of the knee and are often able to walk.

Physical Examination

Patients often have swelling and ecchymosis over the patella and prepatellar bursa. If the fracture is not completely displaced, the patient should still be able to extend his or her knee, although this movement may be limited by pain.

Imaging

The Ottawa or Pittsburgh Knee Rules can be used to evaluate patients with patellar trauma to determine whether diagnostic imaging is necessary.[7,9] Anteroposterior, lateral, and sunrise views all aid in the diagnosis of patellar fractures. Transverse patellar fractures are the most common pattern seen on plain film (**Fig. 3**). Stellate and comminuted fractures are less common. Fracture separation of more than 3 to 4 mm is usually associated with the inability to actively extend the knee, because the quadriceps has essentially lost its connection with the lower leg.[1]

Comparison views with the unaffected knee may be necessary to distinguish between anatomically normal variants and fractures. CT, MRI, or arthroscopy may be needed sometimes if the diagnosis remains in question.

Management

If the fracture is minimally displaced and the extensor mechanism remains intact, the patient may be placed in a long leg cast for 4 to 6 weeks.[43] If the extensor mechanism is damaged and/or the fracture is displaced by more than 2 to 3 mm, then the patient should undergo open reduction with internal fixation.[43] These patients should be placed in a long leg splint until the operation occurs.

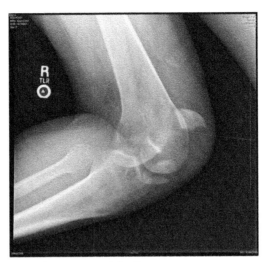

Fig. 3. Transverse patellar fractures on plain film.

TIBIAL PLATEAU FRACTURES

Tibial plateau fractures can be difficult to identify on the initial evaluation of an injured knee, and the failure to diagnose can result in a lifetime of disability.[44] Thus, it is important that clinicians be suspicious for tibial plateau fractures when patients present with concerning history, examination, and plain radiographic findings despite the lack of a clear fracture on the initial radiograph.

History

Tibial plateau fractures are caused by the combination of an axial, compressive load and a varus or valgus force. Common mechanisms of injury include (1) high energy transfer situations such as a vehicle's bumper striking the leg of a pedestrian, downhill skiing crashes, falls from height, and motor vehicle crashes and (2) low energy transfers, with the most common example being ground level falls in osteopenic, elderly patients.[45,46] Patients are usually unable to bear weight on the affected extremity.

Physical Examination

Patients usually have tenderness of the proximal tibia. These fractures are often accompanied by knee joint effusions. Rare complications of tibial plateau fractures include compartment syndrome and neurovascular injuries, and the lower leg should be assessed for the presence of these conditions.[47] Tibial plateau fractures are frequently associated with ACL, PCL, MCL, and meniscal tears[48]; however, evaluation of knee stability may be limited by pain and swelling.

Imaging

When examining a patient with a suspected tibial plateau fracture, use of the Ottawa or Pittsburgh Knee Rules are useful in determining whether radiography is necessary.[7,9,10,49] Plain film evaluation of a suspected tibial plateau fracture should include anteroposterior and lateral views at a minimum. Oblique views can be helpful if the standard views are indeterminate, particularly when CT is unavailable. Tibial plateau fractures most commonly involve the lateral tibial condyle in 60% of cases (**Fig. 4**).

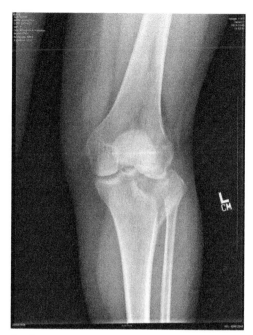

Fig. 4. Tibial plateau fracture.

Bicondilar lesions make up 25% of all tibial plateau fractures, and sole involvement of the medial plateau occurs 15% of the time.[50]

Tibial plateau fractures are often difficult to appreciate with plain radiographic technology, particularly to the nonradiologist. The presence of a lipohemarthosis should raise the clinician's suspicion for a fracture, even if the injury is not appreciated otherwise. In situations where a tibial plateau fracture is suspected despite apparently normal radiographs, CT should be obtained.[51] CT also aids the orthopedist in operative planning.

Management

An orthopedic surgeon should be consulted for all tibial plateau fractures. In cases of minimally displaced fractures, management may be nonoperative with bracing and a non–weight-bearing status. Operative management for more severe injuries may include arthroscopic surgery, external fixation, or internal fixation.[52] Regardless of the initial management strategy, all patients require physical therapy for early, passive range of motion exercises to reduce the risk of arthritis.

KNEE DISLOCATION

Knee dislocations are the result of high-energy trauma and are potentially limb threatening, because vascular disruptions commonly accompany them.[53] If unidentified and left untreated, damage to the vasculature may result in amputation of the lower leg.[54] Occasionally, the dislocation reduces spontaneously, and an unsuspecting medical provider may fail to consider a potential vascular injury. Clinicians must consider the possibility of a knee dislocation with concomitant vascular disruption in all patients presenting after high-energy knee trauma.

History and Injury Mechanism

More than one-half of all knee dislocations occur after motor vehicle collisions. Sports injuries and falls from height are other common mechanisms.[55] Dislocations are classified by the position of the tibia in relation to the femur. The tibia may be displaced anteriorly, posteriorly, medially, or laterally. Anterior dislocations occur approximately 40% of the time, and posterior dislocations are seen in 33% of cases. Lateral and medial dislocations are less common.[56]

In the setting of knee dislocation, the tibia is permitted to disarticulate owing to extensive ligamentous damage, leading to an extremely unstable knee. Usually, at least 3 of the knee ligaments are completely ruptured. The most common combination is an injury to the ACL, PCL, and MCL.[56]

Physical Examination

An unreduced knee dislocation is usually an obvious diagnosis owing to the gross deformity that is inherent with the injury. However, extensive swelling may complicate this, and an x-ray may be needed to confirm the diagnosis. Spontaneously reduced knee dislocations are much more difficult to appreciate, but no less important given the possibility of an underlying neurovascular injury. Damage to the knee ligaments results in gross instability, but this may be difficult to appreciate owing to pain and swelling.

All patients with a known or suspected knee dislocation should have an ankle–brachial index (ABI) measured to assess for damage to the popliteal artery. An ABI of greater than 0.9 has a negative predictive value approaching 100% for ruling out a popliteal artery injury.[57] An ABI of less than 0.9 should prompt further evaluation of the vasculature.

Documentation of peroneal nerve function and an assessment of the compartments of the lower leg should occur. Peroneal nerve injury occurs in approximately one-third of all knee dislocations and is associated with foot drop.[55]

Imaging

Anteroposterior and lateral plain films should be obtained in all cases of suspected knee dislocation. These images confirm the diagnosis and assess for associated fractures (**Fig. 5**). Routine use of angiography or CT angiography to assess the popliteal artery in cases where the ABI is normal and there are no signs of ischemia is controversial.[58] Recent literature suggests that this is unnecessary in patients with palpable distal pulses and an ABI of greater than 0.9.[57,59–61] In cases where the ABI is less than 0.9, angiography and CT angiography are acceptable modalities to access the popliteal artery, although CT is less invasive.[62]

Management

Closed reduction of the dislocation with longitudinal traction should be done immediately. This can be performed before obtaining plain films if the diagnosis is clear. Neurovascular assessment should be done before and after the reduction. A temporary splint should be applied keep the knee in 20° of flexion, because these injuries continue to be unstable.

In cases where a popliteal artery injury is known or suspected, an emergency vascular surgery consultation is necessary. Delay in repair may be associated with an increased risk for amputation, although this has not been established definitively in the literature. If no vascular injury is present, an orthopedic surgeon should be consulted because the patient will require extensive ligamentous repair. This is usually

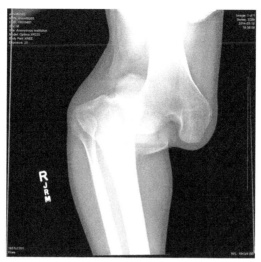

Fig. 5. Dislocated knee.

done at a later time; however, admission for serial vascular and compartment checks is prudent.

SUMMARY

Posttraumatic knee pain is a common ED presentation. The use of clinical decision rules can rule out reliably fractures of the knee and reduce the unnecessary cost and radiation exposure associated with plain radiographs. If ligamentous or meniscal injury to the knee is suspected, the ED physician should arrange for expedited follow-up with the patient's primary care physician or an orthopedic specialist for consideration of an MRI and further management. Patients presenting after high-energy mechanisms are at risk for occult fracture and vascular injuries. ED providers must consider these injuries in the proper clinical setting.

REFERENCES

1. Tintinalli JE, Stapczynski JS, Ma OJ, et al. Tintinalli's emergency medicine: a comprehensive study guide. 7th edition. San Francisco: The McGraw-Hill Companies, Inc; 2011. p. 1056–64.
2. Gilroy AM, Macpherson BR, Ross LM. Atlas of anatomy. New York: Thieme Medical Publishers Inc; 2008. p. 380–92.
3. Perryman JR, Hershman EB. The acute management of soft tissue injuries of the knee. Orthop Clin North Am 2002;33:575–85.
4. Brown JR, Trojian TH. Anterior and posterior cruciate ligament Injuries. Prim Care Clin Office Pract 2004;31:925–56.
5. Broder JS. Diagnostic imaging for the emergency physician. Philadelphia: Saunders – Elsevier Inc; 2011. p. 806–7.
6. Ali F. Clinical examination of the knee. Orthopedics and Trauma 2013;27:50–5.
7. Stiell IG, Wells GA, McDowell I, et al. Use of radiography in acute knee injuries: need for clinical decision rules. Acad Emerg Med 1995;2(11):966–73.
8. Bulloch B, Neto G, Plint A, et al. Validation of the Ottawa Knee Rule in children: a multicenter study. Ann Emerg Med 2003;42:48–55.

9. Seaberg DC, Jackson R. Clinical Decision Rule for knee radiographs. Am J Emerg Med 1994;12:542–3.

10. Cheung TC, Tank Y, Breederveld RS, et al. Diagnostic accuracy and reproducibility of the Ottawa Knee Rule vs. the Pittsburg Decision Rule. Am J Emerg Med 2013;31:641–5.

11. Beutel BG, Trehan SK, Shalvoy RM, et al. The Ottawa Knee Rule: examining use in an academic emergency department. West J Emerg Med 2012;13:366–72.

12. Lee D, Bouffard AJ. Ultrasound of the knee. Eur J Ultrasound 2001;14:57–71.

13. Chiang Y. Application of high resolution ultrasound for examination of the knee joint. J Med Ultrasound 2007;15:203–12.

14. Mustonen AO, Koskinen SK, Kiuru MJ. Acute knee trauma: analysis of multidetector computed tomography findings and comparison with conventional radiography. Acta Radiol 2005;48:866–74.

15. Feller JF, Webster KE. Clinical value of magnetic resonance imaging of the knee. ANZ J Surg 2001;71:534–7.

16. Chissell HR, Keightley A, Allum RL. MRI of the knee: its cost-effective use in a district general hospital. Ann R Coll Surg Engl 1994;76:26–9.

17. Sarraf KM, Sadri A, Thevendran G, et al. Approaching the ruptured anterior cruciate ligament. Emerg Med J 2011;28(8):644–9.

18. Siegel L, Vandenakker-Albanese C, Siegel D. Anterior cruciate ligament injuries: anatomy, physiology, biomechanics, and management. Clin J Sport Med 2012; 22:349–55.

19. Morelli V, Bright C, Fields A. Ligamentous injuries of the knee: anterior cruciate, medial collateral, posterior cruciate, and posterolateral corner injuries. Prim Care Clin Office Pract 2013;40:335–56.

20. Hastings DE. Diagnosis and management of acute knee ligament injuries. Can Fam Physician 1990;36:1169–89.

21. Colvin AC, Meislin RJ. Posterior cruciate ligament injuries in the athlete: diagnosis and treatment. Bull NYU Hosp Jt Dis 2009;67(1):45–51.

22. McAllister DR, Petrigliano FA. Diagnosis and treatment of posterior cruciate ligament injuries. Curr Sports Med Rep 2007;6:293–9.

23. Solomon DH, Simel DL, Bates DW, et al. The rational clinical examination. Does this patient have a torn meniscus or ligament of the knee? Value of the physical examination. JAMA 2001;286(13):1610–20.

24. Phisitkul P, James SR, Wolf BR, et al. MCL injuries of the knee: current concepts review. Iowa Orthop J 2006;26:77–90.

25. DeLee J, Drez D, Miller MD. DeLee & Drez's orthopaedic sports medicine. 3rd edition. Philadelphia: Saunders; 2009. p. 1719–30.

26. Liu SH, Osti L, Henry M, et al. The diagnosis of acute complete tears of the anterior cruciate ligament: comparison of MRI, arthrometry, and clinical examination. J Bone Joint Surg Br 1995;77-B:586–8.

27. O'Shea KJ, Murphy KP, Heekin RD, et al. The diagnostic accuracy of history, physical examination, and radiographs in the evaluation of traumatic knee disorders. Am J Sports Med 1996;24(2):164–7.

28. Larsen LPS, Rasmussen OS. Diagnosis of acute rupture of the anterior cruciate ligament of the knee by sonography. Eur J Ultrasound 2000;12(2):163–7.

29. Spindler KP, Wright RW. Anterior cruciate ligament (ACL) tear. N Engl J Med 2008;359(20):2135–42.

30. Ghosh KM, Dehhan DJ. Soft tissue knee injuries. Surgery 2010;28:494–501.

31. Lee D, Stinner D, Mir H. Quadriceps and patellar tendon ruptures. J Knee Surg 2013;26(5):301–8.

32. Ramseier LE, Werner CM, Heinzelmann M. Quadriceps and patellar tendon rupture. Injury 2006;37(6):516–9.

33. Hak DJ, Sanchez A, Trobisch P. Quadriceps tendon injuries. Orthopedics 2010; 33(1):40–6.

34. Bianchi S, Zwass A, Abdelwahab IF, et al. Diagnosis of tears of the quadriceps tendon of the knee: value of sonography. AJR Am J Roentgenol 1994;162(5): 1137–40.

35. Hall BT, McArthur T. Ultrasound diagnosis of a patellar tendon rupture. Mil Med 2010;175(12):1037–8.

36. Dai LY, Zhang WM. Fractures of the patella in children. Knee Surg Sports Traumatol Arthrosc 1999;7:243–5.

37. Bates DG, Hresko MT, Jaramillo D. Patellar sleeve fracture: demonstration with MR imaging. Radiology 1994;193(3):825–7.

38. Guy SP, Marciniak JL, Tulwa N, et al. Bilateral sleeve fracture of the inferior poles of the patella in a healthy child: case report and review of the literature. Adv Orthop 2011;2011:428614.

39. Hunt DM, Somashekar N. A review of sleeve fractures of the patella in children. Knee 2005;12(1):3–7.

40. Atkin DM, Fithian DC, Marangi KS, et al. Characteristics of patients with primary acute lateral patellar dislocation within the first 6 months of injury. Am J Sports Med 2000;28(4):472–9.

41. Ahmad CS, McCarthy M, Gomez JA, et al. The moving patellar apprehension test for lateral patellar instability. Am J Sports Med 2009;37(4):791–6.

42. Sauli Palmu BM, Kallio PE, Donell ST, et al. Acute patellar dislocation in children and adolescents: a randomized clinical trial. J Bone Joint Surg Am 2008;90(3):463–70.

43. Melvin JS, Mehta S. Patellar fractures in adults. J Am Acad Orthop Surg 2011; 19(4):198–207.

44. Mills WJ, Nork SE. Open reduction and internal fixation of high-energy tibial plateau fractures. Orthop Clin North Am 2002;33(1):177–98.

45. Berkson EM, Virkus WW. High-energy tibial plateau fractures. J Am Acad Orthop Surg 2006;14(1):20–31.

46. Oberant K. Management of fractures in severely osteoporotic bone. New York: Springer; 2000. p. 296–308.

47. Ziran BH, Becher SJ. Radiographic predictors of compartment syndrome in tibial plateau fractures. J Orthop Trauma 2013;27(11):612–5.

48. Shepherd L, Abdollahi K, Lee J, et al. The prevalence of soft tissue injuries in non-operative tibial plateau fractures as determined by magnetic resonance imaging. J Orthop Trauma 2002;16(9):628–31.

49. Tandeter HB, Shvartzman P. Acute knee injuries: use of decision rules for selective radiographic ordering. Am Fam Physician 1999;60(9):2599–608.

50. Fenton P, Porter K. Tibial plateau fractures: a review. Trauma 2011;13(3):181–7.

51. Lee C, Bleetman A. Commonly missed injuries in the accident and emergency department. Trauma 2004;6(1):41–51.

52. Scuderi G, Tria A. The knee: a comprehensive review. Hackensack (NJ): World Scientific Publishing Company; 2010. p. 299–310.

53. Green NE, Allen BL. Vascular injuries associated with injuries of the knee. J Bone Joint Surg Am 1977;59(2):236–9.

54. Wascher DC. High-velocity knee dislocation with vascular injury. Treatment principles. Clin Sports Med 2000;19(3):457–77.

55. Brautigan B, Johnson DL. The epidemiology of knee dislocations. Clin Sports Med 2000;19(3):387–97.

56. Robertson A, Nutton RW, Keating JF. Dislocation of the knee. J Bone Joint Surg Br 2006;88-B:706–11.
57. Mills WJ, Barel DP, McNair P. The value of the ankle-brachial index for diagnosing arterial injury after knee dislocation: a prospective study. J Trauma 2004;56(6):1261–5.
58. Gable DR, Allen JW, Richardson JD. Blunt popliteal artery injury: is physical examination alone enough for evaluation? J Trauma 1997;43(3):541–4.
59. About-Sayed H, Berger DL. Blunt lower extremity trauma and popliteal artery injuries: revisiting the case for selective arteriography. Arch Surg 2002;137(5):585–9.
60. Martinez D, Sweatman K, Thompson EC. Popliteal artery injury associated with knee dislocations. Am Surg 2001;67(2):165–7.
61. Klineburg EO, Crites BM, Flinn WR, et al. The role of arteriography in assessing popliteal artery injury in knee dislocations. J Trauma 2004;56(4):786–90.
62. Inaba K, Potzman J, Munera F, et al. Multi-slice CT angiography for arterial evaluation in the injured lower extremity. J Trauma 2006;60(3):502–6.

Emergency Department Evaluation and Management of Foot and Ankle Pain

Ian Wedmore, MD*, Scott Young, MD, Jill Franklin, MD

KEYWORDS

- Ankle pain • Ankle fracture • Ankle sprain • Malleolar fracture • Talus fracture
- Calcaneus fracture • Lisfranc fracture • Ottowa ankle rules

KEY POINTS

- Ankle and foot pain is a common presenting complaint to the Emergency Department.
- Many patients will not require any imaging for an acute injury, using the Ottawa Foot and Ankle Rules to provide guidance for when imaging is required.
- Most talus and calcaneal fractures require urgent orthopedic consultation.
- The proximal fibula and fifth metatarsal should be examined with any ankle injury.
- Most ankle fractures require urgent orthopedic consultation.
- Immediate surgical intervention is rarely required for acute ankle ligamentous injuries.
- (P)RICE remains the standard treatment for ankle sprains.

FOOT AND ANKLE

Foot and ankle injuries are a frequent cause for a visit to the Emergency Department (ED). Complete evaluation and treatment of these injuries needs to be an area of thorough familiarity for the Emergency Medicine physician.

THE FOOT

The foot is a complex part of the functional human lower extremity. With 28 bones and many more articulations, the foot is a key component to human weight-bearing function. Injury or dysfunction of any of these many moving parts can lead to a presentation to the ED.

Disclosures: None.
Department of Emergency Medicine, Madigan Army Medical Center, 9040 Jackson Avenue, Tacoma, WA 98431, USA
* Corresponding author.
E-mail address: Wedmorei@msn.com

Emerg Med Clin N Am 33 (2015) 363–396
http://dx.doi.org/10.1016/j.emc.2014.12.008
0733-8627/15/$ – see front matter Published by Elsevier Inc.

emed.theclinics.com

Anatomy

The foot can be divided into 3 distinct regions (**Fig. 1**):

- Forefoot: Metatarsals, phalanges, and sesamoids
- Midfoot: Navicular and cuboid bones; medial, middle, and lateral cuneiforms
- Hindfoot: Calcaneus and talus
- Choparts joint: Articulation of the hindfoot with the midfoot
- Lisfranc joint: Articulation of the midfoot with the forefoot

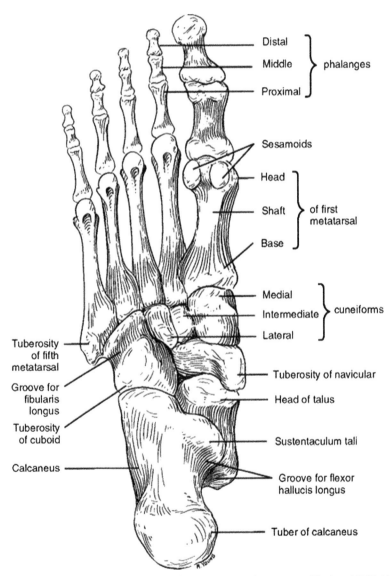

Fig. 1. Plantar view of the bones of the foot. (*From* Jenkins DB, Hollinshead WH. Hollinshead's functional anatomy of the limbs and back, 8th edition. Philadelphia: Saunders, 2002; with permission.)

Other anatomic features that are of clinical importance include

- The peroneus brevis muscle inserts on the head of the fifth metatarsal.
- The plantar fascia inserts on the medial calcaneal tuberosity.
- The posterior tibial nerve provides sensation to the sole of the foot and the heel via the medial and lateral plantar nerves and the medial calcaneal nerve, respectively (**Fig. 2**).
- The deep peroneal nerve, an extension of the L5 nerve root, provides sensory function to the first web space.

History

Determining the exact mechanism of injury is a key factor to making an accurate diagnosis in foot complaints. In addition, providers should ask about injuries or symptoms in all areas along the lower extremity, including the low back, hip, knee, and ankle.

PHYSICAL EXAMINATION

The thorough physical examination for any foot complaint is a 6-step process.

1. Inspection
   - The foot and ankle should be completely exposed, including the unaffected foot for comparison.
   - Ambulation should be observed, if the patient is able.

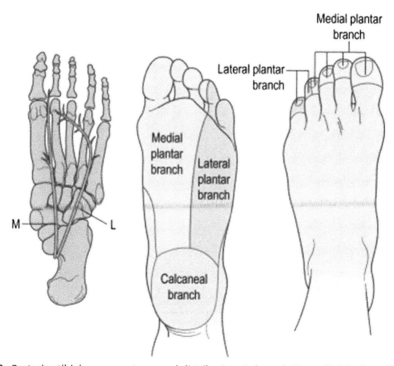

Fig. 2. Posterior tibial nerve anatomy and distribution. L, lateral; M, medial. (*Adapted from* Omer GE, Spinner M. Management of peripheral nerve problems. Philadelphia: Saunders, 1980; with permission.)

2. Palpation: The area of concern should be evaluated last, and the provider should palpate all high-risk areas, including
   - Navicular bone: found on the dorsomedial aspect of the foot at the junction of the anterior tibialis and extensor hallucis longus tendons, best visualized by asking the patient to dorsiflex their foot and great toe (**Fig. 3**)
   - Fifth metatarsal head
   - Calcaneus: best evaluated by the examiner compressing the calcaneus using the heels of both hands with the fingers interlocked
   - Region around the second metatarsal head
3. Range of motion
   - Observe active or passive terminal dorsiflexion, plantar flexion, eversion, and inversion of the ankle joint
4. Strength
   - Provide resistance against all of these ranges of motion
5. Neurovascular function
   - Palpate the dorsalis pedis and posterior tibial pulses
   - Assess sensory function
6. Special tests
   - Midfoot stress test: hold the patient's foot with one hand proximal to the midfoot and one hand distally, each with the operator's palms down. One hand is then turned clockwise while the other is turned counterclockwise, producing a torsional force on the midfoot joint.

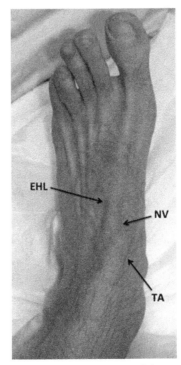

Fig. 3. The navicular bone is found at the intersection of the EHL and the TA tendons on the dorsal surface of the foot. EHL, extensor hallucis longus; NV, navicular; TA, tibialis anterior. (*Courtesy of* S. Young, MD, Tacoma, WA, USA.)

Evaluate the entire lower extremity as well as the lumbar spine in cases of significant mechanisms of injury.

Radiographic Imaging

The Ottawa Foot Rules can help determine the value of plain radiographs in diagnosing fractures with a sensitivity of nearly 100%.[1] To avoid performing radiographs, the patient must meet the following criteria[2]:

1. Able to take 4 steps at the time of injury and at the time of evaluation
2. Have no tenderness over the navicular bone or the fifth metatarsal head

Implementation of these rules can reduce the number of films ordered by 30% to 40%.[1] The major limitations of the Ottawa Foot Rules are that they cannot be used in pregnant patients or children, as those groups were excluded from the original study.

If a plain radiograph is indicated, a weight-bearing view should be obtained when possible. This view can help evaluate for ligamentous injury, even in the absence of fracture. A contralateral view for comparison can be considered if a provider is unclear of the findings on plain radiograph. Common normal variants on foot radiograph include

- Accessory navicular bone: articulates with the navicular bone and may be a source of pain in the uncommon event whereby it is the insertion site for the posterior tibialis tendon[3]
- Os peroneum: ossicle typically found within the peroneus longus tendon and lies just lateral to the cuboid
- Os trigonum: triangular-shaped bone found near the posterior aspect of the talus and present in up to 25% of the population[4]

Plain radiography has been shown to be 78% sensitive for talus fractures, 87% sensitive for calcaneus fractures, and as low as 33% sensitive for navicular fractures.[5] In the case of high clinical suspicion for fracture in one of these bones, computed tomography (CT) should be strongly considered in the presence of a normal plain radiograph.

Key points for examination and imaging
- The navicular bone can be found at the intersection of the tibialis anterior and the extensor hallucis longus.
- The Ottawa Foot Rules require 4 steps at the time of injury and at presentation, and no tenderness at the navicular or fifth metatarsal head to avoid radiographs, with a sensitivity for foot fracture of nearly 100%.
- Common normal variants seen on plain radiograph include accessory navicular, os perineum, and os trigonum.

HINDFOOT INJURIES
Talus

- The talus is divided anatomically into the head, neck, and body (**Fig. 4**).
- Nearly 80% of the surface of the talus is dedicated to articulations with surrounding structures, leaving only a small area for vascular supply from the anterior and posterior tibial arteries.[6–8]
- This unique anatomic feature predisposes the talus to nonunion and avascular necrosis, possible complications with nearly all talar injuries.

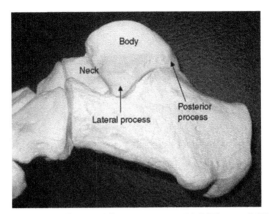

Fig. 4. Anatomy of the talus. (*From* Richter M, Kwon JY, DiGiovanni CW. Foot injuries. In: Browner BD, Jupiter JB, Krettek C, et al., editors. Skeletal trauma: basic science, management and reconstruction. 5th edition. Philadelphia: Saunders, 2015; with permission.)

1. Talar neck fractures
   - One-half of major talar injuries
   - Occur in the coronal plane and secondary to an axial loading force[9]
   - Best seen on radiograph with a Canale view, where the foot is maximally plantar flexed and pronated 15°[10]
   - CT should be considered; the Canale view is not routinely used and may miss some fractures
2. Lateral process fractures
   - Once an uncommon injury, lateral process fractures have become much more prevalent because of their association with snowboarding.[11]
   - Typically the result of loading a dorsiflexed and inverted ankle, a position often encountered in snowboarding.
   - Commonly misdiagnosed as ankle sprains
   - Missing this injury may lead to malunion, nonunion, and degenerative changes of the subtalar joint.[11–14]
   - Physical examination may show point tenderness over the lateral process, which lies near the anterior talofibular ligament (ATFL) just inferior and anterior to the lateral malleolus.
   - Best seen on the ankle mortise view, but avulsion and comminuted fractures can often be visualized on the lateral view (**Fig. 5**).[15]
   - Consider CT if there is clinical concern in the presence of negative plain radiographs.

Closed talar and peritalar dislocations are extremely rare and require emergency reduction. Reduction is performed by flexing the knee to 90°, which relaxes the gastrosoleus complex and provides a source for countertraction. Traction is then applied with manual pressure on the talus opposite the direction of dislocation.[16] Most of these injuries are open and require surgical reduction.

Management of all talus fractures include
- Immobilization
- Non-weight-bearing with crutches

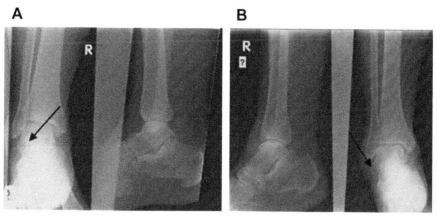

Fig. 5. Lateral process fracture of the talus. *Arrows* indicate the lateral process fractures. (*From* Perera A, Baker JF, Lui DF, et al. The management and outcome of lateral process fracture of the talus. Foot Ankle Surg 2010;16(1):15–20. Figure 2; with permission.)

- Urgent orthopedics consultation because of the high risk of nonunion and avascular necrosis

Calcaneal Fractures

- The calcaneus is the most frequently fractured tarsal bone, accounting for up to 60% of foot fractures.[17]
- The most common mechanism for calcaneal fracture is a fall from height.
- Bilateral fractures occur less than 10% of the time.[18]
- Up to 10% will have a coexisting spinal injury between T12 and L2.[19,20]
- Palpation can be performed by compressing the calcaneus between the heels of both hands rather than using a finger to push on specific areas.

Diagnosis of a fracture begins with standard radiographs of the calcaneus, including measurement of Böhler angle.

- Böhler angle is formed by the intersection of lines drawn from the posterior facet to the anterior process, and from the posterior facet to the anterior tubercle of the calcaneus.
- A normal Böhler angle is 20° to 40°.
- A recent study demonstrated that Böhler angle may have a sensitivity and specificity as high as 100% and 82%, respectively, for an angle less than 25°, and 99% and 99% for an angle less than 21° (**Fig. 6**).[21]
- CT should be considered after a fracture is identified to ensure there is no intra-articular involvement, or if a fracture is not seen on plain radiographs despite high clinical concern.[22]
- Fractures involving the subtalar joint, or intra-articular fractures, have a much worse prognosis than extra-articular fractures and require surgical intervention.[23]

Managing a calcaneal fracture includes

- Detailed evaluation for associated injuries, such as vertebral fracture
- Orthopedic consultation
- Immobilization with a posterior splint
- Non-weight-bearing with crutches
- Compartment syndrome of the foot, noted in up to 10% of acute calcaneal fractures, should be considered in all cases before final disposition.[24]

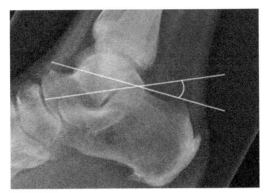

Fig. 6. A normal Boehler angle should be between 25 and 40 degrees. (*From* Willmott H, Stanton J, Southgate C. Bohler's angle - what is the normal in the uninjured British population? Foot Ankle Surg 2012;18(3):187–9. Figure 1; with permission.)

Key points for hindfoot injuries
- Lateral process fractures of the talus can be associated with snowboarding injuries and are often mistaken for lateral ankle sprains.
- CT should be considered in any suspected or confirmed hindfoot fracture because of the potential complications of these injuries.
- Calcaneus fractures are often associated with other injuries, including lower thoracic and lumbar spine fractures.
- Böhler angle of less than 25° has a sensitivity as high as 100% for calcaneus fracture.

MIDFOOT INJURIES
Navicular Fracture

Navicular bone fractures can be divided into 2 general categories: traumatic and stress fractures.

1. Traumatic navicular fracture
   - Crush and twisting forces about the midfoot can result in avulsion, tuberosity, or body fractures of the tarsal navicular.[25]
   - These injuries are difficult to see on plain radiography and are often missed.
   - CT is the imaging study of choice to evaluate for navicular injury.
   - Tarsal navicular fractures resulting from trauma should be splinted in a posterior splint, made non-weight-bearing, and referred to orthopedics.
2. Navicular stress fractures
   - May develop over a period of weeks to months
   - High risk for delayed or nonunion, should be considered in any athlete with midfoot pain[26]
   - Unlikely to show a navicular stress fracture on plain radiographs of the foot[27]
   - CT and technetium bone scanning may be helpful in making the diagnosis, but MRI is the study of choice.

   Management of navicular injuries includes
   - Immobilization
   - Non-weight-bearing with crutches
   - Follow-up with orthopedics or podiatry
   - Any significant displacement, associated dislocation, or open fracture should be addressed urgently in the ED.

Cuboid Fractures

- Typically the result of a fall from height or crush injury
- Often associated with fractures of the talus, calcaneus, or tarsometatarsal region[28]
- Compression injury of the cuboid, termed the "nutcracker" fracture, often associated with horseback riding[29]
- May also occur as an overuse stress injury and will likely present with weeks to months of pain that has acutely worsened
- Should be splinted, made non-weight-bearing on crutches, and discussed with an orthopedist or podiatrist

Lisfranc Injuries

- The Lisfranc joint complex is defined by the proximal first, second, and third metatarsal articulation with the cuneiforms as well as the fourth and fifth metatarsals with the cuboid.
- Lisfranc ligament attaches the base of the second metatarsal to the medial cuneiform, providing a significant amount of stability to the midfoot.
- Lisfranc injuries are typically produced by a high-energy trauma mechanism, but have been increasingly recognized in milder ligamentous sprains.[30,31]
- Injuries typically present with significant pain and inability to bear weight.
- Examination will show tenderness to palpation around the midfoot and pain with the midfoot stress test.

Radiographic evaluation

- Radiographic evaluation includes weight-bearing anteroposterior (AP), lateral, and oblique views of the foot. Weight-bearing views are essential as diastasis of the joint may not be visualized without stress on the midfoot.[32]
- The most consistent radiographic finding of Lisfranc injury is malalignment of the medial borders of the second metatarsal and medial cuneiform (see **Fig. 8**).[33]
- Other findings include widening of the space between first and second metatarsals, increased distance between the medial and middle cuneiforms, and the presence of avulsion fractures (**Fig. 7**).[34]
- CT can be useful in high-energy trauma to evaluate the severity or articular involvement of a fracture, but will not show isolated ligamentous injury.[35]

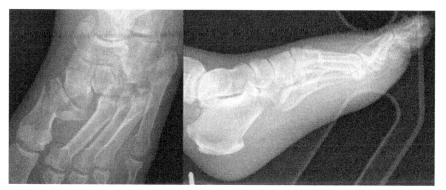

Fig. 7. Lisfranc fracture. (*From* Demirale I, Tecimel O, Celi I, et al. The effect of the Tschene injury pattern on the outcome of operatively treated Lisfranc fracture dislocations. Foot Ankle Surg 2013;19(3):188–93; with permission.)

Management of suspected or confirmed Lisfranc injuries:
- Mild sprains may be managed conservatively, but many cases of Lisfranc injuries will require surgical reduction and fixation.[36]
- Lisfranc injuries should be immobilized with a posterior splint
- Lisfranc injuries should be non-weight-bearing on crutches
- Lisfranc injuries should have orthopedic or podiatry follow-up
- Fracture displacement, associated dislocation, or evidence of compartment syndrome requires emergent intervention.

Key points for midfoot injuries
- When performing plain radiographs to evaluate for midfoot injury, weight-bearing films should be obtained whenever possible.
- Lisfranc injuries do not always involve fractures and may not be visible on plain radiography or CT.
- Any patient with concerns for midfoot injury, even if imaging in the ED is negative, should be made non-weight-bearing and have follow-up with a foot specialist arranged.

FOREFOOT
Metatarsal Injuries

Traumatic metatarsal fractures

- Metatarsal fractures are the most common foot fracture.[37,38]
- Examination will often show widespread swelling and tenderness around the affected metatarsal, sometimes making it difficult to isolate the location of injury.
- Any break in the skin should raise concern for an open fracture.
- Compartment syndrome of the foot is a rare complication of metatarsal fractures and can be associated with severe crush injuries and first metatarsal fractures.[39]
- Concern for compartment syndrome should be raised if there is tense swelling, pain out of proportion to examination findings, and significant symptoms with passive movement of the toes.
- Definitive diagnosis of compartment syndrome can be made with measured resting pressures greater than 30 mm Hg.[40,41]

Management of traumatic metatarsal fractures
- Displacement greater than 4 mm or angulation more than $10°$ may require reduction.[42]
- Any displacement or angulation of a first metatarsal fracture will likely require intervention.
- Traumatic metatarsal fractures should be immobilized in a posterior splint.
- Traumatic metatarsal fractures should be non-weight-bearing with crutches.
- Follow-up with a foot specialist should occur in 3 to 5 days.[41]
- Any evidence of significant fracture displacement, compartment syndrome, or concern for open fracture warrants emergent consultation.

Metatarsal stress fractures

- Metatarsal stress fractures must be differentiated from traumatic fractures because they are generally due to overuse and develop over a longer period of time.
- Flat foot (pes planus), dorsal/plantar flexed metatarsals, and tight gastrocnemius muscles may predispose an individual to metatarsal stress fractures.[43,44]
- The earliest radiographic findings appear after 2 to 6 weeks.[41]
- Physical examination may show a variable amount of swelling, tenderness to palpation, and pain with ambulation.

Management of metatarsal stress fractures

- Correct or modify the offending activity, whether it is overuse or a functional abnormality
- Protect the metatarsal with a walking boot, partial weight-bearing or non-weight-bearing on crutches, depending on which of those implements leads to pain-free ambulation
- Cautious use of nonsteroidal anti-inflammatory drugs, because of controversial use in stress fractures; may be a decision best left to a specialist[45]
- Timely follow-up with an orthopedic, sports medicine, or podiatric specialist

Fifth metatarsal injury

- The proximal one-third of the fifth metatarsal can be anatomically divided into, from proximal to distal, the tuberosity (or "styloid"), metaphysis, and diaphysis.
- The tuberosity and metaphysis are supplied by both metaphyseal blood vessels and branches of the nutrient artery. The proximal diaphysis, however, is only supplied by the nutrient artery and is much more likely to be compromised in a fracture, increasing the risk of nonunion.[46]
- Traditional discussion of the proximal fifth metatarsal fracture has included the term "Jones fracture," referring to Sir Robert Jones, who described a series of proximal diaphyseal metatarsal fractures in 1902.[47]
- To prevent confusing application of this terminology, it is better to separate fifth metatarsal fractures into tuberosity avulsion fractures, proximal diaphyseal fractures (the traditional "Jones fracture"), and stress fractures of the diaphysis (**Fig. 8**).

1. Tuberosity avulsion fractures
   - Often the result of plantar flexed inversion injuries of the ankle
   - Both the peroneus brevis tendon, which originates on the lateral leg, and the lateral band of the plantar fascia insert on the fifth metatarsal tuberosity. These anatomic connections are thought to produce the traction with plantar flexion and inversion that leads to fracture.[48,49]
   - Nondisplaced avulsion fractures can be managed symptomatically, often by a primary care provider.[50]
   - Indications for orthopedic referral include greater than 3 mm of displacement or a step off of more than 2 mm on the articular surface of the cuboid.

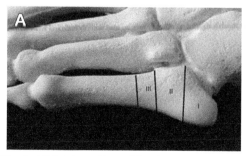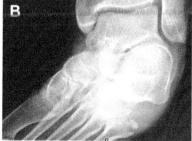

Fig. 8. (*A*) I, tuberosity avulsion fracture; II, acute proximal diaphyseal fracture; III, proximal diaphyseal stress fracture. (*B*) Proximal fifth fracture. (*From* [*A*] Nagar M, Forrest N, Maceachern CF. Utility of follow-up radiographs in conservatively managed acute fifth metatarsal fracture. Foot (Edinb) 2014;24(1):17–20. Figure 1; with permission; and *Courtesy of* [*B*] I. Wedmore, MD, Tacoma, WA.)

- Otherwise, these patients can be placed in a hard-soled shoe or walking boot.
- Patients with severe symptoms may require a partial or non-weight-bearing on crutches.

2. Acute proximal diaphyseal fractures
   - This injury occurs when a significant force is applied to the fifth metatarsal, while the foot is in plantar flexion and the ankle is off the ground.[51]
   - This injury is at high risk for nonunion or delayed union.
   - Management includes a posterior splint, strict non-weight-bearing with crutches, and orthopedic referral for follow-up.

3. Stress fractures of the proximal diaphysis
   - This injury is less common than tuberosity and acute proximal diaphyseal fractures, but has a higher propensity for delayed union and nonunion.[51]
   - This injury often presents after several weeks of worsening pain associated with physical activity.
   - Plain radiographs can differentiate this from acute fractures by the presence of cortical thickening around the fracture site.
   - Management includes a posterior splint, strict non-weight-bearing with crutches and orthopedic referral.

Key points for metatarsal injuries
- A first metatarsal fracture is treated more conservatively than other metatarsal fractures because of its importance in weight-bearing function.
- Compartment syndrome of the foot should be considered in any metatarsal fracture, especially crush injuries.
- Concerns for stress fracture in metatarsals 2 through 4 should prompt protection with a walking boot or non-weight-bearing with crutches, even if plain radiographs are negative.
- Proximal fifth metatarsal tuberosity fractures can be placed in a walking boot, but proximal diaphysis fractures must be made non-weight-bearing on crutches.

Phalangeal injuries

- Toe fractures constitute as much as 9% of all fractures evaluated outside the orthopedic setting.[39]
- Several mechanisms may result in fracture, including axial loading (the "stubbed" toe), crush injuries, and forced abduction (night walker's fracture).
- Physical examination should focus on evidence of an open fracture, deformity, or subungual hematoma.[44]
- The presence of angulation or rotational deformity indicates the need for reduction, which can usually be accomplished by simple traction.

Management of phalangeal fractures
- Splinting is performed using the "buddy taping" method, whereby the injured toe is taped to an adjacent uninjured toe using $1/2$-inch tape, with gauze or other padding in between.
- Subungual hematomas should undergo trephination if they are less than 24 to 48 hours old and are symptomatic.
- The nail should be left in place unless significant nail fold injury has occurred (**Fig. 9**).[52]
- These patients can be placed in a hard-soled shoe if they are having significant pain with ambulation; otherwise, close-toed shoes are recommended to help prevent repeat trauma.
- Primary care follow-up is sufficient for most of these injuries.

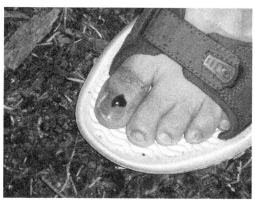

Fig. 9. A just-drained subungual hematoma. (*Courtesy of* I. Wedmore, MD, Tacoma, WA.)

- Open fractures involving the distal phalanx should receive copious irrigation and possibly prophylactic antibiotics depending on wound contamination and comorbidities.
- Open toe fractures not involving the distal phalanx should be referred to a specialist.[39]
- Orthopedic or podiatric referral is indicated in great toe fractures that are displaced, unstable, and intra-articular involving more than 25% of the joint surface, or are associated with a dislocation.[39]

Management of phalangeal dislocations

- Closed toe dislocations not involving the first metatarsophalangeal joint are typically easily reduced with longitudinal traction.
- Open dislocations of the toe warrant specially referral.
- First metatarsophalangeal dislocations can be complicated due to that joint's association with the underlying sesamoid complex.[51,53] Most dislocations are dorsal, and reduction should be performed by initially accentuating the dorsiflexion, followed by traction and plantar flexion of the proximal phalanx.[44] If this fails, surgical reduction may be necessary.

Key points for phalangeal injuries

- Although most toe fractures do not require referral, great toe fractures should be considered for specialty consult, especially if they are displaced, involve greater than 25% of the articular surface, or are associated with a dislocation.
- Subungual hematomas should be evacuated if they are symptomatic and less than 24 to 48 hours old. The nail typically does not need to be removed unless there is significant nail fold injury.
- Great toe dislocations can be complicated because of the underlying sesamoid complex and often require surgical reduction.

SUMMARY

Foot pain is a common chief complaint in the ED. Patients present with a wide range of injuries, from the "stub toe" to the intra-articular calcaneal fracture. Many of the significant injuries at risk for complications such as avascular necrosis and nonunion are not always well visualized by plain radiographs. When in doubt, patients presenting with foot pain and an unclear diagnosis should be placed in a walking boot or made non-weight-bearing on crutches with appropriate follow-up arranged.

THE ANKLE

Ankle injuries are one of the most common sports injuries and extremity complaints presenting to the ED.[54] Inversion injuries alone account for approximately 25% of all musculoskeletal injuries and 50% of sports-related injuries.[55] Although generally benign, 20% or more of these injuries may have a prolonged associated morbidity. Thus, it is incumbent on the emergency physician to accurately diagnose and treat appropriately ankle injuries.

Anatomy

The ankle is composed of the tibia, fibula, and talus, with 3 groups of stabilizing ligaments located laterally, medially, and anteroposteriorly.

Laterally

The joint is stabilized by the following ligaments:
- ATFL, most frequently injured
- Calcaneofibular ligament (CFL)
- Posterior talofibular ligament (PTFL)

These ligaments limit ankle inversion and prevent anterior and lateral subluxation of the talus (**Fig. 10**).[56]

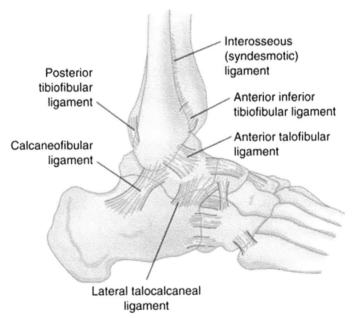

Fig. 10. Anatomy of the lateral syndesmotic ligaments. (*From* Abu-Laban RB, Rose NG. Ankle and foot. In: Marx JA, Hockberger RS, Walls RM, editors. Rosen's emergency medicine, 8th edition. Philadelphia: Saunders, 2014; with permission.)

Medially

The joint is stabilized by the deltoid ligament, which is actually a group of 4 adjoining ligaments:

- Anterior tibiotalar ligament
- Posterior tibiotalar ligament
- Tibionavicular ligament
- Tibiocalcaneal ligaments

The deltoid ligament serves to stabilize the joint during eversion and prevent talar subluxation.[57] These medial ligaments are 20% to 50% stronger than the lateral group (**Fig. 11**).[58]

Anteroposterior

The joint is stabilized by the
- Tibiofibular syndesmosis
- Anterior inferior tibiofibular ligament
- Posterior inferior talofibulra ligament
- Interosseous ligament

This group serves to limit the displacement of the fibula relative to the tibia.

History

The history should determine both the type and the scope of injury. When obtaining the history, one should inquire

- Mechanism of injury
- Ankle and foot position during the injury
- If any sounds were heard at the time of injury

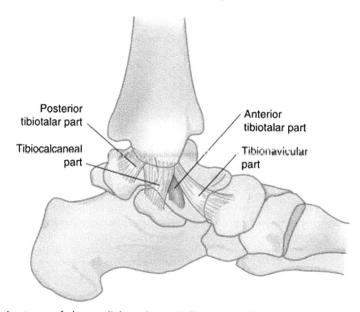

Fig. 11. Anatomy of the medial syndesmotic ligaments. (*From* Abu-Laban RB, Rose NG. Ankle and foot. In: Marx JA, Hockberger RS, Walls RM, editors. Rosen's emergency medicine, 8th edition. Philadelphia: Saunders, 2014; with permission.)

- Previous history of ankle injury
- Associated knee or foot pain
- Degree of function after the event

A low-energy mechanism, such as stepping off a curb, is unlikely to cause significant pathologic abnormality, whereas a hard parachute landing or a fall from great height is likely to result in a fracture. That being said, underlying pathologic abnormality may result in clinically significant injury from a low-energy mechanism. Knowing the vector of injury can suggest which underlying structures are injured. The degree of function after the event is indicative of severity. A history of prior injury predisposes one to subsequent recurrent injury.

Physical Examination

- Inspection
  - Ecchymosis
  - Swelling
- Range of motion
  - 50° plantarflexion
  - 20° dorsiflexion
  - 25° inversion and eversion[59,60]
- Palpation
  - Bones, particularly the proximal fibula and base of fifth metatarsal
  - Individual ligaments
  - Tendons

A thorough evaluation includes the joint above and below. It is important to palpate the entire length of the fibula to ensure not missing a potentially unstable ankle fracture requiring surgical fixation.

Specific tests

The following tests are methods of stressing specific ligaments and should not be performed until radiographs are examined or deemed unnecessary. Tests may be difficult to perform initially secondary to pain and should be repeated once pain and swelling have resolved.

Anterior drawer

- Tests the integrity of the ATFL
- Grasps the heel with one hand
- Applies a posterior force to the tibia with the other hand
- Draws the heel forward
- Laxity is compared with the opposite (uninjured) ankle

Authors differ on the definition of a positive test, with a difference of 2 mm subluxation or greater compared with the opposite side or a visible dimpling of the anterior skin of the affected ankle ("suction sign") indicating significant ATFL injury (**Fig. 12**).[58,61]

Talar tilt

- Tests the integrity of the ATFL and CFL
- Consists of plantar flexing and inverting the patient's foot
- Laxity compared with uninjured foot
- Particularly painful in the acute injury (**Fig. 13**)

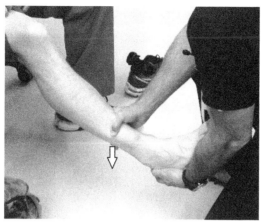

Fig. 12. Ankle draw. One hand is cupped around the heel and the other hand applies posterior force to the tibia (*Arrow*) thus drawing the ankle forward. The amount of laxity is compared to the opposite uninjured ankle. *Courtesy of* Ian Wedmore, MD and Ian May, MD, Tacoma, WA.

Squeeze test

- Tests the integrity of the syndesmotic ligaments
- Place hand 6 to 8 inches below the knee
- Squeezes the tibia and fibula together
- Pain at the ankle indicates an injury to the syndesmotic ligaments (**Fig. 14**)[62]
- Has the highest specificity for syndesmotic injury[63]

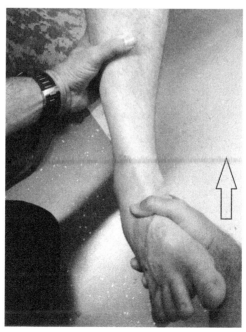

Fig. 13. Talar tilt test. The affected ankle is inverted to determine pain and laxity in the lateral ligaments. *Courtesy of* Ian Wedmore, MD and Ian May, MD, Tacoma, WA.

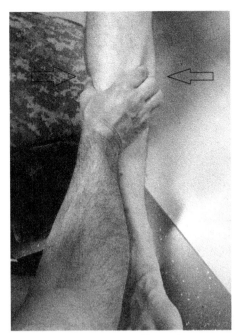

Fig. 14. Squeeze test. The tibia and fibula in the affected leg are grasped approximately 6-8 inches below the knee and the tibia and fibula and compressed together (*Arrows*). *Courtesy of* Ian Wedmore, MD and Ian May, MD, Tacoma, WA.

Thompson test

- Tests the integrity of the Achilles tendon
- Place the patient prone or kneeling
- Squeeze the midcalf
- A positive test indicates the absence of plantar flexion
- Indicates an Achilles tendon rupture[64]

Radiographic Imaging

It was previously standard practice to obtain radiographs of all ankle injuries. As it is, ankle films account for 15% of all traumatic radiographs.[65] The Ottawa Ankle Rules (OAR) were developed to help limit unnecessary radiographs. When properly applied, these rules indicate those who require radiographs without missing any clinically significant injuries. The rules relate that radiographs should be obtained on the following patients:

Ottawa Ankle Rules

1. Those unable to walk more than 4 steps after injury (immediately or in the ED)
2. Those with bony tenderness on the tip of or along the posterior edge of the distal 6 cm of either malleolus,[66] the base of the fifth metatarsal, or the navicular[60]
   There are 2 limitations to these rules
   - Injury must be acute
   - Not intended for pediatric patients[67]

It is also important to note that the absence of a positive OAR does not mean there is not a fracture. It suggests that if negative, clinically significant fractures requiring prolonged immobilization, casting, or surgical fixation are not present. Avulsion fractures may be missed.

Standard ankle radiographs include AP, lateral, and mortise views (**Fig. 15**).[68] Stress views of the ankle are often used to evaluate for significant instability or syndesmotic injury. These views can be particularly helpful to assess for disruption of the ATFL or PTFL.[69]

Adjunctive studies

With improving availability to technology, ultrasound in the acute ankle injury has become more widely used. Ultrasound can significantly reduce the number of people unnecessarily imaged without missing a clinically significant fracture compared with the use of the OAR.[70] Benefits of ultrasound include

- Able to assess for other soft tissue injuries[71–73]
- Relatively inexpensive
- Less painful than plain films

The largest limitation with regard to ultrasound is it relies heavily on the skill of the operator.

Adjunctive studies, such as CT and MRI, have a very limited utility for the emergency physician. Although MRI may be a superior modality for the evaluation of ligamentous and tendon injuries, it should be reserved for a more definitive outpatient workup by a specialist.[62,74]

Key points for physical examination and imaging
- Always examine the proximal fibula and 5th metatarsal with any ankle injury
- Properly applied OAR will save you and the patient unnecessary imaging

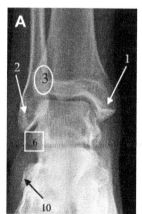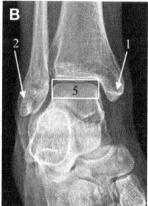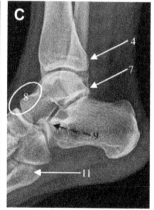

Fig. 15. Approach to reviewing ankle radiographs. (*A–C*), A standard radiographic series of the ankle has 3 views: an AP view (*A*), an internal rotation or mortise view (*B*), and a lateral view (*C*). The following 11 locations should be carefully scrutinized, because they are areas where fractures frequently occur: the medial (1) and lateral (2) malleoli, anterior tibial tubercle (3), and posterior tibial malleolus (4), talar dome (5), lateral talar process (6), tubercles of the posterior talus process (7), dorsal to the talonavicular joint (8), anterior calcaneus process (9), calcaneal insertion of the extensor digitorum brevis (10), and the base of the fifth metatarsal bone (11). (*From* Yu JS, Cody ME. A template approach for detecting fractures in adults sustaining low-energy ankle trauma. Emerg Radiol 2009;16:309; with permission.)

Fractures

Ankle fractures are classified according to several schemes, with the most commonly used being the Lauge-Hansen (L-H) and the Danis-Weber (D-W) classifications. A classification system previously described in this clinic by Hamilton[75] is comparable with the L-H system. The L-H system is based on surgical and cadaveric evaluations of the position of the foot during the injury as well as the direction of force applied to the ankle.[76] The 4 mechanisms are

- Supination-adduction (ankle inversion)
- Supination-lateral (external) rotation
- Pronation-adduction (ankle eversion)
- Pronation-lateral (external) rotation

Each mechanism is then classified by degree of force applied. The accompanying diagram best describes the system (**Fig. 16**). One of its limitations is that radiologists do not use this system because it involves a clinical component. Radiographic modifications to this grading system have been suggested, but communication among different specialists is still challenging.[77]

The L-H system can be cumbersome to use; thus, the D-W system[78] is often preferred. It has 3 fracture types (ie, A, B, C), which are essentially defined by the location of the fibular fracture (**Figs. 17** and **18**). These 3 fracture types are further graded by degree of associated injury. One downfall of the D-W system is there is higher interobserver variability with this classification system.

Treatment

Ankle fractures span the spectrum from simple to open comminuted, but the basics remain as follows:

- Assess neurovascular status of the foot
- Reduce neurovascularly compromised fractures or fracture-dislocations immediately
- Be aware that obtaining radiographs should not delay the reduction[79]
- Attempt to achieve a complete reduction
  - Lateral shift of only 1 mm of the talus results in a 40% reduction in articular contact area in the ankle joint[80]

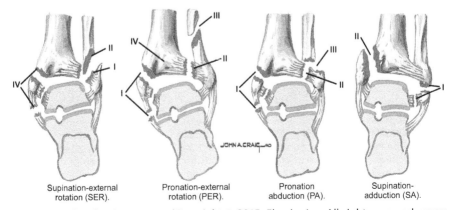

Supination-external rotation (SER).   Pronation-external rotation (PER).   Pronation abduction (PA).   Supination-adduction (SA).

Fig. 16. L-H classification system. (Copyright © 2015, Elsevier Inc. All rights reserved. www.netterimages.com.)

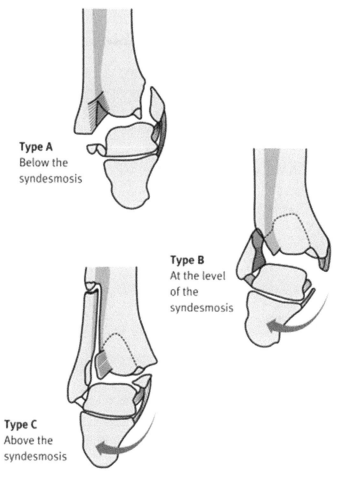

Fig. 17. D-W classification of ankle fractures. (*From* Hopton BP, Harris NJ. Fractures of the foot and ankle. Surgery (Oxford) 2010;28(10):502–7; with permission.)

- Open fractures require emergent orthopedic consultation[81]
  - Obvious contaminants should be removed
  - Intravenous antibiotics should be administered[79,81,82]
  - Tetanus status should be verified or updated
- Significantly displaced, unstable, or fractures involving the intra-articular surface should receive orthopedic consultation in the ED.
- Nondisplaced, stable fractures can be splinted or cast with outpatient follow-up.
- Small chip or avulsion fractures (typically less than 3 mm) can be treated as sprains.[83]

Unimalleolar Fractures

Lateral malleolar fractures are the most common fractures of the ankle. The stability of these fractures depends on their location.

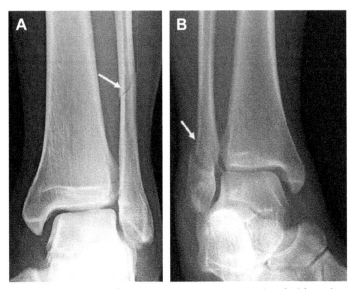

Fig. 18. Radiographs of ankles with common injury patterns associated with syndesmotic injury (*arrows*), demonstrating a pronation-external rotation or Weber type-C fracture (*A*), a supination-external rotation or Weber type-B fracture (*B*). (*Modified from* Van Heest TJ, Lafferty PM. Injuries to the ankle syndesmosis. J Bone Joint Surg Am 2014;96:603–13; with permission.)

- Fractures below the tibiotalar joint tend to be stable.
- Fractures at the tibiotalar joint with medial joint space widening tend to be unstable.[83]
- Fractures proximal to the tibiotalar joint tend to be unstable.

Stable fractures can be splinted or cast with plan for outpatient orthopedic follow-up consultation. Fractures at the tibiotalar joint without concomitant complete deltoid ligament rupture may heal without surgical fixation.[84]

Medial malleolar fractures are often seen in conjunction with other fractures. Their presence should alert one to look carefully for other sites. A truly isolated medial malleolar fracture can be treated by immobilization and outpatient follow-up if nondisplaced. High-functioning individuals may benefit from operative reduction and internal fixation for quicker rehabilitation.

Isolated posterior malleolar fractures are very rare[85] and almost always have other associated injuries. As such, it is recommended that these patients receive orthopedic consultation in the ED.

Bimalleolar and Trimalleolar Fractures

Bimalleolar fractures
- Fracture involving 2 malleoli
- Treatment is controversial
- Obtaining reduction is possible
- There is question as to whether the reduction holds with casting alone
  - May result in up to 10% nonunion rate

Trimalleolar fractures (**Fig. 19**)
- Fracture involving 3 malleoli
- Almost always require open reduction and internal fixation[83]
  - Even small subluxation of the talar articular surface is not tolerated

BEFORE   AFTER

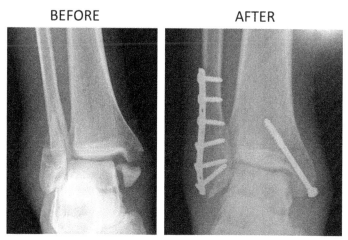

Fig. 19. Trimalleolar fracture. Chaim Mintz under creative commons license. (*Courtesy of* Chaim Mintz.)

Pilon Fractures

These fractures result from a range of energy mechanisms from low-speed rotational to axial load, when the tibia is driven down into the talus ("pilon" is French for pile-driver) (**Fig. 20**). The tibia and fibula are frequently comminuted as a result. The classification system is as follows:

- Type A fractures are extra-articular
- Type B fractures are partially articular
- Type C fractures are complete metaphyseal fractures with articular involvement[86,87]

All types are graded 1 to 3 based on degree of comminution. These pilon fractures require orthopedic consultation in the ED given the articular involvement. A large percentage of these are open fractures, and long-term morbidity is not uncommon.[88]

Talar Dome Fractures

Talar dome fractures are the most common chondral fractures, which are also known as osteochondritis dessicans, transcondral fractures, or flake fractures. These

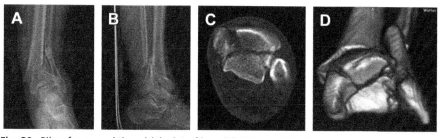

Fig. 20. Pilon fracture. (*A*) and (*B*) plain films, (*C*) CT view, (*D*) CT reconstruction. (*From* Wei SJ, Han F, Lan SH, et al. Surgical treatment of pilon fracture based on ankle position at the time of injury/initial direction of fracture displacement: a prospective cohort study. Int J Surg 2014;12(5):418–25; with permission.)

fractures are often missed initially. These injuries, if not found on initial evaluation, tend to present as a "sprained ankle that did not heal":

- Persistent swelling
- Pain
- Locking of the ankle
- Crepitus

These lesions are classified by stage of development of the osteochondral lesion. Early stage may not be visible on plain films and consists of subchondral compression. The later stage involves the development of loose bodies and a subchondral bone cyst.[89] These patients can be referred for outpatient evaluation for more in-depth imaging. The initial treatment is generally conservative with casting and activity modification as the primary modalities.[90] Treatment ranges from none to arthroscopy for larger fragments, and the course should be determined by the outpatient consultant.[91]

Maissonneuve Fracture

A Maisonneuve fracture is actually a combination of the following:
- Fracture of the proximal fibula
- Disruption of the interosseous membrane and tibiofibular ligament distally
- Medial malleolar fracture or deltoid ligamentous tear (**Fig. 21**)
- Severe instability

Because this fracture represents 1 in 20 ankle fractures,[92] thorough physical examination of the involved extremity is incredibly important. Failure to examine the

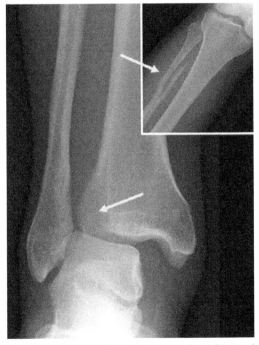

Fig. 21. Maisonneuve fracture. *Arrows* indicate the proximal fibular fracture and area of ligament disruption. (*Modified from* Van Heest TJ, Lafferty PM. Injuries to the ankle syndesmosis. J Bone Joint Surg Am 2014;96:603–13; with permission.)

proximal fibula may result in missing the fracture.[93,94] Treatment depends on the status of the ankle mortise. Most of these fractures require open reduction with internal fixation because of the instability.[95]

Significant points for ankle fractures
- Fractures that are significantly displaced, unstable, or involve the intra-articular surface should receive orthopedic consultation in the ED.
- Bimaleollar fractures often require operative repair.
- Trimalleolar and pilon fractures will require operative stabilization and repair.

Sprains

Ligamentous injuries are extremely common in the ED, with lateral ligamentous injuries making up approximately 85% of injuries.[96]

- Most common mechanism is foot inversion
- ATFL is injured first (60% to 70% of all ankle sprains)
- CFL is injured next
- PTFL is injured last

The last case represents only 0% to 9% of cases referred for surgery. It is usually seen only with a dislocation.[97] Lateral ankle sprains are graded on a scale of 1 to 3, with increasing grade relating to increased anatomic damage.

Most ankle sprains heal well regardless of their grade, and little advantage has been shown with primary surgical repair.[98] That being said, 20% to 40% of ankle injuries progress to chronic ankle instability.[95] Initial care in the ED is similar for all grades. Patients with persistent symptoms after a several-week recovery period can undergo delayed surgical intervention with no detriment to outcome.[99] All sprains are treated with RICEN:

- *Rest*
- *Ice*
- *Compression*
- *Elevation*
- *Nonsteroidal anti-inflammatory drugs*

RICE therapy is considered standard,[100,101] and nonsteroidal anti-inflammatory drugs provide both analgesia and some possible improvement in therapeutic outcome for the patient.[96,102,103] Non-weight-bearing or crutch use depends on the degree of injury and the patient's symptoms. Grade II and III sprains typically benefit from 48 to 72 hours of initial non-weight-bearing.[104]

Immobilization may more quickly reduce pain and swelling; however, early mobilization and proprioception exercises generally improve functional outcome more quickly. The mnemonic PRICE is sometimes used, where the P stands for "protection," meaning the short period of non-weight-bearing, use of an air cast, or other functional splints. All grades can benefit from functional taping or bracing.[104,105] Graded strength training and proprioception exercises through physical therapy may assist in return to full function without the use of external protection.

Lateral Sprains

Grade I

- Minimal to no swelling
- Tenderness only over the ATFL
- Functional treatment results in a full return to activities within 1 week[102]

- Orthopedic intervention is seldom warranted

Grade II

- Involves the ATFL and the CFL
- Localized swelling and more diffuse lateral tenderness
- Period of disability is a few weeks
- Outpatient follow-up care with a specialist (eg, sports medicine specialist, physical therapist, or an orthopedist)

Grade III

- Substantial tears of the lateral ligaments (**Fig. 22**)
- Laxity is demonstrated by a positive drawer or tilt on testing
- Significant swelling, pain, and ecchymosis

Once swelling has occurred, it can be difficult to separate a severe grade II from a grade III on initial examination.[64]

Treatment of these sprains is controversial. Although some advocate early surgical repair,[106,107] one review found that 80% to 90% of grade III injuries did well regardless of treatment used and recommend nonsurgical therapy initially.[108] A meta-analysis concluded that most patients with grade III lateral injuries healed without operative intervention comparably to those with lower grade ankle sprains.[109] Patients with a grade III tear should be referred to a specialist because some 10% to 40% need later definitive therapy.[110] Using immobilization via cast has been shown to be beneficial for the first 10 days after injury.[111,112] Professional athletes may have faster return to play and better overall outcome with early surgical fixation.[113]

Medial Sprains

The strength of the deltoid ligament tends to prevent significant medial sprains. When these occur, it is secondary to an eversion force. They are uncommon, representing only 5% of ankle sprains.[97] These sprains are graded in the same manner as lateral sprains, with similar treatment. Grade III medial ligament injuries with associated injury to syndesmosis ligaments or the lateral ligaments have been shown to have improved outcome with surgical management.[112]

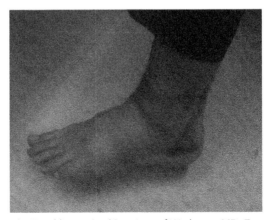

Fig. 22. Authors grade III ankle sprain. (*Courtesy of* Wedmore MD, Tacoma, WA.)

Key Points in Sprains
- Immediate surgical intervention is seldom if ever acutely required for ankle sprains.
- (P)RICE remains the standard treatment for an ankle sprain.
- Higher-grade sprains may benefit from 24 to 48 hours if initial non-weight-bearing.

Syndesmotic Injuries

Initially thought to be uncommon, more recent literature suggests syndesmotic injuries occur in as frequently as 20% to 25%[114–116] of ankle injuries. There is a slight predominance in this injury in youth. They are associated with prolonged disability[67] and a much higher likelihood of chronic pain and instability.[117] The emergency physician must examine patients carefully for their presence. A positive squeeze test result without the presence of a fibular fracture has a high specificity for syndesmotic injury.[118] The ability to hop on the affected foot, the lack of tenderness to palpation along the syndesmotic ligaments, and negative dorsiflexion-external rotation stress are all associated with high sensitivity. Although there is an association with concomitant lateral ligamentous injury, it is not uncommon for there to be a syndesmotic injury without other ligamentous injuries.[118] The ankle should be splinted until the patient receives an outpatient evaluation by a specialist.[78,114]

Tendon Injuries

Achilles tendon rupture

- Sudden dorsiflexion of the foot
- Hearing a "pop"
- Sudden onset of pain over the posterior ankle
- Physical examination with palpable defect of the Achilles tendon

Ruptures of the Achilles tendon are typically seen in middle-aged occasional athletes.[119] The best clinical test is the Thompson test. This test result must be compared with the uninjured contralateral side because weak plantar flexion still can be seen second to the actions of the peroneal and tibialis posterior muscles.[114] If doubt still exists, ultrasonography or MRI can facilitate the diagnosis.[118,120] Although helpful when diagnosis is questionable, it is unnecessary when the Thompson test is positive in the setting of decreased resting tension and a palpable defect.[121] MRI is expensive and could also result in delay of definitive treatment. Optimal therapy remains controversial.

Surgery
- More rapid return to activities
- Lower rerupture rates
- Increase strength and function
- Longer hospitalization
- Associated with wound infections and standard surgical risks[122–124]

The ankle should be splinted with slight plantar flexion and the patient can be referred to a specialist for a discussion of management options.

Peroneal tendon injuries

The anatomic location of the peroneal tendon often results in their injury being mistakenly diagnosed as an ankle sprain.[125,126] The peroneal tendons

- Evert and pronate the foot
- Run through the peroneal sulcus behind and posterior to the lateral malleolus

- Are held in place by the superficial peroneal retinaculum
- Have prevention of the tendons from dislocating by the retinaculum

With sufficient excessive dorsiflexion, the retinaculum's attachment to the fibula can tear, resulting in anterior subluxation of the tendons. Physical examination shows tenderness along the posterior edge of the lateral malleolus, and occasionally, the dislocated tendons themselves can be palpated. A confirmatory test involves holding the foot in dorsiflexion, then attempting to evert the foot. If the tendons subluxate with this maneuver, the test result is positive. As technology advances, ultrasound has begun to replace MRI as the first-line imaging modality to assess for peroneal tendon injuries.[127] The optimal treatment of subluxation is controversial[128–130] and also depends on associated injuries and the activity level of the individual.[130,131] Athletes often require surgical fixation to remain fully functional.[132] ED care involves placing the involved ankle in a stirrup splint and referring the patient for specialty evaluation as an outpatient.

SUMMARY

Because ankle injuries can range from trivial to significant, knowledge of ankle anatomy and specific tests of ankle structures allows proper diagnosis of injuries. Use of the OAR provides a basis for the judicious use of radiographs. Ultrasound use may assist in limiting the amount of radiographs obtained. Fractures that preserve the anatomic alignment of the ankle can be splinted and referred for specialty evaluation on an outpatient basis. Fractures with loss of alignment, significant articular involvement, or instability should be evaluated in the ED by a specialist. Ankle sprains of any grade initially should be treated functionally, with a plan to follow-up on an outpatient basis for further management. Achilles and peroneal tendon injuries may require surgical repair; however, rarely do either require emergent consultation in the ED. These patients can be discharged with splinting and plan for outpatient follow-up for more definitive management.

REFERENCES

1. Bachmann LM, Kolb E, Koller MT, et al. Accuracy of Ottawa ankle rules to exclude fractures of the ankle and mid-foot: systematic review. BMJ 2003; 326:417.
2. Stiell IG, McKnight RD, Greenberg GH, et al. Implementation of the Ottawa ankle rules. JAMA 1994;271(11):827–32.
3. Smith TR. Management of dancers with symptomatic accessory navicular: 2 case reports. J Orthop Sports Phys Ther 2012;42(5):465–73.
4. Karasick D, Schweitzer ME. The os trigonum syndrome: imaging features. AJR Am J Roentgenol 1996;166:125–9.
5. Haapamaki VV, Kiuru MJ, Koskinen SK. Ankle and foot injuries: analysis of MDCT findings. AJR Am J Roentgenol 2004;183(3):615–22.
6. Mulfinger G, Trueta J. The blood supply to the talus. J Bone Joint Surg Br 1970; 52B:160.
7. Canale ST, Kelly FB. Fractures of the neck of the talus. Long-term evaluation of seventy-one cases. J Bone Joint Surg Am 1978;60:143.
8. Schiffer G, Jubel A, Elsner A, et al. Complete talar dislocation without late osteonecrosis: clinical case and anatomic study. J Foot Ankle Surg 2007;46:120–3.
9. Peterson L, Romanus B, Dahlberg E. Fracture of the collum tali–an experimental study. J Biomech 1976;9(4):277–9.

10. Thomas JL, Boyce BM. Radiographic analysis of the Canale view for displaced talar neck fractures. J Foot Ankle Surg 2012;51(2):187.

11. McCrory P, Bladin C. Fractures of the lateral process of the talus: a clinical review of snowboarder's ankle. Clin J Sport Med 1996;6:124–8.

12. Noble J, Royle SG. Fracture of the lateral process of the talus: computed tomographic scan diagnosis. Br J Sports Med 1992;26:245–6.

13. Kirkpatrick DP, Hunter RE, Janes PC, et al. The snowboarder's foot and ankle. Am J Sports Med 1998;26:271–7.

14. Valderrabano V, Perren T, Ryf C, et al. Snowboarder's talus fracture: treatment outcome of 20 cases after 3.5 years. Am J Sports Med 2005;33:871–80.

15. Bonvin F, Montet X, Copercini M, et al. Imaging of fractures of the lateral process of the talus, a frequently missed diagnosis. Eur J Radiol 2003;47:64–70.

16. Nanjayan SK, Broomfield J, Johnson B, et al. Total dislocation of the talus: a case report. Foot Ankle Spec 2014;7(1):71–3.

17. Starosta D, Sacchetti AD, Sharkey P, et al. Calcaneal fracture with compartment syndrome of the foot. Ann Emerg Med 1988;17:144.

18. Janzen DL, Connell D, Munk PL, et al. Intraarticular fractures of the calcaneus: value of CT findings in determining prognosis. AJR Am J Roentgenol 1992; 158(6):1271–4.

19. Stoller DW, Tirman PF, Bredella M, et al. Ankle and foot, osseous fractures, calcaneal fractures. Diagnostic imaging: orthopaedics. Salt Lake City (UT): Amirsys; 2004. p. 70–4.

20. Guerado E, Bertrand ML, Cano JR. Management of calcaneal fractures: what have we learnt over the years? Injury 2012;43(10):1640–50.

21. Isaacs JD, Baba M, Huang P. The diagnostic accuracy of Böhler's angle in fractures of the calcaneus. J Emerg Med 2013;45(6):879.

22. Badillo K, Pacheco JA, Padua SO, et al. Multidetector CT evaluation of calcaneal fractures. Radiographics 2011;31:81–92.

23. Juliano P, Nguyen HV. Fractures of the calcaneus. Orthop Clin North Am 2001; 32:35–51.

24. Germann CA, Perron AD, Miller MD, et al. Orthopedic pitfalls in the ED: calcaneal fractures. Am J Emerg Med 2004;22(7):607–11.

25. Thordarson DB. Fractures of the midfoot and forefoot. In: LM, Myerson MS, editors. Foot and ankle disorders. Orlando (FL): Harcourt; 2000. p. 1265–85.

26. Saxena A, Fullem B. Navicular stress fractures: a prospective study on athletes. Foot Ankle Int 2006;27(11):917–21.

27. Brockwell J, Yeung Y, Griffith JF. Stress fractures of the foot and ankle. Sports Med Arthrosc 2009;17(3):149–59.

28. Jarvis JG, Moroz PJ. Fractures and dislocations of the foot. In: Koval KJ, Beaty JH, editors. Fractures in children. 6th edition. Philadelphia: Lippincott Williams & Wilkins; 2006.

29. Ceroni D, De Rosa V, De Coulon G, et al. Cuboid nutcracker fracture due to horseback riding in children: case series and review of the literature. J Pediatr Orthop 2007;27:557.

30. Hardcastle PH, Reschauer R, Kutscha-Lissberg E, et al. Injuries to the TMT joint. Incidence, classification and treatment. J Bone Joint Surg Br 1982;64:349.

31. Mantas JP, Burks RT. Lisfranc injuries in the athlete. Clin J Sport Med 1994; 13:719.

32. Gupta RT, Wadhwa RP, Learch TJ, et al. Lisfranc injury: imaging findings for this important but often-missed diagnosis. Curr Probl Diagn Radiol 2008;37(3): 115–26.

33. Foster SC, Foster RR. Lisfranc's TMT fracture-dislocation. Radiology 1976; 120:79.
34. Nunley JA, Vertullo CJ. Classification, investigation, and management of midfoot sprains: Lisfranc injuries in the athlete. Am J Sports Med 2002;30:871.
35. Haapamaki V, Kiuru M, Koskinen S. Lisfranc fracture-dislocation in patients with multiple trauma: diagnosis with multidetector computed tomography. Foot Ankle Int 2004;25:614.
36. Meyer SA, Callaghan JJ, Albright JP, et al. Midfoot sprains in collegiate football players. Am J Sports Med 1994;22:392.
37. Hatch RL, Rosenbaum CI. Fracture care by family physicians. A review of 295 cases. J Fam Pract 1994;38(3):238.
38. Saraiya MJ. First metatarsal fractures. Clin Podiatr Med Surg 1995;12:749.
39. Eiff MP, Hatch RL. Fracture management for primary care. Philadelphia: WB Saunders; 2011.
40. McQueen MM, Court-Brown CM. Compartment monitoring in tibial fractures. The pressure threshold for decompression. J Bone Joint Surg Br 1996;78(1):99.
41. Cortina J, Amat C, Selga J, et al. Isolated medial foot compartment syndrome after ankle sprain. Foot Ankle Surg 2014;20(1):e1–2.
42. Armagan OE, Shereff MJ. Injuries to the toes and metatarsals. Orthop Clin North Am 2001;32:1.
43. Simons S. Foot injuries in the runner. In: Wilder RP, O'Connor FG, editors. Textbook of running medicine. New York: McGraw-Hill; 2001. p. 213.
44. DiGiovanni CW, Benirschke SK, Hansen ST. Metatarsal fractures. In: Jupiter JB, Browner BD, Levine AM, et al, editors. Skeletal trauma: fractures, dislocations, ligamentous injuries. Philadelphia: WB Saunders; 2002.
45. Wheeler P, Batt ME. Do non-steroidal anti-inflammatory drugs adversely affect stress fracture healing? A short review. Br J Sports Med 2005;39(2):65–9.
46. Smith JW, Arnoczky SP, Hersh A. The intraosseous blood supply of the fifth metatarsal: implications for proximal fracture healing. Foot Ankle 1992;13:143.
47. Jones R. Fracture of the base of the fifth metatarsal bone by indirect violence. Ann Surg 1902;35:697.
48. Richli WR, Rosenthal DI. Avulsion fracture of the fifth metatarsal: experimental study of pathomechanics. AJR Am J Roentgenol 1984;143:889.
49. Lawrence SJ, Botte MJ. Jones' fractures and related fractures of the proximal fifth metatarsal. Foot Ankle 1993;14:358.
50. Quill GE Jr. Fractures of the proximal fifth metatarsal. Orthop Clin North Am 1995;26(2):353.
51. Jahss MH. Traumatic dislocations of the first metatarsophalangeal joint. Foot Ankle 1980;1:15.
52. Batrick N, Hashemi K, Freij R. Treatment of uncomplicated subungual haematoma. Emerg Med J 2003;20(1):65.
53. Mittlmeier T, Haar P. Sesamoid and toe fractures. Injury 2004;35(Suppl 2):SB87.
54. Garrick JG. The frequency of injury, mechanism of injury and epidemiology of ankle sprains. Am J Sports Med 1977;5:241–2.
55. Czajka CM, Tran E, Cai AN, et al. Ankle sprains and instability. Med Clin North Am 2014;98(2):313–29.
56. Birrer RB. Ankle injuries. In: Sports medicine for the primary care physician. Boca Raton (FL): CRC; 1994. p. 543–60.
57. Hamilton WC. Injuries of the ankle and foot. Emerg Med Clin North Am 1994;361:2.
58. Prins JG. Diagnosis and treatment of injury to the lateral ligament of the ankle: a comparative study. Acta Chir Scand 1978;486:143–9.

59. Rasmussen O. Stability of the ankle joint: analysis of the function and traumatology of the ankle ligaments. Acta Orthop Scand 1985;56:1.
60. Seto JL, Brewster CE. Treatment approaches following foot and ankle injury. Clin Sports Med 1985;13:295.
61. Liu SH, Williams JJ. Lateral ankle sprains and instability problems. Clin Sports Med 1994;793(13):4.
62. Hopkinson WJ, St Pierre P, Ryan JB, et al. Syndesmosis sprains of the ankle. Foot Ankle 1990;10:325–30.
63. Vosseller JT, Karl JW, Greisberg JK. Incidence of syndesmotic injury. Orthopedics 2014;37(3):e226–9.
64. Thompson TC, Doherty JH. Spontaneous rupture of the tendon of Achilles: a new clinical diagnostic test. J Trauma 1962;2:126.
65. Auletta AG, Conway WF, Hayes CW, et al. Role of radiography in ankle trauma. AJR Am J Roentgenol 1991;157:789–91.
66. Steill IG, Greenberg GH, McKnight RD, et al. Decision rules for the use of radiography in acute ankle injuries: refinement and prospective validation. JAMA 1993;269:1127–32.
67. Nelson SW. Some important diagnostic and technical fundamentals in the radiology of trauma, with particular emphasis on skeletal trauma. Radiol Clin North Am 1966;4:241–59.
68. Ho R, Abu-Laban RB. Ankle and foot. In: Rosen P, Barker FJ II, Braen GR, et al, editors. Emergency medicine: concepts and clinical practice, vol. 1, 3rd edition. St Louis (MO): CV Mosby; 1998. p. 821–60.
69. Lee KM, Chung CY, Kwon SS, et al. Relationship between stress ankle radiographs and injured ligaments on MRI. Skeletal Radiol 2013;42(11):1537–42.
70. Hedelin H, Goksör LÅ, Karlsson J, et al. Ultrasound-assisted triage of ankle trauma can decrease the need for radiographic imaging. Am J Emerg Med 2013;31(12):1686–9.
71. Weinfeld SB. Achilles tendon disorders. Med Clin North Am 2014;98(2):331–8.
72. Cheng Y, Cai Y, Wang Y. Value of ultrasonography for detecting chronic injury of the lateral ligaments of the ankle joint compared with ultrasonography findings. Br J Radiol 2014;87:20130406.
73. Bianchi S, Luong DH. Stress fractures of the ankle malleoli diagnosed by ultrasound: a report of 6 cases. Skeletal Radiol 2014;43(6):813–8.
74. Burge AJ, Gold SL, Potter HG. Imaging of sports-related midfoot and forefoot injuries. Sports Health 2012;4(6):518–34.
75. Hamilton WC. Traumatic disorders of the ankle. New York: Springer-Verlag; 1984.
76. Lauge-Hansen N. Fractures of the ankle, I. Combined experimental-surgical and experimental roentgenologic investigations. Arch Surg 1950;60:957.
77. Russo A, Reginelli A, Zappia M, et al. Ankle fracture: radiographic approach according to the Lauge-Hansen classification. Musculoskelet Surg 2013; 97(Suppl 2):S155–60.
78. Daffner RH. Ankle trauma. Radiol Clin North Am 1990;28:395–421.
79. DeSouza IJ. Fractures and dislocations about the ankle. In: Gustilo RB, Kyle RF, Templeton DC, editors. Fractures and dislocations, vol. 2. St Louis (MO): CV Mosby; 1993.
80. Ramsey PL, Hamilton W. Changes in tibiotalar area of contact caused by lateral talar shift. J Bone Joint Surg Am 1976;58A:356.
81. Rosenthal RE. Emergency department evaluation of musculoskeletal injuries. Emerg Med Clin North Am 1984;2:2.

82. Gustilo RB, Anderson JT. Prevention of infection in the treatment of open ankle fractures. Clin Orthop 1989;240:47–52.

83. Michelson JD. Fractures about the ankle. J Bone Joint Surg 1985;67A:67.

84. Koval KJ, Egol KA, Cheung Y, et al. Does a positive ankle stress test indicate the need for operative treatment after lateral malleolus fracture? A preliminary report. J Orthop Trauma 2007;21(7):449–55.

85. Nugent JF, Gale BD. Isolated posterior malleolar ankle fractures. J Foot Surg 1990;29:80.

86. Luk PC, Charlton TP, Lee J, et al. Ipsilateral intact fibula as a predictor of tibial plafond fracture pattern and severity. Foot Ankle Int 2013;34(10):1421–6.

87. Swiontkowski MF, Sands AK, Agel J, et al. Interobserver variation in the AO/OTA fracture classification system for pilon fractures: is there a problem? J Orthop Trauma 1997;11(7):467–70.

88. Bourne RB, Rorabeck CH, MacNab J. Intra-articular fractures of the distal tibia: the pilon fracture. J Trauma 1983;23:591–5.

89. Bernd AL, Harty M. Transchondral fractures (osteochondritis dissecans) of the talus. J Bone Joint Surg Am 1959;41-A:1002.

90. Talusan PG, Milewski MD, Toy JO. Wall EJ3 osteochondritis dissecans of the talus: diagnosis and treatment in athletes. Clin Sports Med 2014;33(2):267–84.

91. Ewing JW. Arthroscopic management of transcondral talar dome (osteochondritis dessicans) and the anterior impingement lesions of the ankle joint. Clin Sports Med 1991;10:677–85.

92. Pankvoich AM. Maisonneuve fracture of the fibula. J Bone Joint Surg 1976;58A: 333–42.

93. Lock TR, Scaffer JJ, Manoli A II. Maisonneuve fracture: a case report of a missed diagnosis. Ann Emerg Med 1987;16:805–7.

94. Taweel NR, Raikin SM, Karanjia HN, et al. The proximal fibula should be examined in all patients with ankle injury: a case series of missed maisonneuve fractures. J Emerg Med 2013;44(2):e251–5.

95. Valderrabano V, Wiewiorski M, Frigg A, et al. Chronic ankle instability. Unfallchirurg 2007;110(8):691–9.

96. Dupont M, Beliveau P, Theriault G. The efficacy of anti-inflammatory medication in the treatment of the acutely sprained ankle. Am J Sports Med 1987;15:41.

97. Brostrom L. Sprained ankles, I. Anatomic lesions in recent sprains. Acta Chir Scand 1964;128:483.

98. Niederman B, Anderson A, Bryde Anderson S, et al. Rupture of the lateral ligaments of the ankle: operation or plaster cast? A prospective study. Acta Orthop Scand 1981;52:579–87.

99. Lassiter TE, Malone TR, Garrett WE. Injury to the lateral ligaments of the ankle. Orthop Clin North Am 1989;20:629–40.

100. Smith RW, Reischel S. Treatment of ankle sprains in young athletes. Am J Sports Med 1986;14:465.

101. Trevino SG, Davis P, Hecht P. Management of acute and chronic lateral ligament injuries of the ankle. Orthop Clin North Am 1994;25:1.

102. McCulluch PG, Holden P, Robson DJ. The value of mobilization and nonsteroidal anti-inflammatory analgesia in the management of inversion injuries of the ankle. Br J Clin Pract 1985;36:69.

103. Moran M. Double-blind comparison of diclofenac potassium, ibuprofen, and placebo in the treatment of ankle sprains. J Int Med Res 1991;19:121.

104. Shapiro MS, Kabo JM, Mitchell PW, et al. Ankle sprain prophylaxis: an analysis of the stabilizing effects of braces and tape. Am J Sports Med 1994;22:1–15.

105. Glick JM, Gordon RB, Nishimoto D. The prevention and treatment of ankle injuries. Am J Sports Med 1976;5:136–41.
106. Brand RL, Collins MD, Templeton T. Surgical repair of ruptured lateral ankle ligaments. Am J Sports Med 1981;9:40–4.
107. Jaskulka R, Fischer G, Schedl R. Injuries of the lateral ligaments of the ankle: operative treatment and long-term results. Arch Orthop Trauma Surg 1988; 107:217–21.
108. Kannus P, Renstrom P. Current concepts review: treatment for acute tears of the lateral ligaments of the ankle. J Bone Joint Surg Am 1991;73:305–12.
109. Petersen W, Rembitzki IV, Koppenburg AG, et al. Treatment of acute ankle ligament injuries: a systematic review. Arch Orthop Trauma Surg 2013;133(8): 1129–41.
110. Gronmark T, Johnson O, Kogstad O. Rupture of the lateral ligaments of the ankle. Foot Ankle 1980;1:84–9.
111. Harris CR. Ankle injuries. In: Ruiz E, Cicero JJ, editors. Emergency management of skeletal injuries. St Louis (MO): CV Mosby; 1995. p. 517–40.
112. McCollum GA, van den Bekerom MP, Kerkhoffs GM, et al. Syndesmosis and deltoid ligament injuries in the athlete. Knee Surg Sports Traumatol Arthrosc 2013;21(6):1328–37.
113. van den Bekerom MP, Kerkhoffs GM, McCollum GA, et al. Management of acute lateral ankle ligament injury in the athlete. Knee Surg Sports Traumatol Arthrosc 2013;21(6):1390–5.
114. Goosens M, DeStoop N. Lisfranc's fracture-dislocations: etiology, radiology, and results of treatment: a review of twenty cases. Clin Orthop 1983;176:154.
115. Roemer FW, Jomaah N, Niu J, et al. Ligamentous injuries and the risk of associated tissue damage in acute ankle sprains in athletes: a cross-sectional MRI study. Am J Sports Med 2014;42:1549–57.
116. Sman AD, Hiller CE, Rae K, et al. Predictive factors for ankle syndesmosis injury in football players: a prospective study. J Sci Med Sport 2014;17: 586–90.
117. Valkering KP, Vergroesen DA, Nolte PA. Isolated syndesmosis ankle injury. Orthopedics 2012;35(12):e1705–10.
118. Kamberger FM, Engel A, Barton P, et al. Injury of the Achilles tendon: diagnosis with sonography. AJR Am J Roentgenol 1990;155:1031.
119. Jozsa L, Kuist M, Balinr BJ, et al. The role of recreational sport activity in Achilles tendon rupture. Am J Sports Med 1989;17:338–43.
120. Pantageas E, Greenberg S, Franklin PD, et al. Magnetic resonance imaging of pathologic conditions of the Achilles tendon. Orthop Rev 1990;19:975.
121. Garras DN, Raikin SM, Bhat SB, et al. MRI is unnecessary for diagnosing acute Achilles tendon ruptures: clinical diagnostic criteria. Clin Orthop Relat Res 2012; 470(8):2268–73.
122. Cetti R, Christensen SE, Ejsted R, et al. Operative vs. nonoperative treatment of Achilles tendon rupture: a prospective randomized study and review of the literature. Am J Sports Med 1993;21:791.
123. Willis CA, Washburn S, Carozzo V, et al. Achilles tendon rupture: a review of the literature comparing surgical vs non-surgical treatment. Clin Orthop 1986; 207:156.
124. Stavrou M, Seraphim A, Al-Hadithy N, et al. Review article: treatment for Achilles tendon ruptures in athletes. J Orthop Surg (Hong Kong) 2013;21(2):232–5.
125. Arrowsmith SR, Fleming LL, Allman FL. Literature comparing surgical vs. nonsurgical treatment. Clin Orthop 1986;207:156.

126. Eckert WR, Davis EA Jr. Acute rupture of the peroneal retinaculum. J Bone Joint Surg Am 1976;58A:670.
127. Bianchi S, Delmi M, Molini L. Ultrasound of peroneal tendons. Semin Musculoskelet Radiol 2010;14(3):292–306.
128. Sammarco GJ. Peroneal tendon injuries. Orthop Clin North Am 1994;25:135.
129. Trevino S, Baumhamer JF. Tendon injuries of the foot and ankle. Clin Sports Med 1992;11:727.
130. Zhenbo Z, Jin W, Haifeng G, et al. Sliding fibular graft repair for the treatment of recurrent peroneal subluxation. Foot Ankle Int 2014;35:496–503.
131. Toussaint RJ, Lin D, Ehrlichman LK, et al. Peroneal tendon displacement accompanying intra-articular calcaneal fractures. J Bone Joint Surg Am 2014; 96(4):310–5.
132. Guillo S, Calder JD. Treatment of recurring peroneal tendon subluxation in athletes: endoscopic repair of the retinaculum. Foot Ankle Clin 2013;18(2): 293–300.

The Emergent Evaluation and Treatment of Hand Injuries

David Hile, MD*, Lisa Hile, MD

KEYWORDS

- Hand injuries • Metacarpal fracture • Phalangeal fracture • Tendon injury
- Emergency physician • Orthopedic injury

KEY POINTS

- A detailed history and physical examination is imperative to correct diagnosis and management of small but important structures of the hand.
- Plain film radiographs remain the standard of care for identifying bony injuries, but ultrasound shows promise in identification of both bony and soft tissue injuries, and can guide reduction.
- An orderly approach to assessment and description of injuries using the NO LOADS mnemonic helps to guide the examiner to appropriate initial and definitive treatment of hand injuries.

BACKGROUND

Hand fractures are among the most common skeletal injuries. Injuries to the hand can be challenging to diagnose and manage owing to the complex anatomy and highly specialized function of this area of the body. Even seemingly minor injuries can inhibit the ability to perform activities of daily living, and lead to devastating infections, chronic pain, and dysfunction. A detailed knowledge of the anatomy of, and common injuries to, bone and soft tissues of the hand is essential to proper diagnosis and management, and thus avoidance of debilitating complications.

EPIDEMIOLOGY

- Fractures of the hand account for 19% to 28% of all fractures.[1]
- Finger fractures are the most common sports-related fractures in adolescents and adults.[2]

Disclosure Statement: The authors have nothing to disclose.
Department of Emergency Medicine, Yale School of Medicine, 464 Congress Avenue, Suite 260, New Haven, CT 06519, USA
* Corresponding author.
E-mail address: David.hile@yale.edu

Emerg Med Clin N Am 33 (2015) 397–408
http://dx.doi.org/10.1016/j.emc.2014.12.009
0733-8627/15/$ – see front matter © 2015 Elsevier Inc. All rights reserved.

emed.theclinics.com

- The small finger ray is the most commonly fractured digit.
- The distal phalanx is the most frequently fractured bone of the hand.[1]
- Dorsal dislocation of the proximal interphalangeal (PIP) joint is the most frequent dislocation in the hand.
- The most common ligament injury in the thumb, and second most common skiing injury overall, is disruption of the ulnar collateral ligament (Skier's thumb).
- An extensor tendon injury overlying the distal interphalangeal joint (Mallet finger) is the most common tendon injury.[3]

HAND ANATOMY

The hand is composed of 5 metacarpals and 14 phalanges. These bones span 4 joints: the carpometacarpal (CMC) joint, the metacarpophalangeal (MCP) joint, the PIP joint, and the distal interphalangeal (DIP) joint. Refer to each digit by name (thumb, index, long, ring, and small) rather than number.

Digital Metacarpals

- The more proximal bones of the hand are the metacarpals. The metacarpals articulate proximally with the distal row of carpal bones, forming the CMC joint.
- The metacarpals form a volar concave arc along their length, with flares at the bases and the necks. The metacarpal head articulates with the base of the proximal phalanx as a condylar joint that permits flexion, extension, and radial and ulnar motion.
- The accepted convention for naming of the fingers is as follows: thumb, index, middle, ring, little. The fingers should be described as such to avoid confusion with numbering.

Phalanges

- Distal to the metacarpals are 3 rows of phalanges, with the exception of the thumb, which has only 2 phalanges.

Soft Tissue Structures

The median, ulnar, and radial nerves and their branches provide motor and sensory innervation to the hand. Although a detailed review of innervation of the hand is important, it is beyond the scope of this article. In brief, the median nerve innervates the muscles involved in fine precision and pinch function of the hand. Its anterior interosseous branch innervates intrinsic muscles of the hand.

The median nerve gives off a palmar cutaneous branch, which provides sensation to the thenar eminence, and a recurrent motor branch, which innervates the thenar muscles. The ulnar nerve innervates the muscles involved in hand grasp. Its palmar cutaneous branch provides sensation to the hypothenar eminence. Its dorsal branch provides sensation to the ulnar portion of the dorsum of the hand. Its superficial branch forms the digital nerves to the small and ring fingers, and its deep motor branch innervates the hypothenar muscles. The radial nerve innervates the wrist extensors (via the deep posterior interosseous branch). The superficial branch provides sensation at the radial aspect of the dorsum of the hand, thumb, index, long, and radial half of the ring fingers.

The flexor tendons of the hand course through sheaths on the volar (palmar) aspect of the fingers. The extensor tendons attach by a tendinous slip to the proximal phalanx. The central tendon, or slip, proceeds dorsally to attach to the base of the middle phalanx, where tension can extend the PIP joint. The lateral bands proceed on either side of the midline and then rejoin before attaching to the distal phalanx. Tension on the lateral bands extends the DIP joint.

EXAMINATION

A complete history must be obtained to include mechanism of injury, because this may suggest other underlying secondary injuries. The history should also include the patient's handedness, functional status, previous hand injuries, occupation, and hobbies. A tobacco use history is also important because smoking can hinder healing of certain fractures.

- Physical examination of the hand begins with adequate lighting and exposure.
  - Use overhead lighting or other hands-free lighting (headlamps) liberally.
- Evaluate skin integrity, including abrasions and lacerations, and localization and extent of any bruising, swelling, or bony deformity.
- Patients with skin injuries require evaluation in as bloodless a field as possible.
  - Use of finger tourniquets if active bleeding is present can be helpful to reduce blood flow into the wound.
  - Anesthetic with epinephrine was considered controversial previously, but has not proven to be harmful to distal tissues with adequate circulation and may aid in diagnosis.
- Evaluate throughout range of motion; ruptured tendons are frequently retracted in tissue and evaluation throughout active and passive range of motion is key to diagnosis.

A neurovascular examination is imperative, paying attention to digits distal to any injury. Light touch, pinprick, and 2-point discrimination should be assessed compared with the unaffected digit and/or limb to evaluate for digital nerve injury. If concern exists for digital artery disruption, obtain Doppler pulses. Again, compare with the unaffected digit. Diminished or absent pulses indicate arterial disruption and the need for an orthopedic hand specialist consultation. Assess and document active and passive ranges of motion. Evaluate digits for shortening or loss of knuckle contour.

A determination of angular and rotational deformity is important and can be subtle when the patient is unable to make a full fist and demonstrate parallel digital alignment. If angular or rotational deformity is suspected as result of fracture, examine end-on the digital pulps and evaluate the planar alignment of the nails with respect to the adjacent digits and the opposite hand. Palpation of the hand is important to determine points of maximal tenderness.

Assess for pinching strength by asking the patient to hold a piece of paper between the thumb and index finger. A patient with normal strength and function will be able to hold onto the paper without difficulty. However, if the patient compensates by flexing the flexor pollicis longus of the thumb to maintain the grip, leading to flexion of the interphalangeal joint of the thumb, as opposed to the natural extension of this joint, this is known as Froment's sign and indicates an ulnar neuropathy that may be owing to a ligamentous injury or fracture of the first metacarpal (**Fig. 1**).[4]

IMAGING

Plain film imaging remains the standard of care for evaluating injuries to the hand.

- Anteroposterior, true lateral, and oblique views of each potentially affected digit are required.

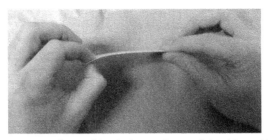

Fig. 1. Froment's sign. Normal use of intrinsic muscles on right side and Froment's sign on left side.

- The lateral view should be obtained so that the other fingers do not obscure the affected digit.
- The oblique view can be particularly helpful in diagnosing fractures of the metacarpal and phalangeal heads.
- Radiographs should be examined for angulation and shortening as well as intra-articular fractures.
- Rotational deformities are usually diagnosed via physical examination rather than radiographic finding.

Once the fracture is reduced and splinted, post-splinting radiographs are taken. There should be no finger rotation and less than 2 mm of displacement or shortening. Bony apposition should approximate 50% or more.[5]

If an intra-articular fracture is suspected but not seen on plain radiograph, computed tomography (CT) can be useful. CT is otherwise rarely necessary in the emergency department (ED).

Ultrasound (US) may also be very helpful to identify fractures. Diagnostic accuracy ranges from 90% to 100% sensitivity and 90% to 98% specificity.[6,7] Preliminary data also show excellent ability to assess accuracy of reduction of finger fractures in the ED.[8]

A small, prospective study evaluated 34 patients with 13 partial or complete tendon ruptures (6 finger injuries, 11 hand injuries, 6 arm injuries, 6 forearm injuries, 5 lower extremity injuries) who had bedside US to evaluate for tendon disruption. US results were compared against findings seen during wound exploration in the ED, in the operating room, or on MRI. Compared with these gold standards, US had a sensitivity of 100%, specificity of 95% (when compared with physical examination, sensitivity was 100% and specificity 76%).[9] A study evaluating accuracy of US to depict tendon, artery, or nerve injuries caused by penetrating wounds of the volar aspect of the hand identified all tendon lesions, and missed 2 arterial lesions, with significantly lower sensitivity for nerve injuries.[10] US may also help to diagnose ligament, nerve, and other soft tissue injuries. Its use for these modalities has been described in the literature, but accuracy not well established. Appropriate imaging should always be ordered after reduction to reassess alignment.

The examination and radiograph findings can be summarized using the NO LOADS mnemonic. Leading with the patient's handedness, the injury can be described as:

- N—Neurovascular intact or deficit.
- O—Open or closed.
- L—Location (fractured bone and location of fracture within that bone).
- O—Orientation of the fractured piece.

- A—Angulation (where is the apex of the triangle formed by the fracture [dorsal, volar, or lateral] and any rotational deformity?).
- D—Displacement (in mm).
- S—Shortening (in mm).

GENERAL TREATMENT

Most hand fractures are well-managed without surgery. However, prolonged immobilization has its risks, including stiffness, pressure sores, and compartment syndrome. Surgery is indicated when early mobilization of soft tissues is critical, when the fracture is otherwise nonreducible, in the presence of an open fracture (other than distal tuft), and in the face of concomitant injury to nerves, vessels, and soft tissue.

Splints should selectively limit motion of injured parts. Fiberglass and other materials may be appropriate for soft tissue injuries and stable fractures, but plaster casting is preferred for unstable fractures. For most fractures, splinting in position of function is optimal.

- The wrist should be in splinted in 0° to 30° of extension (dorsiflexion).[11]
- The MCP joint should be placed in 70° to 90° of flexion.
- The PIP joints should be between 45° to 60°.
- The thumb should be abducted and in opposition and alignment with the pads of the fingers.
- Have the patient hold a large gauze roll during splinting to help ensure functional position.

For some fractures or extensor tendon injuries, the intrinsic plus position is recommended. The position is similar to the provided description, except that the PIP and DIP are splinted in 0° of angulation. Intrinsic plus positions the digits to promote optimal range of motion upon return to mobilization.

FRACTURES
Metacarpals

- Metacarpal fractures comprise approximately 30% of all hand fractures.[12]
- The majority (70%) occur within the second and third decades of life.[13]
- Accidental falls or direct blows to another object or individual, account for most metacarpal fractures, with small finger neck fractures and ring finger shaft fractures among the most common metacarpal fractures.[14]

Thumb metacarpal

The extensive mobility of the thumb provides up to 40% of hand function. The position of the thumb, permitting opposition and prehension, accounts for the dexterity of the human hand, but exposes the thumb to unique injury.

Fractures of the thumb metacarpal are unique and warrant discussion, because of both the digit's importance and the compensatory motion of the adjacent joints. Malrotation and angular deformity are rarely a functional problem owing to the motion of the CMC joint. The strong supporting ligaments allow for the increased mobility of the thumb, but often result in avulsion fractures and injury at either the MCP joint or the CMC joint.[15]

Bennett fracture

- An intra-articular fracture of the thumb metacarpal base that extends into the CMC joint.

- The most common fracture of the thumb metacarpal.
- A single fracture fragment is positioned volar and ulnar to the rest of the meta-carpal base.
- Treatment is typically surgical because of high risk for posttraumatic arthritis.[5]
- Thumb spica splint should be placed while awaiting surgical repair.

Rolando fracture

- Refers to any comminuted intra-articular thumb metacarpal base fracture.
- It is also treated surgically for the best outcomes[5]
- Thumb spica splint should be placed while awaiting surgical repair.

Extra-articular fractures of the thumb metacarpal

- Often managed nonoperatively.
- Up to 30° of lateral angulation is acceptable.[5]

Metacarpal head fractures (of all 5 digits)

- Metacarpal head fractures are rare but challenging to treat, and carry a risk of osteonecrosis.
- For fractures that involve less than 20% of the joint surface, nonoperative management can be undertaken with immobilization in the intrinsic plus position.[13]

Metacarpal neck fractures

- Metacarpal neck fractures are most commonly seen in the small finger and are often referred to as "boxer's fractures," given their typical mechanism of injury.
- Fracture of the volar cortex results in an apex–dorsal angulation fracture pattern with flexion of the metacarpal head.
- The intrinsic muscles of the hand cross the MCP joint and maintain flexion of the metacarpal head, and a pseudoclaw deformity may develop from the imbalance of the extrinsic and intrinsic musculature caused by metacarpal shortening and angulation.
  - When the patient attempts to extend the fingers, the PIP joint flexes and the MCP joint hyperextends, resulting in the claw-like appearance.

Angulation should generally be less than 10°; however, progressively increased angulation is allowed in metacarpal shaft fractures; 10° of angulation is allowable in the index and middle metacarpals, 20° to 30° in the ring, and 30° to 40° in the small metacarpal.[5]

- Once reduced these should be splinted in the intrinsic plus position.

Metacarpal shaft fractures

Metacarpal shaft fractures result from axial loading, torsion, or a direct blow and present as transverse fractures, oblique fractures, or comminuted fractures.

- Injuries that are nondisplaced or minimally displaced, without significant angulation, rotational deformity, or shortening, can be managed conservatively with immobilization.
- Displaced transverse metacarpal shaft fractures are frequently unstable and require operative fixation[5]
- As with MC neck fractures, angulation is better tolerated among the ulnar digits than in the index or middle finger. However, the presence of rotational deformity,

significant metacarpal shortening, and prominent dorsal deformity may require operative intervention.

Metacarpal base fractures

- Intra-articular base fractures of the index through ring fingers metacarpals are uncommon injuries. These fractures are usually a result of a fall on a flexed wrist with the arm in extension and axial loading of the metacarpal.
- Because they are rare in nature, their management is somewhat controversial. Although some have endorsed conservative management, an orthopedic surgeon should be consulted, because there is a growing trend toward operative intervention.[5]

Complications of Metacarpal Fractures

- Healing of metacarpal fractures can be complicated by malunion and nonunion.
- Malunion can occur in the transverse plane with dorsal angulation as the result. Nonunion is a rare complication of metacarpal fractures. This usually can be traced to infection, poor immobilization, or lack of proper reduction of the fracture fragments.[15]

Phalangeal Fractures

Distal phalanx fractures are more common than fractures of the middle or proximal phalanx and are more likely to be isolated injuries.

Distal phalanx

The most common type of distal phalanx fracture is the tuft fracture, a fracture of the fingertip, often with significant associated soft tissue injury. Because the mechanism is often a crush injury, there is frequently associated injury to the nearby tissues, namely the fingernail and nail bed.

- If the fracture is complicated by a subungual hematoma but the nail is intact, the nail should be left in place and the hematoma should be drained if it covers greater than 50% of the nail bed.
- If the nail is damaged it should be removed, and the nail bed repaired, taking care to avoid the matrix. The nail or a protective covering should then be placed, covering the nail bed and anchored between the cuticle and the matrix.
- Once the soft tissue injury has been adequately treated, these can be splinted by use of a single finger splint, or buddy taped, in position of function.

Middle phalanx

Middle phalangeal fractures angulate dorsally with fractures proximal to the flexor digitorum superficialis (FDS) insertion and volarly with fractures distal to the FDS insertion.

- Middle (and proximal) phalanx fractures are classified as intra-articular or extra-articular.
- Intra-articular fractures should be referred to a hand specialist.

Proximal phalanx

- Proximal phalangeal fractures typically produce a volar apex angulation because of tension on the central slip distally and the lumbrical proximally.
- Angulation of more than 25° in adults produces loss of flexion and extension.[16]

Nonunion of phalangeal fractures can occur and is associated with soft tissue injuries, smoking, and infection. Phalanx fractures typically heal within 4 weeks. When tenderness disappears, therapy can be advanced to range of motion exercises.[16] Some studies have evaluated early range of motion with positive results.[17] Proximal phalanx fractures, when shortened or angulated, can lead to laxity by disrupting the extensor and flexor tendon balance.[16]

Refer to a hand specialist if greater than 30% of the volar intra-articular surface is involved, or if the PIP joint demonstrates subluxation or instability.[18]

- Middle and proximal phalanx fractures should be splinted in a position of function.

DISLOCATIONS

Dislocations occur at the MCP, PIP, or DIP joints. Dislocations may occur in the dorsal, volar, or lateral planes, and are described in relation of the more distal bone as compared with the more proximal bone.

- Dislocations are most common at the PIP joint because the greater range of motion of this joint makes it more vulnerable to injury. Of the PIP dislocations, most are dorsal. Volar dislocations of the PIP joint are much less common, more difficult to reduce, and associated with more complications.
- Before reduction, obtain a radiograph to evaluate for fracture. Attempt to reduce a dorsal PIP dislocation by applying traction and volar pressure on the middle phalanx at the PIP joint. Reduction of the PIP can often be performed without anesthesia. However, an intra-articular block or digital block may facilitate reduction.
- Splint reduced dorsal dislocations in position of function.
- Splint reduced volar dislocations in full extension.
- DIP joint dislocations are also uncommon, almost always dorsal, and often associated with fractures and tissue injury.
- In addition to PIP and DIP joint dislocations, MCP and CMC joint dislocations occur occasionally.
- The MCP joint of the 4 fingers usually dislocates dorsally.
- CMC joint dislocation is a disabling injury, which is usually dorsal and may be associated with fractures of the bases of the metacarpals.[5]

LIGAMENT INJURIES

The most clinically important ligament injury in the hand is the ulnar collateral ligament (UCL) of the thumb MCP joint. This is frequently an acute injury owing to forced radial distraction of the thumb and is known as skier's thumb. Although the name is often misapplied to an acute injury, gamekeeper's thumb more accurately refers to chronic laxity of the MCP joint owing to injury of this ligament.

- Evaluate for ligamentous damage by applying pressure at the radial aspect of the MCP and attempting to distract the thumb radially, while the thumb is held in extension and again in 30° of flexion at the MCP (**Fig. 2**).
  - While 30° of laxity of the affected MCP, or a 15° difference between affected and unaffected MCP joints has been cited as cutoff for complete UCL tear, some experts feel that lack of a firm endpoint on MCP joint testing may be the most reliable clinical indicator of a complete UCL tear.[19]
- Treatment of suspected or confirmed ulnar collateral ligament injuries:
  - Partial or suspected tears (less than 30° of laxity when applying valgus stress in either extension or 30° of flexion at the MCP) are treated nonoperatively by immobilization of the MCP joint in a thumb spica splint.

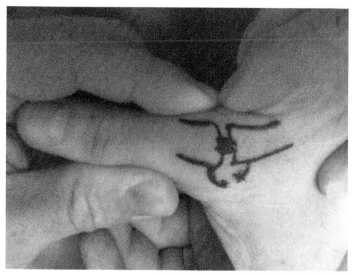

Fig. 2. Ulnar collateral ligament testing.

○ Complete tears, and those associated with a displaced avulsion fragment, are treated with operative management. These patients should be splinted and orthopedic follow-up arranged for operative assessment.

Thumb radial collateral ligament injuries account for a significant minority (up to 42%) of collateral ligament injuries at the MCP joint. These may be associated with avulsion fractures of the thumb as well, and may lead to chronic instability. However, there is no clear difference in outcome between primary repair of radial collateral ligament tears as opposed to cast immobilization and conservative treatment.[20]

TENDON INJURIES

This section describes the diagnosis and treatment of common tendon injuries in the hand.

Extensor Tendon Injuries

Mallet finger is a common fingertip injury owing to disruption of the extensor mechanism at its terminal insertion that results in inability to actively extend the DIP. This injury is usually caused by forced flexion of an extended fingertip. The result may be an isolated soft tissue injury or may include a bony avulsion of the dorsal base of the distal phalanx. Subluxation can occur when more than 50% of the articular surface is affected. When untreated, this injury can lead to osteoarthritis at the DIP and, potentially, a swan neck deformity (**Figs. 3** and **4**).[21]

- Mallet fingers without associated fracture are treated conservatively with splinting in extension or slight hyperextension.
- Surgical referral is recommended when an associated fracture includes more than one-third of the articular surface or when palmar subluxation is present on examination.[21]

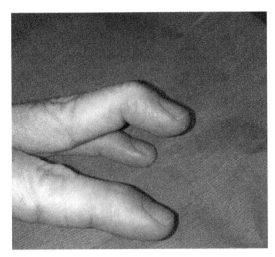

Fig. 3. Mallet finger.

Boutonniere Deformity

Traumatic injury of the extensor digitorum central slip results from forced flexion of the PIP joint, palmar dislocation of the middle phalanx, or a direct blow to the dorsum of the hand. Untreated, this leads to development of the boutonniere deformity over time (**Fig. 5**). The lateral bands of the tendon displace palmar to the PIP joint axis, resulting in tension placed on the terminal tendon at the DIP joint. This leads to DIP extension.[22,23] Early identification and management of the injury can avoid this complication. The patient may have swelling about the PIP joint, ecchymosis, and tenderness. If this diagnosis is suspected, splinting in extension should be performed.

Flexor Tendon Injuries

Jersey finger refers to an injury classically caused by an athlete grabbing for the jersey of another with the DIP in flexion. This mechanism causes forced hyperextension of the DIP joint while it is actively flexed. This results in avulsion of the flexor digitorum profundus tendon at the base of the distal phalanx.[22] The patient presents with pain on the palmar surface of the distal phalanx and weakened or absent flexion at the DIP joint, but preserved flexion at the PIP and MCP joints. Early surgical referral is recommended because any delay in treatment leads to retraction of the torn tendon.[22]

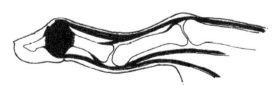

Fig. 4. Swan-neck deformity.

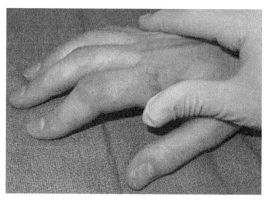

Fig. 5. Boutonniere deformity.

SUMMARY

Injuries to the hand account for a significant percentage of all injuries that present to the ED. The identification of injuries takes time and care, because small injuries can manifest significant changes in functional abilities. A knowledge and understanding of injury patterns and treatment principles is vital to providing excellent care for patients with these injuries.

REFERENCES

1. Meals C, Meals R. Hand fractures: a review of current treatment strategies. J Hand Surg 2013;38(5):1021–31 [quiz: 1031].
2. Wood AM, Robertson GA, Rennie L, et al. The epidemiology of sports-related fractures in adolescents. Injury 2010;41(8):834–8.
3. Chauhan A, Jacobs B, Andoga A, et al. Extensor tendon injuries in athletes. Sports Med Arthrosc 2014;22:45–55.
4. Richardson C, Fabre G. Froment's sign. J Audiov Media Med 2003;26(1):34.
5. Diaz-Garcia R, Waljee JF. Current management of metacarpal fractures. Hand Clin 2013;29(4):507–18.
6. Tayal VS, Antoniazzi J, Pariyadath M, et al. Prospective use of ultrasound imaging to detect bony hand injuries in adults. J Ultrasound Med 2007;26:1143–8.
7. Heiner JD, Baker BL, McArthur TJ. Ultrasound detection of simulated long bone fractures by U.S. Army Special Forces Medics. J Spec Oper Med 2010;10(2): 7–10.
8. McManus JG, Morton MJ, Crystal CS, et al. Use of ultrasound to assess acute fracture reduction in emergency care settings. Am J Disaster Med 2008;3(4): 241–7.
9. Wu TS, Roque PJ, Green J, et al. Bedside ultrasound evaluation of tendon injuries. Am J Emerg Med 2012;30(8):1617–21.
10. Soubeyrand M, Biau D, Jomaah N, et al. Penetrating volar injuries of the hand diagnostic accuracy of US in depicting soft-tissue lesions. Radiology 2008; 249(1):228–35.
11. Gillen G, Goldberg R, Muller S, et al. The effect of wrist position on upper extremity function while wearing a wrist immobilizing splint. J Prosthet Orthot 2008;20(1): 19–23.

12. Chung KC, Spilson SV. The frequency and epidemiology of hand and forearm fractures in the United States. J Hand Surg 2001;26(5):908–15.
13. Stanton JS, Dias JJ, Burke FD. Fractures of the tubular bones of the hand. J Hand Surg Eur Vol 2007;32(6):626–36.
14. Soong M, Got C, Katarincic J. Ring and little finger metacarpal fractures: mechanisms, locations, and radiographic parameters. J Hand Surg 2010;35(8): 1256–9.
15. McNemar TB, Howell JW. Management of metacarpal fractures. J Hand Ther 2003;16:143–51.
16. Markiewitz AD. Complications of hand fractures and their prevention. Hand Clin 2013;29(4):601–20.
17. Figl M, Weninger P, Hofbauer M, et al. Results of dynamic treatment of fractures of the proximal phalanx of the hand. J Trauma 2011;70(4):852–6.
18. Calfee RP, Sommerkamp TG. Fracture-dislocation about the finger joints. J Hand Surg 2009;34(6):1140–7.
19. Ritting AW, Baldwin PC, Rodner CM. Ulnar collateral ligament injury of thumb metacarpophalangeal joint. Clin J Sport Med 2010;20:106–12.
20. Kottstorfer J, Hofbauer M, Krusche-Mandl I, et al. Avulsion fracture and complete rupture of the thumb radial collateral ligament. Arch Orthop Trauma Surg 2013; 133(4):583–8.
21. Bloom JM, Khouri JS, Hammert WC. Current concepts in the evaluation and treatment of mallet finger injury. Plast Reconstr Surg 2013;132(4):560e–6e.
22. Scalcione LR, Pathria MN, Chung CB. The athlete's hand: ligament and tendon injury. Semin Musculoskelet Radiol 2012;16(4):338–49.
23. Schoffl V, Heid A, Kupper T. Tendon injuries of the hand. World J Orthop 2012; 3(6):62–9.

Evaluation and Treatment of the Elbow and Forearm Injuries in the Emergency Department

Katja Goldflam, MD

KEYWORDS

- Trauma • Elbow injury • Forearm injury ulnar and radius fracture • Dislocated elbow

KEY POINTS

- Neurologic and vascular status should be assessed in any patient with elbow and/or forearm injuries.
- Significantly displaced fractures and dislocations of the elbow and forearm may require urgent operative intervention and urgent consultation is warranted.
- Early range of motion in nondisplaced fractures may decrease stiffness of the joint and concurrent morbidity.
- Elbow dislocations should be reduced expeditiously and this is within the purview of the emergency physician.

BACKGROUND

Injuries to the elbow and forearm result most commonly from either a direct blow to the area or from a fall on outstretched hand (FOOSH). The elbow may be injured if it is locked at the time of impact. Elbow or forearm bone dislocations may occur alone or in conjunction with fractures and generally require reduction to minimize future morbidity. The primary goal of management is to achieve anatomic reduction of any fracture or dislocation, while allowing for early range of motion (ROM) to minimize future morbidity, including in particular elbow stiffness.[1] Generally, earlier intervention is preferred to minimize complications and surgery is usually performed within 24 hours of initial injury whenever possible.[2–4]

Disclosures: None.
Department of Emergency Medicine, Yale School of Medicine, 464 Congress Avenue, New Haven, CT 06511, USA
E-mail address: katja.goldflam@yale.edu

Emerg Med Clin N Am 33 (2015) 409–421
http://dx.doi.org/10.1016/j.emc.2014.12.010
0733-8627/15/$ – see front matter © 2015 Elsevier Inc. All rights reserved.

EPIDEMIOLOGY

Elbow fractures are more common in elderly females and younger males; however, each fracture pattern had as a unique epidemiology, often depending on the mechanism of injury. Fractures involving the elbow account for about 5% of all fractures with distal humerus fractures specifically make up about 2% of all fractures.[5,6] Of forearm fractures, radial head fractures make up about 20% to 56%,[7–9] whereas olecranon and radial neck fractures make up about 10 to 20% of forearm fractures each.[10] Combined radius and ulna fractures make up the remaining 4% of forearm fractures.[5,11] Sports injuries and fall from standing are the most common etiologies of injury, with penetrating trauma being exceedingly rare. For this reason, the vast majority of injuries are closed injuries.[5]

Elbow dislocations are second only to shoulder dislocations in the adult population and are the most common dislocation in the pediatric population.[12,13] The incidence of elbow dislocations is thought to be about 6 to 8 per 100,000 people annually.[14–16] Of these, 10% to 50% are thought to be sports related.[17]

ELBOW AND FOREARM ANATOMY

The elbow is a complex joint with 3-dimensional mobility. For this reason, any limitation in its function significantly restricts ROM and even minimal impairment or posttraumatic stiffness of the joint may impact day-to-day utility.

Elbow

The elbow consists of 3 joints at the intersection of 3 bones—the humerus, the radius, and the ulna (**Fig. 1**). The joints include the ulnohumeral and radiocapitellar joint, both ginglymus or hinge joints, and the proximal radioulnar joint (PRUJ), a trochoid or pivot joint. The medial trochlea articulates with the greater sigmoid notch of the proximal ulna, and the capitellum articulates with the radial head.

- The elbow complex is stabilized by the bones themselves and the adjacent capsules and ligaments.
- The ulnohumeral joint provides a greater proportion of static elbow stability than the radiocapitellar joint and thus disruption of this hinge is generally a more devastating injury.[12,18,19] It is also involved primarily in flexion and extension, whereas the radiocapitellar and radioulnar joints guide pronation and supination of the forearm.
- The static ligamentous stabilizers of the joint include the medial collateral ligament complex, the lateral collateral ligament complex, and the anterior capsule.
- Dynamic stabilization is provided by the muscles that cross the elbow joint. These are the elbow flexors (biceps, brachialis, and brachioradialis) and extensors (triceps), as well as the forearm extensors and forearm flexor–pronators.[12,20,21]

Forearm

The radius and ulna are connected at the proximal and distal radioulnar joints (DRUJs), as well as longitudinally through the interosseous membrane (IOM) between them. The PRUJ is maintained by the annular, oblique, and quadrate ligaments, whereas the DRUJ is supported by the triangular fibrocartilage complex. During pronation and supination, the ulna remains relatively immobile, and the radius rotates the wrist relative to the forearm. The IOM provides stability to their alignment. The anatomic bow of

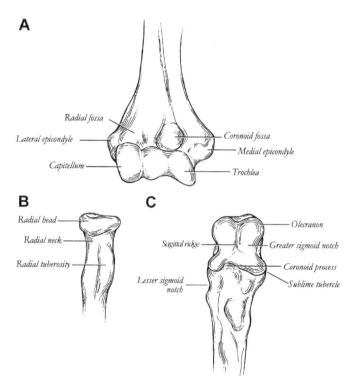

Fig. 1. Elbow anatomy. (*A*) Humerus, (*B*) Radius, (*C*) Ulna. (*From* Armstrong AD, King GJ, Yamaguchi K. Total elbow arthroplasty design. In: Williams GR, Yamaguchi K, Ramsey ML, et al., editors. Shoulder and elbow arthroplasty. Philadelphia: Lippincott Williams & Wilkins, 2005. p. 301; with permission.)

the radius provides the arc of motion of the radius around the ulna. Maintaining this shape is critical to preserving functionality of the forearm.

IMAGING

Initial imaging of the elbow and forearm generally includes plain radiographs to assess for fractures, dislocations, and bony malalignment. As in the evaluation of most joints and long bones, at least 2 orthogonal views of the relevant anatomy should be obtained. The standards views for the elbow are the anteroposterior view, the lateral view, and the oblique view.

Anteroposterior View

The elbow is held extended and imaging is obtained head on.

Lateral View

The elbow is held in 90° of flexion. Two lines can be drawn on the radiograph to check for radiocapitellar alignment. The first runs along the anterior cortex of the distal humerus and should intersect the capitellum in its middle third.[22] The second line is drawn along the longitudinal axis of the proximal radial neck and bisects the capitellum (**Fig. 2**). Although these concepts have been described for use in pediatric radiography, they are applied frequently to adult films as well.

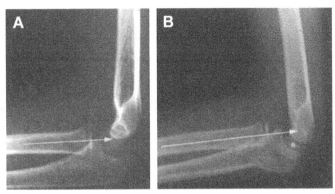

Fig. 2. Radiocapitellar alignment. The line (*arrow*) is drawn along the longitudinal axis of the radius. (*A*) In normal alignment the line should intersect the capitellum at any degree of flexion. (*B*) Abnormal radiocapitellar aligment. The radiocapitellar line should intersect the capitellum (*asterisk*). (*From* Perron AD, Hersh RE, Brady WJ, et al. Orthopedic pitfalls in the ED: Galeazzi and Monteggia fracture-dislocation. Am J Emerg Med 2001;19(3):225–8; with permission.)

Oblique View

Also called the radial head view, this provides improved imaging of the radial head, coronoid process, and capitellum, allowing visualization of more subtle, often nondisplaced fractures. The x-ray beam is angled at 45° to the radial head to minimize overlap of other osseous structures.[23]

Nondisplaced or minimally displaced fractures are often difficult to identify on plain radiographs. Subtle signs suggestive of injury, including anterior or posterior fat pads seen on the lateral view, may be the only findings. These findings result from displacement of the fat pads by a joint effusion or hemarthrosis. The anterior fat pad sign, or "spinnaker sail sign," consists of a convex contour along the anterior humerus. The posterior fat pad is not normally seen, unless an effusion pushes it outward and posterior to the humerus. When the joint capsule is disrupted these radiographic findings may disappear, because the effusion is no longer contained within in the joint space.[24,25]

CT has greater utility in the preoperative planning of patient care, rather than the acute setting. Similarly, MRI may be beneficial in more detailed evaluation of ligamentous and other soft tissue injuries.

In patients with forearm injuries where there is concern for DRUJ or PRUJ instability, wrist and elbow films should be obtained in addition to forearm films.

Forearm

Imaging includes an anteroposterior view and a lateral view to evaluate the radius and ulna. Additionally, patients should generally undergo imaging of the joint above and below the injury. Radiographs of the elbow and wrist are used to exclude alignment of the elbow joint and DRUJ, respectively.

SIMPLE ELBOW DISLOCATIONS

Simple dislocations do not have fractures associated with them (**Fig. 3**). Posterolateral dislocations are the most common injuries, making up at least 90% of dislocations.[17]

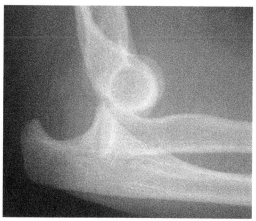

Fig. 3. Elbow dislocation. (*From* Lowden C, Garvin G, King GJ. Imaging of the elbow following trauma. Hand Clin 2004;20(4):353–61; with permission.)

These generally occur from a FOOSH or sports-related injuries.[15,20,26–28] Anterior dislocations are much less common and occur usually in combination with fractures. They result primarily from a blow to the posterior forearm when it is held in a partially flexed position. As the ulna is pushed out of its articulation with the trochlea, the lateral collateral ligament and anterior capsule are disrupted by the force. This leads to ligamentous instability and laxity of the joint.

Evaluation

Neurovascular status must be ascertained before any manipulation of the dislocated elbow, because the brachial artery and ulnar and median nerves may be entrapped. Serial examinations may be beneficial in patients where compartment syndrome may be a consideration. Anteroposterior view and lateral view radiographs should be obtained to evaluate the joint for any fractures associated with a suspected dislocation. Elbow instability is graded in stages as described by O'Driscoll[29]:

1. Posterolateral rotatory subluxation, which reduces spontaneously;
2. Perched, an incomplete posterolateral dislocation; and
3. Dislocated, with tearing of the capsule and ligamentous stabilizers.

Treatment

Simple dislocations can usually be treated nonoperatively with closed reduction.

- Perched dislocations may be reduced using only intra-articular anesthesia. The elbow is held supine in partial extension, and axial distraction with direct gentle pressure over the olecranon is applied.
- Complete dislocations generally require conscious sedation to optimize relaxation of the associated muscle spasm. Anterior pressure is placed on the olecranon as gentle longitudinal traction on the supine forearm is performed and the elbow is slowly brought into flexion. Countertraction on the upper arm facilitates the maneuver. Initial hyperextension of the joint may risk medial nerve entrapment and should be avoided.[30] Placing a patient in the prone position during reduction has also been successful.[13,28]

- After relocation of the joint, it should be ranged through its complete arc to ensure stability; an intact neurovascular status should be reconfirmed and post-reduction radiographs should be obtained to confirm bony alignment.
- Open reduction is usually unnecessary; however, it may be required if several attempts at closed reduction fail, are contraindicated, or if significant instability remains.
- Simple dislocations without postreduction instability should be immobilized in a posterior splint in just under 90° flexion. Full ROM should be resumed after a maximum of 5 to 7 days. Patients should be referred for orthopedic follow-up, especially if any remaining joint instability is noted after reduction. If joint instability is noted after reduction, supervised rehabilitation is indicated, rather than free unrestricted motion.

ELBOW FRACTURES

As a general rule, a complete neurovascular examination should be performed in every patient.

Distal Humerus Fracture

Distal humerus fractures can be supracondylar, as are commonly found in children, or transcondylar, as occur more frequently in the elderly population. The Orthopedic Trauma Association categorizes these fractures into 3 types[31]:

- Type A: extra-articular (supracondylar) fractures;
- Type B: fractures with partial articular involvement (transcondylar, single column); and
- Type C: complete disruption of the articular surface (transcondylar, both columns).

Extra-articular fractures with no or minimal displacement may be managed conservatively, including splinting and early ROM. Generally, however, the literature favors operative fixation for the majority of distal humerus fractures, especially when the articular surface is involved. Outcomes after fixation are positive generally, although ulnar nerve dysfunction and loss of ROM were noted in about 11% of patients in 1 cohort.[32,33] Orthopedic consultation should be initiated for type B and C fracture patterns, any open fractures, evidence of compartment syndrome, or any concern for neurovascular compromise. Capitellar fractures are managed similarly, with displaced fractures requiring orthopedic referral and likely operative intervention.

Olecranon Fracture

Fractures of the proximal tip of the ulna may occur via a fall or direct blow to the olecranon or from an avulsion by the triceps tendon that inserts on the posterior one-third of the olecranon process. Excluding avulsion fractures, olecranon fractures are generally intra-articular, and as such alignment of the original contour of the articular surface is critical in maintaining joint integrity. The Mayo classification system takes this into account by focusing on displacement, comminution and stability of the fracture[34]:

- Mayo type I: undisplaced (<2 mm) fractures, with or without comminution;
- Mayo type II: stable, displaced (>3 mm) fractures with or without comminution; and
- Mayo type III: unstable, displaced fractures with dislocation, with or without comminution.

Mayo type I nondisplaced fractures can be treated nonoperatively, whereas type II and III fractures all require fixation. Nonoperative care involves a long arm cast for immobilization in 90°flexion for up to a month, followed by protected ROM.[35,36]

Radial Head Fractures

Radial head fractures occur most commonly from axial loading of the radius during FOOSH injuries, when the elbow is held in pronation and slightly flexed, and are the most common elbow fracture. Radial head fractures may also have concomitant ligamentous or bony injuries, such as olecranon or coronoid fractures, in up to 30% of cases.[37,38] Patients present with pain and swelling over the lateral elbow. Tenderness over the radial head and pain or crepitus with ranging of the elbow through pronation and supination is suggestive of injury. The forearm and wrist should also be examined to evaluate for associated injuries, including the medial collateral ligament and the IOM. The elbow joint should be ranged through its entire arc, including flexion–extension and pronation–supination. Motion may be blocked owing to pain from a hemarthrosis. The joint should be aspirated to reduce pressure within the joint capsule and local anesthetic should be injected. Any motion block persisting after this is suggestive of a fracture fragment within the joint and requires surgical referral.[39] Orthopedics should also be consulted for any open fracture, fracture–dislocations, or when there is concern for neurovascular compromise.

Mason[8] provided the original classification scheme for radial head fractures, which was modified by Hotchkiss[40] to provide a more management-based categorization.

- Type 1: nondisplaced or minimally displaced fractures without mechanical block to motion;
- Type 2: fractures displaced greater than 2 mm;
- Type 3: comminuted fractures; and
- Type 4: fractures with associated elbow dislocation.

The goal of treatment in each case is to provide stabilization of the fracture fragments and promote early ROM of the elbow.[41] Mason type 1 fractures with normal ROM may be splinted for comfort or placed in a sling for 24 to 48 hours.[42,43] After this, active ROM exercises should be started as tolerated by the patient. Most Mason type 2 and 3 fractures, any open fractures, and any fractures with mechanical block from bony fragments in the joint space require operative fixation.[36,39] Decision as to the surgical technique used depends on a variety of factors, including number of bony fragments, amount of displacement, impaction, and quality of the bone involved.[38,39] In the acute setting, they can be splinted or placed in a sling with urgent orthopedic follow-up. Mason type 4 fractures should be reduced as soon as possible and intact neurovascular status confirmed after manipulation.

Coronoid Process Fractures

The ulnar coronoid process provides critical stability to the elbow as part of the ulnohumeral joint. Additionally, it serves as the attachment site for the medial collateral ligament and a portion of the anterior capsule. Large fractures, therefore, result in significant instability and require operative fixation. These fractures occur most frequently in association with other injuries, such as elbow dislocations, and a coronoid fracture should suggest the need to look for other signs of injury to the joint.[44] They are a result of shear forces of the distal humerus on the coronoid process.[45] The Regan and Morrey classification system describes fractures in 3 categories[46]:

- Type I: fracture of the tip of the coronoid process;
- Type II: fracture involving 50% or less or the coronoid process; and
- Type III: fracture involving more than 50% of the coronoid process.

Higher grade fractures were associated with poorer outcomes. Type I fractures in isolation may be considered for nonoperative treatment; short immobilization is followed by early active ROM. Type II or III fractures or type I fractures with joint instability should be managed operatively and require orthopedic referral in the acute setting.

The Terrible Triad

The triple threat of a radial head fracture, coronoid process fracture, and elbow dislocation has been named the "terrible triad" because it is difficult to treat and has generally poor outcomes, including significant stiffness of the elbow joint and persistent, long-term instability.[18,47,48] Injuries may result from high-energy impacts, such as falls from height and vehicular accidents, or from lower energy falls from standing. The elbow dislocation may reduce spontaneously in some cases, leaving only secondary signs of the episode of joint instability. On plain radiographs, the oblique view provides visualization of the radial head and coronoid process. The anteroposterior view may demonstrate an avulsion fracture of the lateral epicondyle, suggesting lateral ulnar collateral ligament injury.

If the dislocation has not reduced spontaneously, closed reduction must be performed expeditiously. Postreduction films should be obtained. If radial head and coronoid fractures are known to be present, no further ROM testing should be performed, because this may exacerbate the injury.[18] A posterior splint is used to hold the elbow in approximately 90° of flexion, with the forearm in neutral position. Rarely, fracture fragments within the joint may prevent successful reduction. Open reduction may then be indicated.[18] After splinting, the patient should be referred for expeditious follow-up with an orthopedic specialist for definitive management by operative fixation.

FOREARM FRACTURES
Diaphyseal Radius and Ulna Fractures

Diaphyseal radius and ulna fractures can occur as isolated or combined "both bone" fractures and frequently lead to functional defects if appropriate alignment and interosseous spacing are not maintained. Isolated midshaft ulnar fractures, also known as nightstick fractures, may occur from direct trauma of an arm raised to protect from an overhead blow.[49] Open fractures are common, whereas neurovascular injuries are more rare. Pain with passive extension of fingers on examination should raise the concern for compartment syndrome and a complete neurovascular examination should be performed.

Isolated single bone fractures with minimal displacement and angulation and no evidence of instability at the PRUJ or DRUJ can generally be immobilized in a long arm cast for 4 to 6 weeks.[50] Using finger traps may help in reducing significantly displaced fractures. The forearm should be held in neutral position with the elbow in 90° of flexion. These fractures are frequently unstable during casting and good alignment should be confirmed on postreduction radiographs.

Fractures that are unstable, displaced by more than 50%, or angulated more than 10°, or those involving the proximal one-third of the ulna, should undergo operative fixation. For the radius in particular, maintenance of the anatomic bow is critical for functionality after healing.

Both bone fractures are an indication for operative fixation, because high rates of nonunion, malunion or cross-union occur in injuries managed with closed reduction.[49]

Monteggia Lesions

This eponym denotes a fracture of the proximal one-third of the ulna associated with a dislocation of the radial head at the radiocapitellar joint and the PRUJ, through a disruption of the annular and quadrate ligaments (**Fig. 4**).[51–53] Most commonly, patients have a FOOSH while the forearm is held in the pronated position. There is limited ROM of the elbow with pain and swelling at the joint. Owing to the proximity of the radial nerve to the radial head, radial nerve injuries may occur in association with the Monteggia injury. This may result in weakness of extension of the fingers, which are innervated by the posterior interosseous branch of the radial nerve.[54,55] Radiographs easily show the ulna fracture. To identify subtle dislocations, a line can be drawn along the axis of the radius, which should intersect the capitellum.[56]

Adults suffer predominantly from posterior radial head dislocations that usually require open reduction. Children are more prone to anterior dislocations that may occasionally be reduced nonoperatively and cast in supination.[51,57] Because the IOM and the triangular fibrocartilage complex remain mostly intact, a reduction of the dislocation reinstates stability and congruity of the joint in the majority of cases.[52] Open or unstable fractures always require operative intervention. In the acute setting, an orthopedist should be consulted if available. Synostosis may occur in poorly managed fractures, significantly limiting rotational ability of the forearm.[36]

Galeazzi Fracture–Dislocations

Galeazzi fracture–dislocations consist of a fracture of the middle to distal third of the radius and a concomitant dislocation of the distal ulna or instability of the DRUJ (**Fig. 5**).[58] The mechanism of injury is not well understood, but is thought to be owing to FOOSH in pronation, similar to the Monteggia injury.[59] Patients have pain at the site of the radius fracture, as well as tenderness at the wrist. Peripheral nerve injuries are relatively rare.[59,60] A high level of suspicion must be maintained for the possible

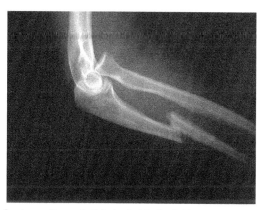

Fig. 4. Monteggia fracture. (*From* Eathiraju S, Mudgal CS, Jupiter JB. Monteggia fracture-dislocations. Hand Clin 2007;23(2):165–77, v; with permission.)

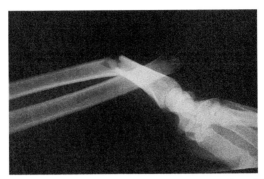

Fig. 5. Galeazzi fracture. (*From* Giannoulis FS, Sotereanos DG. Galeazzi fractures and dislocations. Hand Clin 2007;23(2):153–63, v; with permission.)

dislocation of the DRUJ, because the Galeazzi fracture may seem to be a simple radial fracture on plain radiographic imaging. Comparison films of the opposite wrist may be beneficial to distinguish subtle changes. Anteroposterior films may show a relatively shortened radius (>5 mm) and a widened interspace (>1–2 mm) between the radioulnar articulation at the DRUJ. Lateral films show the dorsally angulated radius fragment with a dorsally angulated ulna. A fractured ulnar styloid may also suggest an avulsion injury.[61,62] Successful treatment relies on recognition of the lesion, because it generally requires operative reduction of the fracture in adults, with realignment of the distal joint anatomy. Rarely, children may be managed conservatively with closed reduction and splinting.[59] Whenever available, an orthopedist should be consulted in the acute setting.

Essex–Lopresti Injuries

An Essex–Lopresti injury complex consists of the combination of a fractured radial head, disruption of the DRUJ, and a torn IOM.[63] Often these injuries go unrecognized, because attention is focused on the obvious radial head fracture, the pain of which frequently overshadows the pain in the more distal forearm. If the Essex–Lopresti lesion is not diagnosed in the acute setting, the radius migrates proximally and the ruptured IOM results in instability of the forearm. The longitudinal compressive force of a high-impact FOOSH is transmitted along the length of the forearm, rupturing the ligamentous components as the radial head fractures. The combination of wrist and elbow pain or the radiographic finding of a comminuted radial head fracture (suggesting a high impact force) should raise the suspicion for this injury. Patients may have ecchymoses along the path of the IOM, as well as tenderness along the distal ulna. In a patient with the correct mechanism and suggestive symptoms the possibility of an Essex–Lopresti injury should be considered, even if radiographs show only a radial head fracture. Ultrasound and/or MRI may be considered as adjunct imaging in this setting.[64,65] Essex–Lopresti injuries should be managed operatively, with the goal being to realign bony anatomy at both the radiocapitellar joint and DRUJ.

REFERENCES

1. Kuntz DG Jr, Baratz ME. Fractures of the elbow. Orthop Clin North Am 1999; 30(1):37–61.
2. Constant CR. Injuries to the elbow. J R Coll Surg Edinb 1990;35(6 Suppl):S31–2.

3. Plancher KD, Lucas TS. Fracture dislocations of the elbow in athletes. Clin Sports Med 2001;20(1):59–76.

4. O'Driscoll SW. Optimizing stability in distal humeral fracture fixation. J Shoulder Elbow Surg 2005;14(1 Suppl S):186S–94S.

5. Court-Brown CM, Caesar BC. Overview of epidemiology of fractures. In: Bucholz RW, Court-Brown CM, Tornetta P, et al, editors. Rockwood and Green's fracture in adults. Philadelphia: Lippincott Williams and Wilkins; 2006. p. 95–113.

6. Asprinio D, Helfet DL. Fractures of the distal humerus. In: Levine AM, editor. Orthopaedic knowledge update: trauma. Rosemont (IL): American Academy of Orthopedic Surgeons; 1996.

7. Harrington IJ, Tountas AA. Replacement of the radial head in the treatment of unstable elbow fractures. Injury 1981;12(5):405–12.

8. Mason ML. Some observations on fracture of the head of the radius with a review of one hundred cases. Br J Surg 1954;42:123–32.

9. Black WS, Becker JA. Common forearm fractures in adults. Am Fam Physician 2009;80(10):1096–102.

10. Rommens PM, Kuchle R, Schneider RU, et al. Olecranon fractures in adults: factors influencing outcome. Injury 2004;35(11):1149–57.

11. Simon RR, Koenigsknecht SJ. Fractures of the distal humerus. In: Medina M, Noujaim S, Holton B, editors. Emergency orthopedics - the extremities. St Louis (MO): McGraw-Hill; 2001. p. 234.

12. Bryce CD, Armstrong AD. Anatomy and biomechanics of the elbow. Orthop Clin North Am 2008;39(2):141–54, v.

13. Kuhn MA, Ross G. Acute elbow dislocations. Orthop Clin North Am 2008;39(2):155–61, v.

14. Conn J, Wade P. Injuries of the elbow: a ten-year review. J Trauma 1961;1:248–68.

15. Josefsson PO, Nilsson BE. Incidence of elbow dislocation. Acta Orthop Scand 1986;57(6):537–8.

16. Josefsson PO, Johnell O, Wendeberg B. Ligamentous injuries in dislocations of the elbow joint. Clin Orthop Relat Res 1987;(221):221–5.

17. Hobgood ER, Khan SO, Field LD. Acute dislocations of the adult elbow. Hand Clin 2008;24(1):1–7.

18. Dodds SD, Fishler T. Terrible triad of the elbow. Orthop Clin North Am 2013;44(1):47–58.

19. Morrey BF. Current concepts in the management of complex elbow trauma. Surgeon 2009;7(3):151–61.

20. Sheps DM, Hildebrand KA, Boorman RS. Simple dislocations of the elbow: evaluation and treatment. Hand Clin 2004;20(4):389–404.

21. Funk DA, An KN, Morrey BF, et al. Electromyographic analysis of muscles across the elbow joint. J Orthop Res 1987;5(4):529–38.

22. Rogers LF, Malave S Jr, White H, et al. Plastic bowing, torus and greenstick supracondylar fractures of the humerus: radiographic clues to obscure fractures of the elbow in children. Radiology 1978;128(1):145–50.

23. Greenspan A, Norman A, Rosen H. Radial head-capitellum view in elbow trauma: clinical application and radiographic-anatomic correlation. AJR Am J Roentgenol 1984;143(2):355–9.

24. Schaeffeler C, Waldt S, Woertler K. Traumatic instability of the elbow - anatomy, pathomechanisms and presentation on imaging. Eur Radiol 2013;23(9):2582–93.

25. Norell HG. Roentgenologic visualization of the extracapsular fat pad; its importance in the diagnosis of traumatic injuries to the elbow. Acta Radiol 1954;42(3):205–10.

Emergency Department Evaluation and Treatment of Pediatric Orthopedic Injuries

Matthew D. Thornton, MD[a], Karen Della-Giustina, MD[b,*], Paul L. Aronson, MD[c]

KEYWORDS

- Pediatric orthopedics • Salter-Harris • Physis • Growth plate • Fracture

KEY POINTS

- The pediatric skeleton is unique compared with adults because of the growth plates, strong periosteum, and dynamic growth state.
- Fractures involving the physis (growth plate) must be evaluated thoroughly to avoid interfering with bone growth.
- Supracondylar fractures are high-risk injuries that may be associated with brachial artery injury and potential ischemia or compartment syndrome of the forearm.
- The child with hip pain requires a thorough evaluation to rule out septic arthritis.
- Always consider nonaccidental trauma as the source of the child's injuries with a focus on those high-risk injuries.

INTRODUCTION: NATURE OF THE PROBLEM

Orthopedic injuries in children are unique because of the dynamic state of growth and development of children. The biochemical and physiologic differences of the child's skeleton from that of the adult lead to distinctly different mechanisms of injury, fracture patterns, healing, and treatment needs that are crucial for the emergency medicine practitioner to understand. Moreover, infants and children of different ages are susceptible to unique fracture patterns. In this country, unintentional injuries are the leading cause of death and disability in children, and up to one-half of all Emergency Department (ED) -related visits are orthopedic in nature.[1] In the ED, providers should know how to diagnose and treat children with orthopedic injuries, with particular attention to the age, growth, and development of the child.

The authors have no financial disclosures.
The authors have no conflicts of interest.
[a] Department of Emergency Medicine, Bay State Medical Center, 759 Chestnut Street, Springfield, MA 01199, USA; [b] Department of Emergency Medicine, Bridgeport Hospital, 267 Grant Street, Bridgeport, CT 06610, USA; [c] Department of Pediatric Emergency Medicine, Yale New Haven Childrens Hospital, 100 York Street, Suite 1F, New Haven, CT 06511, USA
* Corresponding author. 15 Skyview Road, Orange, CT 06477.
E-mail address: karendg@me.com

Emerg Med Clin N Am 33 (2015) 423–449
http://dx.doi.org/10.1016/j.emc.2014.12.012

PEDIATRIC ORTHOPEDIC BASICS

Children's bones have structural properties that allow them to withstand greater force. In addition, fractures in children heal more rapidly than those in adults. The child's remarkable remodeling potential allows for some longitudinal misalignment and greater degrees of angulation. New bone remodels according to local forces, especially in the plane of motion of the joint. If a child has at least 2 years of growth remaining, a fracture adjacent to a hinged joint will remodel acceptably if the angulation is less than 30° in the plane of motion.[2] Precise anatomic reduction is required, however, for fractures with rotational deformities, excessive degrees of angulation, or those that are intra-articular and displaced. The pediatric periosteum is thicker and stronger than mature periosteum, which results in diminished fracture displacement, fewer open fractures, and more stability as well as an osteogenic potential that makes nonunion rare.

The more porous and pliable pediatric bone allows for 4 unique types of fractures seen in children: (1) plastic deformity, (2) torus (buckle) fractures, (3) greenstick fractures, and (4) fractures involving the physis. In plastic deformity, the bone is deformed beyond its ability to recoil, but not to the point at which an actual fracture occurs. The remainder of the fracture types is described later.

PHYSEAL FRACTURES

The most significant difference between the skeleton of a child and an adult is the presence of the physis or growth plate. Composed of cartilage, the physis represents the "weak link" in pediatric bone. The physis will separate or fracture before disruption or "spraining" of an adjacent strong and flexible ligament. Injuries that produce sprained ligaments or even joint dislocations in adults usually result in physeal injuries in children. Physeal injuries, which are most common during times of rapid growth, represent up to 18% of pediatric fractures.[2]

Although physeal injuries generally heal in one-half of the time of long-bone injuries, they are the fractures in which anatomic alignment is most critical for optimal growth and minimal deformity. If the injured child is tender at the physis, the physician should suspect a fracture and not a sprain, even in the presence of normal radiographs.

In 1963, Robert B. Salter and W. Robert Harris[3] classified epiphyseal plate (physis) injuries in terms of clinical treatment and prognosis. Salter-Harris fractures are numbered I through V, with the higher numbers corresponding to an increased risk for growth disturbances.

Salter-Harris Classification

Type I

- This injury involves a fracture through the physis only (**Fig. 1**).
- If the radiographs appear normal, the injury can be a nondisplaced fracture.
- Point physeal tenderness on examination is the most common finding.
- If the patient has point tenderness over the physis, even in the presence of an otherwise normal examination (including radiographs), one should treat this with cast or splint immobilization.
- The prognosis for this fracture is excellent.[3]

Type II

- This injury is a fracture through the physis and metaphysis, with a fragment of the metaphysis remaining attached to the epiphysis.

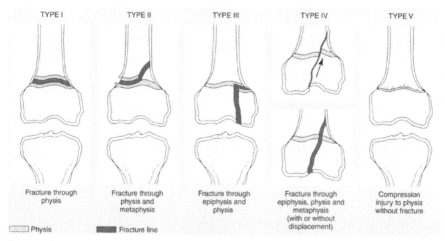

Fig. 1. Salter-Harris classification. *Arrow* pointing to the physis. (*From* Deeney VF, Arnold JA, Moreland MS, et al. Orthopedics. In: Zitelli BJ, McIntire SC, Nowalk AJ, editors. Zitelli and Davis' atlas of pediatric physical diagnosis. 7th edition. Philadelphia: Saunders/Elsevier, 2012; with permission.)

- This triangular metaphyseal fragment is commonly referred to as the Thurston-Holland sign.
- This injury is the most common type of physeal fracture.
- This injury requires treatment with cast or splint immobilization.
- The prognosis for this type fracture is also excellent.[3]

Type III

- This fracture involves a fracture line that begins intra-articularly and travels through the epiphysis into the physis.
- Because this is an intra-articular fracture, precise anatomic reduction is imperative to minimize future joint and growth abnormalities, as well as posttraumatic arthritis.
- With appropriate reduction, the prognosis for this injury is good.[3]

Type IV

- This fracture involves a fracture line that begins intra-articularly and travels through the epiphysis, physis, and the metaphysis.
- Precise anatomic reduction is imperative.
- This fracture commonly requires surgical fixation to maintain the reduction.
- This injury has a significant incidence of growth disturbance.[3]

Type V

- The physis is crushed without any other injury.
- This injury is often difficult to diagnose, because the initial radiographs are usually unremarkable.
- A careful history revealing a mechanism with significant axial load is a key factor to identifying the diagnosis.
- The prognosis is poor, owing to the premature cessation of growth.[3]

TREATING THE ORTHOPEDICALLY INJURED CHILD
History

Obtaining a history from an injured child can be challenging. The often-tense environment may make it difficult to obtain an accurate history from parents and children alike. In addition, the child may be preverbal or unable to localize pain because of age. Finally, pain often limits the completeness of the history taking in the setting of injury. A calm approach in addition to the proper use of analgesia can aid in obtaining the history.

Physical and Diagnostic Evaluation

By keeping in mind a child's fear, pain, and developmental level, a gentle and systematic approach may improve evaluation and treatment. Administering appropriate analgesia will not only reduce the child's pain and anxiety, but also aid in examining the injured area. Before palpating the injured area, one should examine the skin carefully for any breaks. Next, evaluate the neurovascular status of the limb carefully, especially before and after reduction and splinting. Finally, one should examine the injury by first palpating the areas away from the area of complaint rather than going directly to the area of injury.

The injured region should be radiographed using plain radiography in at least 2 different planes. There are some areas, such as the elbow or wrist, where oblique views may also be obtained. The radiographs should include the joint above and below the injury if there is any suspicion for secondary injury.

UPPER EXTREMITY INJURIES
Clavicle

The clavicle is the most frequently fractured bone in the pediatric population.[1,4] Fractures most often occur between the middle and outer thirds of the bone. Because of its subcutaneous location, a fractured clavicle is often simple to detect. Although often fractured at birth, a clavicle fracture in a newborn may be diagnosed in the ED, when the new parents detect the palpable callus of healing after the baby's discharge from the nursery.[5] Older children usually sustain clavicle fractures from short falls onto an extended arm.

The child with a clavicle fracture will have pain with arm and neck movement. Local swelling and crepitus are often present, and one may see displacement of the affected shoulder downward and inward. The examining physician should perform a careful neurovascular examination to detect damage to the underlying vessels and structures. For diagnosing a clavicle fracture, an anteroposterior (AP) radiograph is usually sufficient.

Ordinarily, newborns, who have sustained a clavicle fracture during birth, require no further treatment. However, the parents should be educated about the fracture and the probability of a detectable callus developing over the following weeks. In older children and adolescents with a simple clavicle fracture, immobilization with a sling and swath for 4 to 6 weeks is generally sufficient.[5] Older adolescents with significant displacement or shortening of the clavicle should receive orthopedic follow-up.

Shoulder Dislocations

Glenohumeral shoulder dislocations, which are rare in young children, are more commonly seen in adolescents. In most of these cases, the dislocation is anterior. These dislocations are usually reducible by the emergency physician in the ED and require orthopedic evaluation within 1 week.

Humerus

The proximal humeral epiphysis is responsible for 80% of the longitudinal growth of the humerus.[4] In newborns and preschoolers, the typical injury is a Salter-Harris type I fracture, whereas children who are 11 to15 years old typically sustain Salter-Harris II fractures.

The history is often that of a fall backward onto an extended arm. A midshaft humerus fracture, a severe fracture of the humeral head, or one in which the history is inconsistent with the injury should raise suspicion of abuse, especially in very young children.

The entire shoulder girdle should be radiographed after the neurovascular examination. The physician should pay particular attention to possible axillary nerve damage with resulting abnormal deltoid function and paresthesia or anesthesia over the lateral shoulder.

Most children can be treated with a sling and swath if the angulation is less than 40°, there is less than 50% displacement, and there is no malrotation.[1,4] In children less than 5 years old, up to 70° of angulation and 100% displacement may be acceptable.[6] An orthopedic surgeon should reevaluate the child within 24 to 48 hours.

Supracondylar Fractures

Supracondylar fractures are the most common elbow fracture in pediatric patients. They typically occur between ages 5 and 10 years.[7] The typical history is a fall onto an extended arm, which forces the distal fragment upward and posteriorly. The child will hold the arm in pronation and resist elbow movement because of pain. These fractures require emergent treatment because flow through the brachial artery can be affected at the site of injury.[8]

The physician who suspects a supracondylar fracture should do a careful neurovascular examination, checking for the 5 "Ps" of arterial injury: pain, pallor (poor perfusion), weak radial pulse (to pulselessness), paralysis, and paresthesias.[4] Worsening pain or pain with passive extension of the fingers are also symptoms concerning for ischemia. An orthopedic surgeon must immediately evaluate and reduce a supracondylar fracture with any sign of ischemia. Compartment syndrome of the volar forearm can develop in less than 12 hours, with subsequent necrosis and fibrosis of the involved musculature. This ischemia/infarction can lead to Volkman ischemic contracture.[9] If no orthopedic surgeon is available and there is evidence of arterial injury or ischemia, then the emergency physician must reduce the fracture. The technique for fracture reduction is placement of the forearm in supination, then applying longitudinal traction and direct pressure to the displaced fragment in a downward and anterior direction.[4] Oblique fractures usually require open reduction.

In a child without neurovascular compromise, radiographs of the AP view in extension and a lateral view in 90° of flexion should be obtained. Because the fracture line is often difficult to visualize, one can use the anterior humeral line and pathologic "fat pads" as indirect evidence of subtle fractures. The anterior humeral line is a line that is visualized on the lateral view, being drawn down the anterior margin of the humerus. This line should intersect the capitellum in its posterior two-thirds. If this line intersects the anterior one-third of the anterior capitellum or appears anterior to the capitellum, it is strongly suggestive of a supracondylar fracture with posterior displacement of the distal fragment (**Figs. 2** and **3**).

In addition, one can use the fat pads as nonspecific indicators of elbow joint effusion or hemorrhage of an occult elbow fracture. Both fat pads are visualized on the lateral

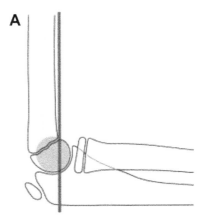

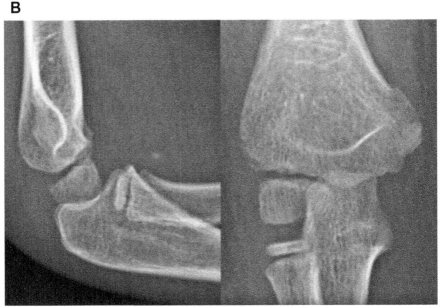

Fig. 2. Anterior humeral line (on lateral). (*A*) Normal alignment: When drawn along the anterior cortex of the humerus, in most normal patients at least one-third of the ossifying capitellum lies anterior to this line. Be careful: in very young children the ossification within the cartilage of the capitellum might be minimal (ie, normal and age related), and so is insufficiently calcified and does not allow application of the above rule. This line helps to detect a supracondylar fracture with posterior displacement. (*B*) The abnormal anterior humeral line suggests a supracondylar fracture. (*From* Raby N, Berman L, Morley S, et al. Paediatric elbow. In: Raby N, Berman L, de Lacey G, editors. Accident and emergency radiology: a survival guide. 3rd edition. Philadelphia: Elsevier, 2015; with permission.)

elbow view. The posterior fat pad is recognized as a radiolucency posterior to the distal humerus adjacent to the olecranon fossa; the presence of a posterior fat pad is always pathologic and indicative of elbow effusion. The anterior fat pad, which can be seen in normal children, is an area of radiolucency located superior to the radial head and anterior to the distal humerus. The anterior fat pad is considered pathologic when it "sails" anteriorly from its normal position (**Fig. 4**).

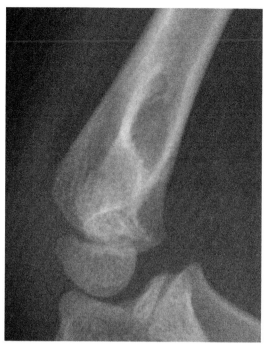

Fig. 3. This patient has an abnormal anterior humeral line that does not intersect the capitellum. (*From* Raby N, Berman L, Morley S, et al. Paediatric elbow. In: Raby N, Berman L, de Lacey G, editors. Accident and emergency radiology: a survival guide. 3rd edition. Philadelphia: Elsevier, 2015; with permission.)

A nondisplaced type I supracondylar fracture that has no signs of neurovascular compromise does not require urgent orthopedic evaluation in the ED; these can be placed in a long arm splint or cast with the elbow flexed at 90°, with the forearm splinted in either pronation or a neutral position.[10] One must always evaluate the neurovascular status of the forearm, wrist, and hand following splinting. These patients should be evaluated by an orthopedist within 24 hours. Type II or III supracondylar fractures need emergent evaluation by an orthopedic surgeon, because most type II and all type III supracondylar fractures require operative repair.

Elbow Injuries

Radiographs should be obtained for children with elbow tenderness, deformity, or swelling in the setting of trauma. At least 2 views of the elbow should be obtained, with a third view, the lateral oblique, which can be helpful in diagnosing subtle lateral condyle fractures and displacements.[10]

ANATOMY

It is imperative to be familiar with the anatomy and radiographic features of the skeletally immature elbow. The elbow joint contains 6 ossification centers that can be easily mistaken for fractures. These ossification centers appear in a fairly predictable order that does not vary. A helpful acronym for remembering the order of appearance of the ossification centers is CRITOE, with each letter of the mnemonic representing an ossification center (**Fig. 5**, **Table 1**).

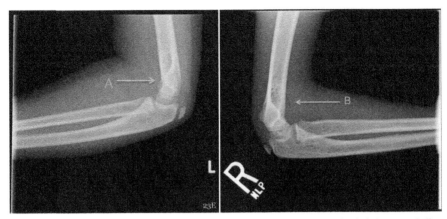

Fig. 4. Physiologic versus pathologic anterior fat pads. The image on the left (*arrow A*) illustrates a smooth anterior fat pad, a normal physiologic variant, in an 8 year old. The image on the right (*arrow B*) demonstrates a "sail sign," which is represents a pathologic fracture, in a 9 year old. (*Courtesy of* C. Silva, MD, Yale Department of Diagnostic Radiology, Yale New Haven Hospital, New Haven, CT; with permission.)

Although they appear earlier in girls than boys, one can approximate the timing of appearance by remembering that there is a 2-year progression of the above ossification centers. Most experts remember this as 1, 3, 5, 7, 9, 11 years old, for the appearance of the capitellum to the external (lateral) epicondyle, respectively.[11] It is worth noting that radiographs of the contralateral elbow may be helpful to assess the developmental stage of the patient, when an injury is suspicious for a fracture.

Radial Head Subluxation

Radial head subluxation, commonly known as nursemaid's elbow, is seen frequently in the ED because of parental concern over a child's refusal to move his or her arm. This injury occurs primarily in toddlers, but can appear in the infant or preschooler. Often, the history is difficult to obtain because the caretaker may not realize the cause of the injury. The typical mechanism is abrupt longitudinal traction on the child's pronated wrist or hand. This action forces the annular ligament over the radial head, lodging it between the radial head and the capitellum. Usually, the child refuses to move the affected arm, holding it close to his or her body.

After carefully examining the child's arm and shoulder girdle, the physician who is confident of the diagnosis of radial head subluxation can attempt reduction without obtaining any radiographs. If there is focal bony tenderness on examination, one should obtain plain radiographs to rule out a fracture. The 2 most popular techniques for reduction are supination/flexion and hyperpronation. Both methods are highly effective, with hyperpronation proving slightly superior in a meta-analysis of randomized control trials.[12] In one study, hyperpronation was perceived as less painful than supination/flexion to caretakers and nurses, while physicians perceived no difference.[13]

With both methods, the examiner supports the child's arm at the elbow and places moderate pressure with a finger on the radial head. In hyperpronation, the examiner grips the distal forearm and hyperpronates the arm. In the supination/flexion method, the examiner holds the forearm and gives gentle traction and then fully supinates the forearm and flexes the elbow in one motion. In many cases, there is a palpable click

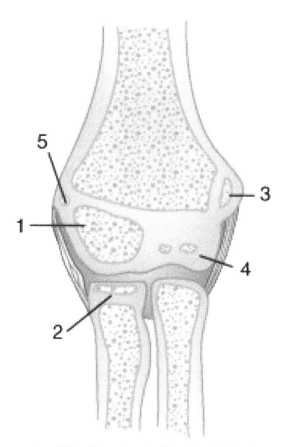

Fig. 5. Ossification centers of the elbow: 1, capitellum; 2, radial head; 3, inner (medial) epi-condyle; 4, trochlea; 5, external (lateral) epicondyle. (*From* Marx JA, Hockberger RS, Walls RM, editors. Rosen's emergency medicine-concepts and clinical practice. 8th edition. Philadelphia: Saunders/Elsevier; 2013.)

Table 1
Secondary ossification centers of the elbow and the age of appearance based on sex

Secondary Ossification Center	Average Age of Appearance in Girls	Average Age of Appearance in Boys
Capitellum	5 mo	7 mo
Radial head	4 y	5 y
Inner (medial) epicondyle	5 y	7 y
Trochlea	8 y	9 y
Olecranon	9 y	10 y
External (lateral) epicondyle	11 y	12 y

From Bachman D, Santora S. Orthopedic trauma. In: Fleisher G, Ludwig S, editors. Textbook of pe-diatric emergency medicine. Philadelphia: Lippincott Williams & Wilkins; 2006. p. 1538; with permission.

over the child's radial head when the annular ligament is reduced. A younger child should start to move his arm in about 10 minutes. If the child fails to move his or her arm in that period, then another attempt at reduction can be repeated. If repeated attempts at reduction are unsuccessful, then one should obtain radiographs and place the child in a posterior elbow splint. These children should be followed up in 24 to 72 hours. Fortunately, most reduction attempts are successful. Because many parents do not realize the harm in lifting a child's entire body from the hand or wrist, the physician should caution against lifting the child in this manner.

Elbow Fractures

Condylar fractures

Although supracondylar fractures are much more common than condylar fractures, lateral condylar fractures account for up to 15% of pediatric elbow fractures.[10,14] The peak age for these fractures is 6 years, and early recognition and management are essential to avoid elbow deformity and to maintain proper function.[14,15] Medial condylar fractures are much less common.[15] A fall on outstretched hand (FOOSH) is the typical mechanism of injury for both medial and lateral condylar fractures. Patients with these types of fractures generally present with pain on the medial or lateral elbow, and limited range of motion.[8] Serious neurovascular compromise is rare with condylar fractures.

Unlike supracondylar fractures, which can often be adequately visualized without oblique radiographs, condylar fractures may require 2 oblique views to be fully characterized.[15] Comparison views of the contralateral elbow may be helpful to detect subtle fractures. Lateral and medial condylar fractures extend from the metaphysis through the physis and into the epiphysis, giving them characteristics similar to Salter-Harris IV physeal fractures.

Initial treatment of condylar fractures consists of pain management, splinting, and elevation of the extremity.[10] Prompt orthopedic consultation should be obtained for any patient with an open fracture, neurovascular compromise, or a condylar fracture with greater than 2 mm of displacement.[16] If diagnosed and managed in a timely manner, the long-term prognosis for patients with a condylar fracture is excellent.

Forearm Fractures

Forearm fractures represent approximately 40% to 50% of all pediatric fractures.[17,18] Seventy-five percent of these involve the distal third of the radius and/or ulna.[19] In general, these fractures are also the result of an FOOSH.[20] AP and lateral radiographs of the injured forearm should be obtained. Careful examination of the wrist and elbow must be performed.

Because pediatric bones are more porous and flexible than their adult counterparts, they tolerate more bending and deformation before a fracture. Thus, comminuted fractures are rare.

Nondisplaced and incomplete fractures can generally be stabilized with splinting in the emergency department and referred for outpatient evaluation by an orthopedist.

Certain distal forearm fractures require immediate orthopedic consultation (**Box 1**)[18]:

Physeal Fractures

With respect to forearm fractures, the type of fracture, based on Salter-Harris classification, and the degree of displacement determine the treatment. Patients with a nondisplaced Salter-Harris type I fracture should receive immobilization with a sling and volar splint for 3 to 4 weeks. Those with a Salter-Harris type II fracture should receive

> **Box 1**
> **Distal forearm fractures that require immediate orthopedic consultation**
>
> Open fractures
>
> Fractures with neurovascular compromise
>
> Displaced Salter I or II physeal fractures
>
> Salter III, IV, or V physeal fractures
>
> Single displaced radius fractures with intact ulna where a difficult reduction is anticipated
>
> Forearm fractures complicated by wrist or elbow dislocation or supracondylar fracture (seen with up to 5% of forearm fractures[21])
>
> Angulated and/or complete fractures, if clinician is not experienced in fracture reduction
>
> Bowing fracture of the radius and ulna
>
> *Data from* Rodriguez-Merchan EC. Pediatric fractures of the forearm. Clin Orthop Relat Res 2005;(432):65–72.

a sugar tong splint or cast for the same duration.[22] Orthopedic follow-up should occur within 1 week. Patients with persistent tenderness over the radial or ulnar physis in the setting of a normal radiograph should be treated as a nondisplaced Salter-Harris type I fracture.

In the acute care setting, nondisplaced Salter-Harris type I or II fractures can be immobilized and splinted or casted as described above. These fractures must be reduced within 1 week, as the growth plate heals quickly and reduction thereafter increases risk of growth arrest.[20] Prompt reduction leads to an excellent prognosis for healing and normal subsequent growth.

Salter-Harris type III, IV, and V fractures require prompt orthopedic consultation. Because Salter-Harris type III fractures involve the joint surface, they commonly necessitate open reduction to maintain joint stability.[23] Salter-Harris type IV fractures are unstable, and because perfect reduction is essential for a good outcome, open reduction internal fixation (ORIF) is usually required. Salter-Harris type V fractures, which can initially be difficult to identify and are later followed by premature growth plate closure and growth arrest months later, also require ORIF.[23]

Complete Fractures

Complete fractures extend through both cortices of the distal metaphysis of the radius and/or ulna. These fractures are caused by high-energy FOOSH and often result in displacement.[17] These fractures do not result in disruption of the growth plate. The position of the bony fracture segments is dictated by the forces exerted on the bones by their attached muscles.[17,24] As a result, overlapping fracture segments often result in shortening of the arm.[22]

Complete metaphyseal fractures of one or both bones with minimal or no displacement have significant remodeling potential because of their proximity to the distal growth plate. Isolated metaphyseal fractures with up to 20° of angulation can be placed in a sugar tong splint or casted without reduction in patients less than 10 years of age.[19,22] Isolated distal radius diaphyseal fractures with less than 2 mm of lateral shift, dorsal angulation of less than 10°, and shortening of less than 2 mm and minimal or no displacement can be safely casted without reduction.[25] Closed reduction is required for all displaced fractures and those with greater than 20° of angulation. All complete fractures merit orthopedic follow-up within 1 week of splinting or casting.[22]

Buckle (Torus) Fractures

The buckling of the bony cortex due to compression failure causes torus fractures. These fractures typically occur at the distal metaphysis, where young bones are most porous.[18] Clinical examination of patients with buckle fractures reveals bony tenderness. Findings on radiograph may be very subtle. These fractures most commonly affect the dorsal surface of the radius, but both bones may be involved.

Buckle fractures are stable, and treatment is geared toward pain relief and prevention of further injury to the bone using a short arm cast or a splint. Multiple clinical trials have shown preference for immobilization with a removable splint, rather than a short arm cast.[19,26–28] Two randomized controlled trials demonstrated that patients with buckle fractures who were splinted had a mildly increased duration of pain, but had a faster return to normal function (**Fig. 6**).[26,28]

Greenstick Fractures

A greenstick fracture is a complete fracture of the tension side of the cortex of the radius or ulna, and a plastic deformation (buckling) of the compression side of the same bone.[20] A greenstick fracture of one forearm bone is often accompanied by a fracture of the other bone.

Patients with greenstick fractures of the forearm generally require immobilization in a long arm cast for 3 to 4 weeks, followed by short arm cast for 2 to 3 weeks.[29] Greenstick fractures with mild or no displacement may be splinted without reduction in the ED, with orthopedic follow-up.[17,22] The degree of angulation that can be treated without reduction is age-dependent. Generally, children under 5 years of age can

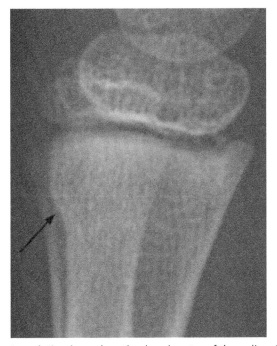

Fig. 6. Slight bulge/angulation (*arrow*) on the dorsal cortex of the radius. A torus (or greenstick) fracture. (*From* Raby N, Berman L, Morley S, et al. Paediatric elbow. In: Raby N, Berman L, de Lacey G, editors. Accident and emergency radiology: a survival guide. 3rd edition. Philadelphia: Elsevier, 2015; with permission.)

tolerate 10 to 35° of angulation on lateral radiograph and up to 10° of angulation on AP view, whereas children 5 to 10 years old can have 10 to 25° of angulation on lateral and up to 10° of angulation on AP films without need for reduction. Children older than 10 years old can tolerate 5 to 20° of angulation on lateral radiograph as long as there is no angulation on the AP view.[22] Patients with greenstick fractures that have moderate to severe displacement must undergo prompt reduction by an experienced clinician or orthopedist. Greenstick fractures that have been casted in the acute setting can be followed by an orthopedist in 7 days (**Fig. 7**).[22]

Ulnar Styloid Fractures

An ulnar styloid fracture is a distal avulsion fracture at the site of the triangular fibrocartilage complex (TFCC) or the ulnocarpal ligament attachment. These fractures are usually accompanied by a radial fracture, which dictates management. The exception to this is a displaced fracture that occurs at the base of the ulnar styloid, which may warrant surgical intervention if there is a disruption in the TFCC.[30]

LOWER EXTREMITY INJURIES
Hip Pain

Hip pain in children is disturbing for both parents and physicians. The causes of hip pain are numerous, so it is prudent for the physician to become familiar with the

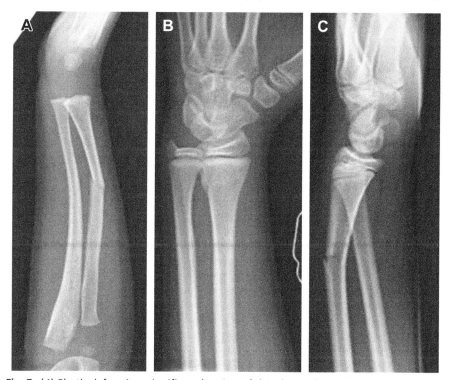

Fig. 7. (*A*) Plastic deformity—significant bowing of the ulna without disruption of the cortex. (*B*) Buckle fracture—the cortex of the distal radius is deformed but intact. (*C*) Greenstick fracture—disruption of dorsal cortex of the radius with plastic deformity of its volar cortex in this forearm fracture involving both bones. (*From* Browner BD, Fuller R. Musculoskeletal emergencies. Philadelphia: Elsevier Saunders; 2013; with permission.)

significant features and epidemiology of the common and potentially serious causes of hip pain in children.

Transient Synovitis Versus Septic Arthritis

For the child with fever and limp, the clinician must emergently differentiate between transient, or "toxic," synovitis and septic arthritis of the hip. Transient synovitis is a self-limited inflammatory process that occurs most commonly in children 1.5 to 7 years old, with a peak between the ages of 3 and 6 years.[31] This entity, which occurs more frequently in boys than girls, is the most common hip disorder that causes atraumatic limp in children.[32,33] The onset, which is generally acute, often follows a viral upper respiratory illness or mild trauma. Transient synovitis has a good clinical outcome in most patients.

The major concern is the differentiation of transient synovitis from septic arthritis of the hip, which can cause severe hip destruction with delay in diagnosis, especially when treatment is undertaken more than 4 days after symptom onset.[34,35] Although children with septic arthritis usually have a fever and refuse to bear weight on the affected leg, children with transient synovitis may have a low-grade or no fever and may limp but bear some weight.[36] Because of hip effusion, a child with either condition may hold the affected hip in flexion, abduction, and external rotation to widen the joint space and can have pain with passive hip movement.[31,37] Classically, children with septic arthritis of the hip will have pain with micromotion on internal rotation of the hip joint. In a young child, one examination technique to assess micromotion pain is for the examiner to internally and externally rotate the child's affected leg using the foot. In addition, a child with an irritable hip may complain of thigh or knee pain that is referred from the hip.

The first step in evaluation is often radiographs of the affected hip, although the utility is low in children with acute atraumatic limp, particularly those younger than 9 years old.[32] Ultrasound examination of the hip is highly sensitive in detection of hip effusions and septic arthritis, but cannot reliably differentiate septic arthritis from transient synovitis.[35,38,39] Caution should be used in children with symptoms for less than 24 hours when a small hip effusion may not be detected on ultrasound.[39] Laboratory investigation, including C-reactive protein (CRP), erythrocyte sedimentation rate (ESR), and peripheral white blood cell (WBC) count, is often undertaken to distinguish septic arthritis from transient synovitis. Although CRP has better test characteristics than ESR and peripheral WBC count in differentiating septic arthritis from other causes of joint effusion, no single laboratory test is predictive of septic arthritis.[40,41]

Because clinical features often overlap, ultrasound cannot distinguish between septic arthritis and transient synovitis, and because individual laboratory tests are not diagnostic of either condition, researchers have attempted to develop a prediction rule to differentiate septic arthritis from transient synovitis of the hip in children. Kocher and colleagues[42] performed the first study that identified 4 independent predictors of septic arthritis that have become known as the "Kocher criteria" (**Box 2**).

In Kocher's initial retrospective study of children who underwent arthrocentesis for an irritable hip, no patients with 0/4 predictors had septic arthritis.[42] The probability of septic arthritis increased with the number of predictors present, to 99.6% with 4/4 predictors.[42] Kocher and colleagues[43] performed a follow-up, prospective validation study in 2004 and reported that the criteria performed similarly well in prediction of septic arthritis, although patients with 0/4 predictors had a 2% probability of septic arthritis. However, Luhmann and Luhmann[44] reported that children with 4/4 predictors only had a 59% probability of septic arthritis, likely influenced by the high prevalence of transient synovitis in their cohort.

Box 2
Kocher criteria for differentiation of septic arthritis from transient synovitis of the hip in children

History of fever greater than 38.5

Non-weight-bearing

ESR ≥40 mm/h

Peripheral WBC count greater than 12,000 cells/mm³

CRP greater than 2 mg/dL[a]

[a] Added to criteria by Caird and colleagues.[36]

Data from Kocher MS, Zurakowski D, Kasser JR. Differentiating between septic arthritis and transient synovitis of the hip in children: an evidence-based clinical prediction algorithm. J Bone Joint Surg Am 1999;81(12):1662–70; and Caird MS, Flynn JM, Leung YL, et al. Factors distinguishing septic arthritis from transient synovitis of the hip in children. A prospective study. J Bone Joint Surg Am 2006;88(6):1251–7.

Caird and colleagues[36] added CRP to the prediction rule and reported favorable test characteristics of the prediction rule, because patients with 5/5 predictors had 97.5% probability of septic arthritis and no patients with transient synovitis had a fever. Importantly, though, 12% of patients with septic arthritis had 0 or 1 predictors. Similar to the Luhmann study, Sultan and Hughes[45] reported the 5 predictors to be substantially less accurate in differentiating septic arthritis from transient synovitis. In summary, the Kocher criteria are a useful adjunct to physical examination, but should not be used in isolation to predict septic arthritis. Patients with 0/5 predictors are low, but not zero, risk for septic arthritis. Thus, a period of close observation may be warranted.

If septic arthritis is suspected, arthrocentesis of the hip should be performed under ultrasound guidance.[46] Synovial fluid should be sent for cell count, Gram stain, and bacterial culture. Although the literature definition of septic arthritis is a synovial fluid WBC of 50,000/μL, this synovial WBC has a sensitivity for septic arthritis of only 62%.[47] Patients who have an irritable hip with synovial WBC greater than 50,000/μL are likely to have septic arthritis, as the specificity is 92% for septic arthritis (99% for WBC of 100,000/μL).[47] Gram strain is positive in only 29% to 50% patients with septic arthritis.[47] Even with synovial cell counts less than 50,000/μL and a negative Gram stain, if septic arthritis is highly suspected clinically, the clinician should consider initiation of therapy for septic arthritis.

Treatment of transient synovitis includes symptomatic relief with rest and nonsteroidal anti-inflammatory drugs (NSAIDs). The duration of symptoms is 1 week or less in 67% of patients, and less than 1 month in an additional 21% of patients.[48] Close follow-up is important for children with a diagnosis of transient synovitis to monitor for development of symptoms or signs that are more consistent with septic arthritis.

Therapy for septic arthritis includes urgent surgical drainage and intravenous antibiotics. Empiric intravenous antibiotics should be given in the ED after successful arthrocentesis. The most common pathogen is *Staphylococcus aureus*, followed by *Streptococcus pneumoniae*.[36,43,49] Given the frequency of community-acquired methicillin-resistant *S aureus* (CA-MRSA) in causing septic arthritis and its association with worse outcomes, empiric antibiotic therapy should include coverage for both methicillin-sensitive *S aureus* and CA-MRSA.[49,50] Gram-negative antibiotic therapy with a third-generation cephalosporin should be added in neonates and in adolescents when disseminated gonorrhea is suspected and considered in young children because of the presence of *Kingella kingae* as a pathogen in septic arthritis.[51] Lyme testing and empiric Ceftriaxone should be considered in Lyme-endemic areas.[52]

Legg-Calvé-Perthes Disease

Legg-Calvé-Perthes Disease (LCPD) is an idiopathic avascular necrosis of the femoral head with subsequent reossification. This disorder is more common in boys and has a peak incidence between 3 and 12 years of age. Of note, children with LCPD often have delayed bone age and a history of low birth weight.[53] The ratio of affected white to African American children is 10:1. The incidence of LCPD in patients with siblings who have LCPD is 1 in 35.[54] The incidence of bilateral involvement is reported to be 10% to 20%.[53]

Children with LCPD frequently present with limp and have limited internal rotation and abduction of the hip. Children often complain of either no pain or pain that is referred to thigh or knee. AP and frog leg lateral radiographs should be obtained if there is a clinical suspicion for LCPD. Radiographic stages in LCPD follow a progression.

1. Early in the illness, the radiographs may be normal.
2. Radiographs demonstrate a small femoral head with a widened medial joint space.
3. A crescent-shaped radiolucent line ("crescent sign") appears along the proximal femoral head.[31,54]
4. The ossific nucleus of the femoral head becomes more radiopaque with subsequent fragmentation and collapse of the epiphysis as avascular bone is resorbed (**Fig. 8**).[31] This point is usually when the symptoms are the most prominent.
5. Reossification occurs last.
6. Residual deformities, such as an abnormal femoral head and acetabular configuration, may persist.

If the child's radiographs appear normal but LCPD is suspected, MRI or bone scan can be the next helpful step in diagnosis.[55,56]

Treatment includes orthopedic referral, restriction of activity, and NSAIDs. Age at the onset of the symptoms is the best predictor of outcome. Those patients with

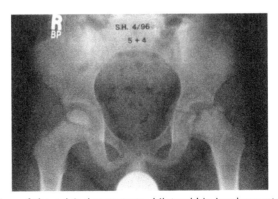

Fig. 8. This AP view of the pelvis demonstrates bilateral hip involvement with Legg-Calvé-Perthes disease. The right hip demonstrates early signs of the avascular stage with diminished femoral head size. The left hip demonstrates the fragmentation stage. (*From* Koop S, Quanbeck D. Three common causes of childhood hip pain. Pediatr Clin North Am 1996;43:1059; with permission.)

the symptoms occurring before the age of 6 years have the best outcome, whereas those aged 8 years or older have the worst prognosis.[53,57]

Slipped Capital Femoral Epiphysis

Slipped capital femoral epiphysis (SCFE) is a disorder in which there is disruption through the capital femoral physis (**Fig. 9**). The term SCFE is actually a misnomer, because the epiphysis remains in the normal position in the acetabulum, whereas the femur distal to the physis displaces anterolaterally and superiorly. SCFE typically occurs during adolescence, and the male-to-female ratio is approximately 1.5:1.[31] Obesity is also a factor in this disorder, although it has also been reported in tall, thin, rapidly growing adolescents.[31,58]

SCFE can be classified either in terms of duration of symptoms or in the severity of the displacement. If the symptoms have been present for less than 3 weeks, it is considered an acute slip, whereas when symptoms last longer than 3 weeks, it is considered chronic. It is possible for a child with a chronic slip to experience an acute slippage, however, sometimes known as an "acute on chronic" slip.[31] Mild slips can demonstrate displacement up to one-third of the metaphyseal width. Moderate slips occupy from one-third to one-half the metaphyseal slips, whereas severe slips have a slippage of greater than one-half of the metaphyseal width.[31]

Children with SCFE usually have a limp and hip pain that is often referred to the thigh, knee, or deep in the groin. Physical examination usually shows loss of internal rotation of the affected hip, decreased flexion, and perhaps shortening of the affected limb.

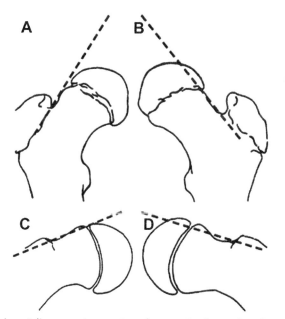

Fig. 9. SCFE, AP view. A line superimposed on the superior femoral neck normally intersects part of the head (*B* and *D* are normal). With a slipped epiphysis, the line does not intersect the femoral head (*A* and *C*). Occasionally, the frog-leg view (*C* and *D*) is needed to show the slip. (*From* Farber AJ, Wilckens JH, Jarvis CG. Pelvic pain in the athlete. In: Seidenberg PH, editor. The sports medicine resource manual. Philadelphia: WB Saunders; 2008; with permission and *Adapted from* Behrman RE, Kleigman R, Jenson HB. Nelson textbook of pediatrics. 17th edition. Philadelphia: WB Saunders; 2004.)

Radiographic studies of children suspected of having SCFE should include AP pelvis and lateral view of both hips. On the AP view, a line drawn along the superior margin of the femoral neck cortex (Klein line) is useful for demonstrating subtle slips. The line should intersect or fall within the epiphysis, usually by at least 20%.[31] In patients with SCFE, the line passes along or outside the epiphysis. In subtle cases, the more remarkable finding will be an asymmetry from the normal hip. Because the slip in most cases of SCFE is usually posterior, the lateral view may reveal the slip better than AP view.

The physician making the diagnosis of SCFE should prescribe no weight bearing for the child and obtain immediate orthopedic consultation. Many of these patients will be admitted to the hospital for surgical pinning before discharge. Studies have shown that surgical pinning in situ provides the best results.[59]

Bilateral SCFE can occur in 37% to 61% of children.[60,61] Thus, one must examine the opposite hip closely and inform the patient and his or her parents of the potential for this problem. Interestingly, 88% of subsequent slips occur within 18 months of diagnosis of the first slip.[60] The prognosis of SCFE is based on the chance of developing avascular necrosis or chondrolysis with the subsequent arthritis. These problems are less likely to occur when there has been a short duration of symptoms, when the slip is mild, and when the slip is surgically fixed in situ, rather than attempted reduction and then fixation.[31,62]

Toddler's Fracture

The toddler's fracture is a nondisplaced oblique fracture of the distal tibia.[63] This fracture most commonly occurs in children 1 to 4 years old and is often precipitated by only minor trauma such as tripping while walking or running, a fall from a relatively low height, or a twisting mechanism.[64,65] A history of trauma may not even be elicited in some cases.[63] The child with a toddler's fracture presents with limp or refusal to bear weight on the affected extremity. Although tenderness may be present on physical examination, swelling and deformity are often not observed.[64] The examiner may also elicit pain with gentle twisting of the tibia.

The characteristic radiographic finding is a subtle oblique lucency through the distal tibia that terminates medially (**Fig. 10**).[64] The fracture is most easily seen on the AP view and is often not noted on the lateral radiograph.[64] An internal oblique film is very sensitive for toddler's fracture and may be required to identify the fracture.[64] In some cases, the fracture is missed on initial radiography and is not identified until follow-up examination.[64,65]

A toddler's fracture is most often nondisplaced and heals well with 3 to 4 weeks of immobilization.[63–65] Importantly, a toddler's fracture occurs in the distal half to distal third of the tibia. This location is distinct from a midshaft spiral fracture of the tibia, which is more consistent with child abuse.[64,65]

Tillaux and Triplane Fractures

Tillaux and triplane fractures are transitional fractures, named for their occurrence during the 18-month period when the distal tibia physis transitions from open to closed.[66] Full closure of the physis occurs around age 14 in girls and age 16 in boys, so most fractures occur between ages 12 and 16.[67,68] Closure of the physis begins centrally, followed by closure of the anteromedial portion, and last, lateral physeal closure.[66] During this transition period, the lateral distal tibia physis is weak and external rotation of a supinated foot can cause fracture and separation of the anterolateral portion of the epiphysis.[69] Approximately 7% to 15% of adolescent ankle fractures are transitional fractures.[70]

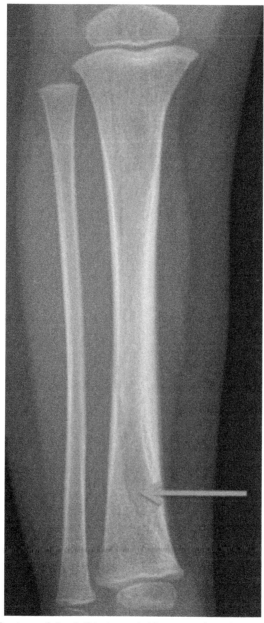

Fig. 10. Toddler's fracture of distal tibia (*arrow*). (*Courtesy of* C. Silva, MD, Yale Department of Diagnostic Radiology, Yale New Haven Hospital, New Haven, CT; with permission.)

A Tillaux fracture is a Salter-Harris type III fracture of the distal tibia that occurs horizontally through the physis and vertically through the epiphysis of the distal tibia, with a resultant intra-articular fracture (**Fig. 11**).[66] The anterior tibiofibular ligament causes avulsion of the lateral epiphysis and potential displacement of the fracture fragment.[66]

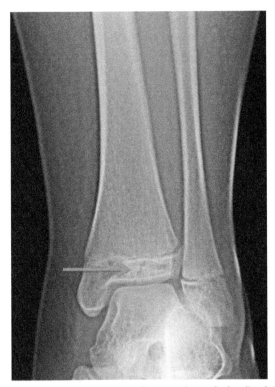

Fig. 11. Tillaux fracture, a Salter-Harris type III fracture through the distal tibial epiphysis (*arrow*). (*Courtesy of* C. Silva, MD, Yale Department of Diagnostic Radiology, Yale New Haven Hospital, New Haven, CT; with permission.)

A triplane fracture is a Salter-Harris type IV fracture with fracture lines in 3 planes that traverse the physis of the distal tibia. A triplane fracture involves fractures through the epiphysis in the sagittal plane, the physis in the transverse plane, and the tibial metaphysis in the coronal plane (**Fig. 12**).[68] In both types of transitional fractures, the patient will usually not bear weight on the affected extremity and will have swelling, ecchymosis, and tenderness over the anterior ankle.[66]

Plain radiographs should include AP, lateral, and mortise views, as multiple radiographs are needed to identify all components of a triplane fracture.[68] Although the degree of fracture fragment displacement can be determined with plain radiography alone, computed tomography can better delineate fracture configuration and its use is associated with improved outcomes.[71,72] Tillaux and triplane fractures with less than 2 mm of epiphyseal fragment displacement can be immobilized with a long leg cast with good outcomes.[73] Fractures with greater degrees of displacement require closed or open reduction, and functional outcomes are generally excellent if displacement less than 2 mm is achieved.[74]

CHILD ABUSE

A recent report on the incidence of child maltreatment estimates that nearly 1.25 million cases or 1 in 58 children are abused annually in the United States.[75] The Department of Health and Human Services defines 4 main types of maltreatment in the Fourth National Incidence Study of Child Abuse and Neglect Report to Congress as physical abuse,

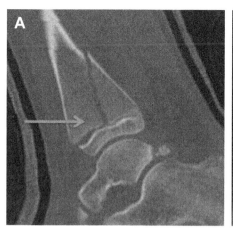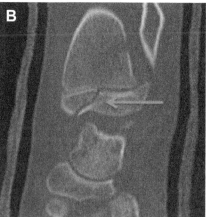

Fig. 12. Triplane fracture. Computed tomography demonstrates fractures through the (*A*) distal tibial metaphysis and physis, and (*B*) epiphysis. *Arrow* pointing to the fractures. (*Courtesy of* C. Silva, MD, Yale Department of Diagnostic Radiology, Yale New Haven Hospital, New Haven, CT; with permission.)

sexual abuse, neglect, and emotional abuse. Of the children who are abused, 58% have sustained some physical abuse.[75] Fractures are the second most common injury caused by physical abuse, with bruising being the most common.[76]

In infants and toddlers, nonaccidental trauma (NAT) is the cause of 12% to 20% of the fractures. About 80% of fractures caused by child abuse occur in children younger than 18 months of age.[77] However, patients older than 18 months who present with long bone fractures generally have injuries that are more likely to be related to accidental trauma than child abuse.[78] Thus, fractures from child abuse tend to occur in very young children, but can occur at any age and in any socioeconomic group. When evaluating an orthopedic injury in a child, the provider needs to carefully consider the history, the development and age of the child, the type and location of the fracture, the age of the fracture, and mechanism for the type of fracture.[79]

Diagnosis

History

After any necessary resuscitative efforts are completed, the physician should obtain a detailed history from the child's caretaker. Suspicion should be raised if the stated mechanism of injury is inconsistent with the child's developmental stage. For example, a femoral or humeral fracture in a child who is not yet walking should raise suspicion for abuse.[79] Furthermore, if the caregiver changes the history of the injury or gives no history for the injury, suspicion for abuse should be raised. In addition, if the age of the fracture is not consistent with the history or if there are multiple factures in different stages of healing, the provider should strongly consider abuse. Likewise, if the historian is evasive, inappropriately angry, or obviously lying, suspicion should be raised. If the child is verbal, the experienced physician should ask him about the injury with open-ended questions in a nonthreatening manner, without the presence of the caregiver. A social history should be included as well. It should be noted who cares for the child, any other children in the household, Child Protective Services involvement with the family, and history of domestic or substance abuse in the child's living situation.

Physical Examination

A thorough and gentle approach is best. The child should be examined completely, head to toe, including the genitalia. Any scarring, ecchymosis, lacerations, burns, or other lesions should be documented carefully. The skeletal examination should be complete, considering that multiple fractures may be present.

Radiography

A complete skeletal survey should be done on all physically abused children less than 2 years of age and on infants suffering from neglect. In addition, if the clinical situation necessitates, the provider should consider obtaining a skeletal survey in children ages 2 to 5 years.[77] Highly detailed radiographs are essential and should follow the guidelines set forth by the American College of Radiology.[80] A "babygram" or an AP view of the entire child on one film is an unacceptable alternative.

Radiographic Features of Child Abuse

The American Academy of Pediatrics has published a clinical report that categorizes fractures in children as "High Specificity for Abuse," "Moderate Specificity for Abuse," and "Common, but Low Specificity for Abuse."[77] The fractures, especially in infants, which have High Specificity for Abuse, are sternal fractures, scapula fractures, spinous process fractures, rib fractures—especially posteromedial, and classic metaphyseal lesions (CMLs). A CML is a disk-like fragment of bone and calcified cartilage that is wider on the outer edge than it is centrally.

This fracture is transmetaphyseal through the primary spongiosa and leaves the disk-like fragment attached to the epiphysis (**Fig. 13**).[81] Classic metaphyseal lesions have been termed "corner" or "bucket handle" fractures in the past and are the same entity viewed in different planes. Although these fractures appear relatively benign in terms of healing, it is their clear association with NAT that providers need to understand. The CMLs are specific for abuse due to the mechanism that causes them: traction and torsion forces, rather than falling.

Fractures that are Moderate Specificity for Abuse include multiple fractures, especially bilaterally, fractures of different ages, epiphyseal separations, vertebral body fractures

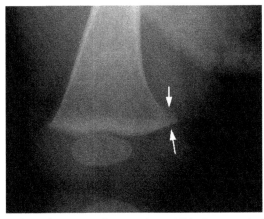

Fig. 13. Classic metaphyseal "corner" fracture in a child. *Arrow* pointing to the fracture fragment. (*Courtesy of* J.G. Smirniotopoulos, Uniformed Services University of Health Sciences, Bethesda, MD.)

and subluxations, digital fractures, and complex skull fractures.[77] Factures, which have Low Specificity for Abuse, include long bone fractures, clavicle fractures, subperiosteal new bone formation, and linear skull fractures.[77] It is, however, important for the providers to keep in mind that a single long bone diaphyseal fracture is the most common fracture pattern identified in abused children.[78] With all of these injuries, the provider needs to take into consideration that the history of injury, the child's age and development, the patient's past medical history as well as an understanding of the mechanism of injury and forces that need to be applied to sustain the injury are all imperative.

SUMMARY

The emergency physician will inevitably encounter child abuse if their practice includes the care of children. The possibility for abuse needs to be considered by providers when caring for children with skeletal injuries, especially the very young child. Taking into consideration all of the factors of the case, including the history, age of the child, type of fracture, and understanding the specificity for abuse and mechanism of injury, are all important for determining suspicion for child abuse.

REFERENCES

1. England SP, Sundberg S. Management of common orthopedic fractures. Pediatr Clin North Am 1996;43:991–1012.
2. Greenfield R. Orthopedic injuries: pediatric emergency medicine. In: Strange G, Ahrens W, editors. Pediatric emergency medicine. New York: McGraw-Hill; 1996. p. 113–8.
3. Salter RB, Harris WR. Injuries involving the epiphyseal plate. J Bone Joint Surg Am 1963;45A:587–621.
4. Joffe M. Upper extremity. In: Strange G, Ahrens W, editors. Pediatric emergency medicine. New York: McGraw-Hill; 1996. p. 340–54.
5. Eiff MP, Hatch RL, Calmbach W. Clavicle and scapula fractures. In: Eiff MP, Hatch RL, Calmbach W, editors. Fracture management for primary care. Philadelphia: WB Saunders; 2002. p. 198.
6. Beaty JH. Fractures of the proximal humerus and shaft in children. Instr Course Lect 1992;41:369–72.
7. Kasser JR, Beaty JH. Supracondylar fractures of the distal humerus. In: Beaty JH, Kasser JR, editors. Rockwood and Wilkins' fractures in children. Philadelphia: Lippincott Williams & Wilkins; 2001. p. 577.
8. Baratz M, Micucci C, Sangimino M. Pediatric supracondylar humerus fractures. Hand Clin 2006;22(1):69–75.
9. Wu J, Perron AD, Miller MD, et al. Orthopedic pitfalls in the ED: pediatric supracondylar humerus fractures. Am J Emerg Med 2002;20(6):544–50.
10. Carson S, Woolridge DP, Colletti J, et al. Pediatric upper extremity injuries. Pediatr Clin North Am 2006;53(1):41–67, v.
11. Bachman D, Santora S. Orthopedic trauma. In: Fleisher G, Ludwig S, editors. Textbook of pediatric emergency medicine. Philadelphia: Lippincott Williams & Wilkins; 2006. p. 1538.
12. Krul M, van der Wouden JC, van Suijlekom-Smit LWA, et al. Manipulative interventions for reducing pulled elbow in young children. Cochrane Database Syst Rev 2012;(1):CD007759.
13. Green DA, Linares MY-R, Garcia Peña BM, et al. Randomized comparison of pain perception during radial head subluxation reduction using supination-flexion or forced pronation. Pediatr Emerg Care 2006;22(4):235–8.

14. Gogola GR. Pediatric humeral condyle fractures. Hand Clin 2006;22(1):77–85.
15. Beaty JH, Kasser JR. The elbow: physeal fractures, apophyseal injuries of the distal humerus, avascular necrosis of the trochlea, and T-condylar fractures. In: Beaty JH, Kasser JR, editors. Rockwood and Wilkins' fractures in children. Philadelphia: Lippincott Williams & Wilkins; 2001. p. 625.
16. Mirsky EC, Karas EH, Weiner LS. Lateral condyle fractures in children: evaluation of classification and treatment. J Orthop Trauma 1997;11(2):117–20.
17. Price CT, Flynn JM. Management of fractures. In: Morrissey RT, Weinstein SL, editors. Lovell and Winter's pediatric orthopaedics. Philadelphia: Lippincott; 2006. p. 1463.
18. Rodriguez-Merchan EC. Pediatric fractures of the forearm. Clin Orthop Relat Res 2005;(432):65–72.
19. Abraham A, Handoll HH, Khan T. Interventions for treating wrist fractures in children. Cochrane Database Syst Rev 2008;(2):CD004576.
20. Rang M, Stearns P, Chambers H. Radius and ulna. In: Rang M, Pring ME, Wenger DR, editors. Rang's children's fractures. Philadelphia: Lippincott Williams & Wilkins; 2005. p. 135.
21. Roposch A, Reis M, Molina M, et al. Supracondylar fractures of the humerus associated with ipsilateral forearm fractures in children: a report of forty-seven cases. J Pediatr Orthop 2001;21(3):307–12.
22. Waters PM, Bae DS. Fractures of the distal radius and ulna. In: Beaty JH, Kasser JR, editors. Rockwood and Wilkin's fractures in children. Philadelphia: Lippincott Williams & Wilkins; 2010. p. 292.
23. Pizzutillo PD. Pediatric orthopaedics. In: Griffin YL, editor. Essentials of musculoskeletal care. Rosemont (IL): American Academy of Orthopaedic Surgeons; 2005. p. 863.
24. Noonan KJ, Price CT. Forearm and distal radius fractures in children. J Am Acad Orthop Surg 1998;6(3):146–56.
25. Stoffelen D, Broos P. Minimally displaced distal radius fractures: do they need plaster treatment? J Trauma 1998;44(3):503–5.
26. Oakley EA, Ooi KS, Barnett PL. A randomized controlled trial of 2 methods of immobilizing torus fractures of the distal forearm. Pediatr Emerg Care 2008;24(2):65–70.
27. Davidson JS, Brown DJ, Barnes SN, et al. Simple treatment for torus fractures of the distal radius. J Bone Joint Surg Br 2001;83(8):1173–5.
28. Plint AC, Perry JJ, Correll R, et al. A randomized, controlled trial of removable splinting versus casting for wrist buckle fractures in children. Pediatrics 2006;117(3):691–7.
29. Randsborg PH, Sivertsen EA. Distal radius fractures in children: substantial difference in stability between buckle and greenstick fractures. Acta Orthop 2009;80(5):585–9.
30. Abid A, Accadbled F, Kany J, et al. Ulnar styloid fracture in children: a retrospective study of 46 cases. J Pediatr Orthop B 2008;17(1):15–9.
31. Koop S, Quanbeck D. Three common causes of childhood hip pain. Pediatr Clin North Am 1996;43(5):1053–66.
32. Baskett A, Hosking J, Aickin R. Hip radiography for the investigation of nontraumatic, short duration hip pain presenting to a children's emergency department. Pediatr Emerg Care 2009;25(2):78–82.
33. Fischer SU, Beattie TF. The limping child: epidemiology, assessment and outcome. J Bone Joint Surg Br 1999;81(6):1029–34.
34. Fabry G, Meire E. Septic arthritis of the hip in children: poor results after late and inadequate treatment. J Pediatr Orthop 1983;3(4):461–6.

35. Zamzam MM. The role of ultrasound in differentiating septic arthritis from transient synovitis of the hip in children. J Pediatr Orthop B 2006;15(6):418–22.

36. Caird MS, Flynn JM, Leung YL, et al. Factors distinguishing septic arthritis from transient synovitis of the hip in children. A prospective study. J Bone Joint Surg Am 2006;88(6):1251–7.

37. Lawrence LL. The limping child. Emerg Med Clin North Am 1998;16(4):911–29, viii.

38. Zawin JK, Hoffer FA, Rand FF, et al. Joint effusion in children with an irritable hip: US diagnosis and aspiration. Radiology 1993;187(2):459–63.

39. Gordon JE, Huang M, Dobbs M, et al. Causes of false-negative ultrasound scans in the diagnosis of septic arthritis of the hip in children. J Pediatr Orthop 2002; 22(3):312–6.

40. Levine MJ, McGuire KJ, McGowan KL, et al. Assessment of the test characteristics of C-reactive protein for septic arthritis in children. J Pediatr Orthop 2003; 23(3):373–7.

41. Li SF, Cassidy C, Chang C, et al. Diagnostic utility of laboratory tests in septic arthritis. Emerg Med J 2007;24(2):75–7.

42. Kocher MS, Zurakowski D, Kasser JR. Differentiating between septic arthritis and transient synovitis of the hip in children: an evidence-based clinical prediction algorithm. J Bone Joint Surg Am 1999;81(12):1662–70.

43. Kocher MS, Mandiga R, Zurakowski D, et al. Validation of a clinical prediction rule for the differentiation between septic arthritis and transient synovitis of the hip in children. J Bone Joint Surg Am 2004;86-A(8):1629–35.

44. Luhmann JD, Luhmann SJ. Etiology of septic arthritis in children: an update for the 1990s. Pediatr Emerg Care 1999;15(1):40–2.

45. Sultan J, Hughes PJ. Septic arthritis or transient synovitis of the hip in children: the value of clinical prediction algorithms. J Bone Joint Surg Br 2010;92(9): 1289–93.

46. Tsung JW, Blaivas M. Emergency department diagnosis of pediatric hip effusion and guided arthrocentesis using point-of-care ultrasound. J Emerg Med 2008; 35(4):393–9.

47. Margaretten ME, Kohlwes J, Moore D, et al. Does this adult patient have septic arthritis? JAMA 2007;297(13):1478–88.

48. Haueisen DC, Weiner DS, Weiner SD. The characterization of "transient synovitis of the hip" in children. J Pediatr Orthop 1986;6(1):11–7.

49. Young TP, Maas L, Thorp AW, et al. Etiology of septic arthritis in children: an update for the new millennium. Am J Emerg Med 2011;29(8):899–902.

50. Vander Have KL, Karmazyn B, Verma M, et al. Community-associated methicillin-resistant staphylococcus aureus in acute musculoskeletal infection in children: a game changer. J Pediatr Orthop 2009;29(8):927–31.

51. Basmaci R, Lorrot M, Bidet P, et al. Comparison of clinical and biologic features of Kingella kingae and Staphylococcus aureus arthritis at initial evaluation. Pediatr Infect Dis J 2011;30(10):902–4.

52. Glotzbecker MP, Kocher MS, Sundel RP, et al. Primary Lyme arthritis of the pediatric hip. J Pediatr Orthop 2011;31(7):787–90.

53. Wenger DR, Ward WT, Herring JA. Legg-Calve-Perthes disease. J Bone Joint Surg Am 1991;73(5):778–88.

54. Chung SM. Diseases of the developing hip joint. Pediatr Clin North Am 1986; 33(6):1457–73.

55. Dillman JR, Hernandez RJ. MRI of Legg-Calve-Perthes disease. AJR Am J Roentgenol 2009;193(5):1394–407.

56. Uno A, Hattori T, Noritake K, et al. Legg-Calve-Perthes disease in the evolutionary period: comparison of magnetic resonance imaging with bone scintigraphy. J Pediatr Orthop 1995;15(3):362–7.

57. Canavese F, Dimeglio A. Perthes' disease: prognosis in children under six years of age. J Bone Joint Surg Br 2008;90(7):940–5.

58. Chung S. Diseases of the developing hip joint. Pediatr Clin North Am 1977;24(4):857–70.

59. Carney BT, Weinstein SL, Noble J. Long-term follow-up of slipped capital femoral epiphysis. J Bone Joint Surg Am 1991;73(5):667–74.

60. Loder RT, Aronson DD, Greenfield ML. The epidemiology of bilateral slipped capital femoral epiphysis. A study of children in Michigan. J Bone Joint Surg Am 1993;75(8):1141–7.

61. Hagglund G, Hansson LI, Ordeberg G, et al. Bilaterality in slipped upper femoral epiphysis. J Bone Joint Surg Br 1988;70(2):179–81.

62. Chung SM. Identifying the cause of acute limp in childhood. Some informal comments and observations. Clin Pediatr (Phila) 1974;13(9):769–72.

63. Dunbar JS, Owen HF, Nogrady MB, et al. Obscure tibial fracture of infants–the toddler's fracture. J Can Assoc Radiol 1964;15:136–44.

64. Tenenbein M, Reed MH, Black GB. The toddler's fracture revisited. Am J Emerg Med 1990;8(3):208–11.

65. Mellick LB, Milker L, Egsieker E. Childhood accidental spiral tibial (CAST) fractures. Pediatr Emerg Care 1999;15(5):307–9.

66. Wuerz TH, Gurd DP. Pediatric physeal ankle fracture. J Am Acad Orthop Surg 2013;21(4):234–44.

67. Johnson EW Jr, Fahl JC. Fractures involving the distal epiphysis of the tibia and fibula in children. Am J Surg 1957;93(5):778–81.

68. Rosenbaum AJ, DiPreta JA, Uhl RL. Review of distal tibial epiphyseal transitional fractures. Orthopedics 2012;35(12):1046–9.

69. El-Karef E, Sadek HI, Nairn DS, et al. Triplane fracture of the distal tibia. Injury 2000;31(9):729–36.

70. Karrholm J. The triplane fracture: four years of follow-up of 21 cases and review of the literature. J Pediatr Orthop B 1997;6(2):91–102.

71. Liporace FA, Yoon RS, Kubiak EN, et al. Does adding computed tomography change the diagnosis and treatment of Tillaux and triplane pediatric ankle fractures? Orthopedics 2012;35(2):e208–12.

72. Kim JR, Song KH, Song KJ, et al. Treatment outcomes of triplane and Tillaux fractures of the ankle in adolescence. Clin Orthop Surg 2010;2(1):34–8.

73. Cooperman DR, Spiegel PG, Laros GS. Tibial fractures involving the ankle in children. The so-called triplane epiphyseal fracture. J Bone Joint Surg Am 1978;60(8):1040–6.

74. Rapariz JM, Ocete G, González-Herranz P, et al. Distal tibial triplane fractures: long-term follow-up. J Pediatr Orthop 1996;16(1):113–8.

75. Sedlak AJ, Mettenburg J, Basena M, et al. Fourth national incidence study of child abuse and neglect (NIS-4). Washington, DC: U.S. Department of Health and Human Services, Administration for Children and Families; 2010. Available at: http://www.acf.hhs.gov/programs/opre/research/project/national-incidence-study-ofchild-abuse-and-neglect-nis-4-2004-2009.

76. Loder RT, Feinberg JR. Orthopaedic injuries in children with nonaccidental trauma: demographics and incidence from the 2000 kids' inpatient database. J Pediatr Orthop 2007;27(4):421–6.

77. Flaherty EG, Perez-Rossello JM, Levine MA, et al. Evaluating children with fractures for child physical abuse. Pediatrics 2014;133(2):e477–89.

78. Pandya NK, Baldwin K, Wolfgruber H, et al. Child abuse and orthopaedic injury patterns: analysis at a level I pediatric trauma center. J Pediatr Orthop 2009; 29(6):618–25.

79. Hui C, Joughin E, Goldstein S, et al. Femoral fractures in children younger than three years: the role of nonaccidental injury. J Pediatr Orthop 2008;28(3): 297–302.

80. Radiology, ACO. ACR–SPR Practice guideline for skeletal surveys in children. Amended 2014, Resolution 39. 2013. Avaialble at: http://www.acr.org/~/media/9bdcdbee99b84e87baac2b1695bc07b6.pdf.

81. Nimkin K, Kleinman PK. Imaging of child abuse. Pediatr Clin North Am 1997; 44(3):615–35.

Orthopedic Emergencies

A Practical Emergency Department Classification (US-VAGON) in Pelvic Fractures

Hao Wang, MD, PhD[a], Paolo T. Coppola, MD[b],
Marco Coppola, DO[c],*

KEYWORDS

- Orthopedics • Emergency department • Classification • Pelvic fractures

KEY POINTS

- The traditional classifications of pelvic fractures are summarized to show their poor value for emergency physicians in the initial evaluation and treatment of patients with pelvic fractures in the emergency department (ED).
- The ED classification of pelvic fractures is divided into 2 main types: unstable (U) and stable (S) pelvic fractures. Unstable fractures are evaluated and treated according to Advanced Trauma Life Support guidelines.
- Once pelvic fractures are stabilized, they are further classified into 5 categories based on the risks of potential severe complications, including hemorrhagic/vascular (Va), genitourinary or gastrointestinal (G), orthopedic (O), neurologic (N), and uncomplicated pelvic fractures. Therefore, this ED classification refers to them as the US-VAGON classification.

Trauma is one of the leading causes of death before the age of 40 years and approximately 5% of patients with trauma who require hospital admission have pelvic fractures.[1-3] Among all patients with pelvic fractures, about 60% result from vehicular trauma (eg, automobile, motorcycle, bicycle); 30% from falls; and 10% from crush injuries, athletic injuries, or penetrating trauma.[4,5] Although the mortality of trauma victims with pelvic fractures has decreased significantly in the past 10 years, it is still the third most commonly seen injury in fatalities caused by motor vehicle accidents, with a 5% to 16% mortality.[6-8] However, these rates have increased to 25% to 45% in patients with a pelvic fracture who present hemodynamically unstable to the emergency department (ED).[9,10] In addition, pelvic fractures pose a complex challenge to

Disclosures: None.
[a] Department of Emergency Medicine, John Peter Smith Health Network, 1500 South Main Street, Fort Worth, TX 76104, USA; [b] STAT-Health, 519 W Jericho Turnpike, Smithtown, NY 11787, USA; [c] University of North Texas Health Science Center, 3500 Camp Bowie Boulevard, Fort Worth, TX 76107, USA
* Corresponding author. Premier One Emergency Centers, Frisco, TX 75034.
E-mail address: drmarcocoppola@gmail.com

emergency physicians (EPs) because they are often associated with life-threatening hemorrhage, deformity, and associated internal injuries.

TRADITIONAL CLASSIFICATIONS OF PELVIC FRACTURES

Pelvic fractures include pelvic ring disruptions and sacral, acetabular, and avulsion fractures. Pelvic fractures are usually divided into 2 major types based on the amount of energy impacted. Injuries with low-energy mechanisms can result in isolated fractures of individual bones, avulsion fractures, and acetabular fractures in the elderly. However, injuries with high-energy mechanisms can result in pelvic ring disruptions, sacral fractures, and acetabular fractures in younger patients. These patients can quickly become hemodynamically unstable and rapid stabilization and aggressive treatment are required on the patients' arrival in the ED. EPs should be mindful that patients with pelvic fractures have associated multiorgan injuries. Each type of pelvic fracture has a different classification based on the mechanisms, anatomic locations, or other associated injuries to predict the severity, the clinical outcome, or the indications for any surgical intervention. However, these traditional classifications were developed by trauma or orthopedic surgeons and have limited practical value for EPs in the initial evaluation and treatment of patients presenting to the ED with pelvic fractures.

Two most commonly used classifications of pelvic ring fractures are the Tile and Pennal and the Young and Burgess classifications. The Tile and Pennal classification is based on the integrity of the posterior sacroiliac complex, whereas the Young and Burgess classification is based on the mechanism of injury. Although previous studies showed some correlation with the type of pelvic ring fractures and the risk of hemorrhage by using both of these classifications, they have failed to show a consistent correlation between injury type and severity and/or mortality among patients with pelvic fractures.[11–14]

Sacral fractures are commonly associated with pelvic ring fractures (30%–45%) caused by high-energy mechanisms of injury, but occasionally can be isolated. Approximately 25% to 30% of these sacral fractures are associated with neurologic injury. Patients can initially present as neurologically intact and physicians frequently miss subtle sacral fractures.[15,16] There are several classification systems for sacral fractures and the most commonly used are the Denis 3-zone classification and Isler lumbosacral junction classification.[17,18] The Denis classification divides sacral fractures into 3 different zones (lateral to the sacral neural foramina, through the sacral foramina, and medial to the sacral foramina). The Isler classification assesses lumbosacral injury by the location of the pelvic ring fracture relative to the L5-S1 facet joint. These classifications assist physicians predicting neurologic injury and can also affect management if properly used.[16–19] In addition, the Frankel classification, which identifies spinal cord injury, and the Gibbons classification, which was designed specifically to grade the sacral neurologic injuries in patients with sacral fractures, are also used by spinal surgeons.[15,20]

Because of the complex acetabular anatomy, various classifications have been suggested. The classification derived by Letournel and Judet is by far the most wildly used and accepted by orthopedic surgeons.[21] Letournel and Judet[21] classifies acetabular fracture into 10 major fracture patterns consisting of 5 elementary and 5 complex patterns. The Tiles classification is a modification of the Letournel classification and consists of 4 different types based on the involvement of anterior or posterior wall column and its stability.[22] These classifications correlate well with the surgical approach and fracture reduction tactics. With the development of advanced computed tomography

(CT) technique, Harris and colleagues[23] simplified acetabular fractures into 4 categories (wall fracture only, 1 column fracture, 2 column fractures, and floating acetabulum), which are easily understandable by both radiologists and orthopedic surgeons. All these classifications are based on the anatomic fracture location and provide surgical guidance. However, because acetabular fractures are so complex, none of these classifications can accurately predict outcome.

To be useful, a fracture classification should show clinical relevance, be thorough, provide guidance for treatment, predict outcome, and be easily remembered and understood by all physicians involved in the diagnosis and treatment. Many classification schemes have been proposed to try to simplify or organize the many types of pelvic fractures, as mentioned earlier. However, most of these classifications are used as a guideline to help orthopedic trauma surgeons consider proper surgical management preoperatively. These guidelines have limited value for the EP owing to their complexity, and offer little for the immediate ED management of patients. In order to efficiently and appropriately manage these patients with pelvic fractures by EPs, early recognition and evaluation of the severity of this injury and its potential associated complications is essential, especially in hemodynamically stable patients. Therefore, ED physicians benefit more from a classification that attempts to classify pelvic fractures into categories that correlate with the potential risk of complications and other associated instabilities.

EMERGENCY DEPARTMENT CLASSIFICATION OF PELVIC FRACTURES

In this new classification, pelvic fractures are initially divided into stable and unstable groups. Patients with traumatic injuries and unstable pelvic fractures are managed following advanced trauma life support (ATLS) guidelines. EPs should consider the potential complications of pelvic fractures and rule out any potential life-threatening/limb-threatening events before definitive treatment of pelvic fractures is undertaken.

UNSTABLE PELVIC FRACTURES

Patients with pelvic fractures that are clinically unstable most often present to the ED with hypovolemia. However, relying exclusively on the systolic blood pressure might be misleading. Early significant blood loss may present only as tachycardia, narrowed pulse pressure, or poor skin turgor before the blood pressure decreases. A base deficit with metabolic acidosis can also be obtained quickly via arterial blood gas analysis, which is useful to determine the severity of hypovolemic shock.[24]

The initial evaluation should include the ABCs (airway, breathing, circulation) of trauma evaluation described in the ATLS protocols. Usually these unstable pelvic fractures are caused by high-energy mechanisms. All patients complaining of symptoms in the pelvis with unstable vital signs or who are unconscious should be considered to have an unstable pelvic fracture until proved otherwise.

Physical examination of the pelvis should begin with visual inspection for contusions, abrasions, bleeding, or deformities. The Destot sign, which is a superficial hematoma in the scrotum or perineal area, can be noted and indicates a pelvic fracture. A rotational deformity of the pelvis or lower extremities, or the presence of leg-length discrepancies, may also be present with pelvic fractures. The practice of compressing the iliac wings to determine pelvic stability lacks specificity and should be avoided. Blood at the urethral meatus indicates urethral or bladder injury. Rectal or vaginal bleeding alerts the clinician that puncture injuries may be caused by a pelvic fracture. On rectal examination, rectal tone and position of the prostate should be noted. High-riding prostate displacement can indicate a rupture of the membranous urethra. The Earle sign is present if a large hematoma, bony prominence, or fracture line is palpated on rectal examination.

All unstable patients must receive resuscitative fluid (ie, crystalloid, blood) by large-bore intravenous access, and ATLS efforts should be continued. The pneumatic antishock garment (PASG) or medical antishock trouser (MAST) may benefit patients in the prehospital setting, and, if already applied, can continue to tamponade and support the fractured pelvis during the early phases of resuscitation. However, randomized trials have not shown a survival benefit for their use.[25–27] In addition, placement is time consuming, can further destabilize the fracture, and is difficult to perform in the environment of resuscitation. It is also inappropriate to use MAST for long periods of time because of the risk of compartment syndrome.[28,29] Therefore, the role of PASG and MAST currently is limited. Circumferential pelvic binders or sheets are now the choice of immediate external stabilization because these binders are noninvasive, inexpensive, and simple to apply in the prehospital setting.

Once a pelvic fracture has been identified, all efforts to identify the cause of hemodynamic instability must continue per ATLS protocol. These efforts are followed by an evaluation for intra-abdominal bleeding, with a focused assessment with sonography for trauma examination. The pelvis can be externally fixated once a fracture has been radiographically identified and is determined to be a possible cause of the patient's hemodynamic instability. External fixation or the pelvic C clamp can be applied in 15 to 30 minutes by an orthopedic surgeon or a physician credentialed in this procedure (see **Fig. 5**).[4] These methods reduce the relative volume of a fractured pelvis by 10% to 20% and reduce pelvic fractures as well. However, emergency external fixation and the pelvic C clamp used to control hemorrhage are not supported by the available literature. If the patient remains hemodynamically unstable despite the resuscitative efforts listed earlier, continued efforts in the ED are unlikely to be successful. Patients therefore should undergo angiographic embolization or be brought to the operating room for surgical intervention.[29] Angiography for control of hemorrhage has an important role in the treatment of patients with pelvic fractures. Pelvic angiography with embolization can be performed bilaterally if needed and can be repeated to control bleeding.[30,31] Retroperitoneal pelvic packing is effective in controlling hemorrhage when used as a salvage technique after angiographic embolization.[32]

STABLE PELVIC FRACTURES

Once pelvic fractures are stabilized, they are classified with respect to potential life-threatening events or potential severe complications requiring subspecialty further evaluation and treatment. The associated injury complications include potential hemorrhagic/vascular, genitourinary (GU)/gastrointestinal (GI), orthopedic, and neurologic instabilities. This pelvic fracture classification helps EPs to initiate proper work-up, rule out the associated injuries, consult appropriate subspecialty services, determine management, and predict the outcome of these patients. In order to easily remember this classification, we refer to the US-VAGON classification, in which US indicates initially unstable and stable pelvic fracture classification and VAGON indicates potential vascular (class I, VA), GU/GI (class II, G), orthopedic (class III, O), and neurologic (class IV, N) complications in stable pelvic fractures.

Class I. Potential Hemorrhagic/Vascular Complications

1. Any pelvic fractures with 5 mm or more displacement
2. Open-book injury/pelvis dislocation
3. Open pelvic fracture

Class II. Potential Genitourinary or Gastrointestinal Complications

1. Pubic symphysis subluxation
2. Straddle fracture
3. Malgaigne fracture/Bucket handle fracture
4. Open-book injury/pelvis dislocation

Class III. Potential Orthopedic Complications

1. Double breaks in the pelvic ring

Class IV. Potential Neurologic Complications

1. Sacral fracture
2. Acetabular fracture

Class V. Uncomplicated

1. Avulsion fractures
2. Single pubic and ischial rami and double unilateral rami fractures
3. Iliac wing fracture (Duverney fracture)
4. Coccyx fracture
5. Ischial body fractures

Class I Fractures (Potential Hemorrhagic Complications)

The pelvic fractures listed here can cause potential life-threatening hemodynamic instability. Hemorrhage is the leading cause of death in patients with major pelvic fractures. Bleeding associated with pelvic fractures can come from the presacral and lumbar venous plexus, iliac or femoral vessels, or directly from the fracture sties.[5,33] Of these deaths, 20% are the result of injury to the iliac or femoral vessels.[33] It is imperative that EPs immediately identify patients at risk for vascular injury.

Any pelvic fracture with 5 mm or more displacement

In 1988, Cryer and colleagues[34] identified the correlation between significant hemorrhage and the displacement of 5 mm or more at any fracture site in the pelvic ring and acetabulum. The displacement is measured on the anteroposterior (AP) pelvis radiograph. Any pelvic (eg, Malgaigne, Duverney, straddle) or acetabular fracture with a displacement of 5 mm or more should be considered as high risk for significant bleeding and vascular instability. Therefore, aggressive treatment should be initiated immediately. A previous study on 1891 patients with trauma showed that a displaced pelvic fracture is one of the major risk factors for massive transfusion (more than 10 units of red blood cell transfusion within 24 hours).[35] Sagi and colleagues[36] reported that even minimally displaced pelvic fractures could become unstable, and Weaver and colleagues[37] found that bilateral pubic rami fractures, complete comminuted fractures of the sacrum, and crescent fractures warrant further evaluation because of high risk of pelvic hemorrhage and instability. Blackmore and colleagues[38] found that major hemorrhage could occur in patients with displaced obturator ring fractures and pubic symphyseal wide diastases. Overall, the sensitivity and specificity of predicting massive hemorrhage in displaced pelvic fractures are still uncertain. It is worthwhile for EPs to be vigilant to rule out any hemorrhagic potential in any patient with displaced pelvic fractures.

Open-book injury/pelvic dislocation

An anterior compressive force against the anterior superior iliac spine (ASIS) is usually the cause of an open-book injury or sprung pelvis. An open-book injury is defined as a separation of the pubic symphysis with a corresponding posterior injury (**Fig. 1**). Cryer

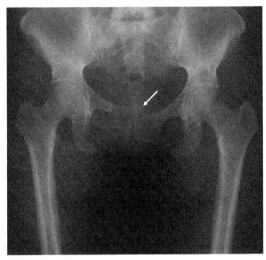

Fig. 2. Fracture of the body of the pubis with subluxation. Note symphysis is intact. *Arrow* indicate fracture location.

which had 24 times higher risk of urethral injury than any other type of pelvic fractures.[59] Patients sustaining straddle fractures present with inability to urinate, hematuria, or perineal ecchymosis and tenderness.

Malgaigne fracture and bucket handle fracture

In 1859, Malgaigne described fractures of the pelvis caused by vertical shear mechanisms. The vertical force required to produce this fracture usually results from a fall onto the lower extremities that fractures both the anterior and posterior pelvis. The anterior component is usually a longitudinally oriented fracture through either ipsilateral ischiopubic rami, or diastasis of the pubic symphysis, potentially resulting in a bladder or urethral injury. The posterior component includes fracture of the ipsilateral ilium, sacrum, or disruption of the SI joint (**Fig. 4**). The Malgaigne fracture is associated with a high rate of morbidity and mortality and is seen in about 21% of patients sustaining a fatal motor vehicle accident.[40] Because these fractures are usually the result of severe trauma, concomitant head and thoracic injuries are often seen.[4] A study on Malgaigne fractures found that it was the second most common pelvic fracture (other than straddle fracture) that could cause urethral injuries.[59,60] The bucket handle

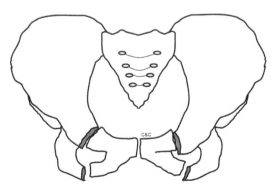

Fig. 3. Straddle fracture.

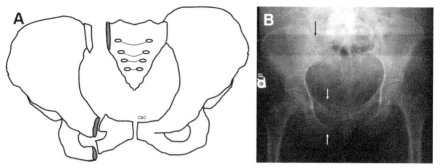

Fig. 4. (*A, B*) Malgaigne fracture. *Arrows* indicate fracture locations.

fracture occurs when a lateral compressive force with an upward rotatory component is applied to the pelvis (**Fig. 5**). It is similar to the Malgaigne fracture, except that the posterior element of the fracture is contralateral to the pubic rami fractures.

The posterior SI complex is important because it maintains the stability of the pelvic ring. Thus, a classification scheme based on the stability of the posterior lesion was developed. In this classification, the pelvic ring is stable in type A fractures. The pelvic ring in type B fractures is partially stable, such as in bucket handle fractures or some types of open-book fractures caused by external or internal rotation forces that could have a high risk of GU/GI injuries. Type C fractures refer to complete disruption of the posterior SI complex resulting in a displaced, unstable pelvic ring.[61,62]

Open-book fracture/pelvic dislocation
This fracture has previously been discussed as a potential cause of hemorrhage (see **Fig. 1**). Because of its higher association with injuries to the GU/GI tract, this fracture pattern is included in this category. In addition, the mortality can be more than 50% in patients with open pelvic fracture if rectal injury was missed initially.[63–66]

Emergency department management of class II fractures (potential genitourinary/gastrointestinal complications)
Patients with signs of GU/GI trauma must be scrutinized for GU/GI injury. Foley catheterization must be delayed until urethral injury is ruled out. Digital rectal examination is indicated to evaluate for the presence of blood or bony fragments caused by rectal perforation.[67] Vaginal examination with a speculum should be performed in women with pelvic fractures to exclude an open fracture. The perineum should be inspected for external lacerations to rule out open pelvic fracture.

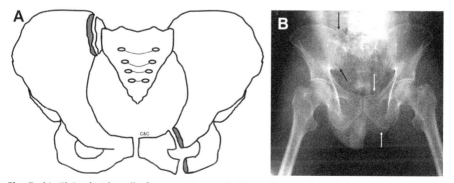

Fig. 5. (*A, B*) Bucket handle fracture. *Arrows* indicate fracture locations.

Retrograde urethrography is a simple procedure easily performed in the ED to rule out urethral injury. After obtaining a scout kidney ureter bladder, 60 mL of contrast material is injected slowly into the urethra. The syringe must be snug onto the meatus to prevent spillage of the contrast dye because this can result in false-positive findings. During the injection of the last 10 mL, a radiograph is obtained. Extravasation indicates a urethral rupture and should be further managed by the urologist (**Fig. 6**). Once urethral injury is ruled out, a Foley catheter is placed and retrograde cystography should be performed. A maximum of 400 mL of contrast dye is instilled by gravity through the Foley catheter. Positive findings for bladder injury include extravasation, indicating rupture or laceration, or mucosal defects, indicating a possible hematoma. It is also recommended to obtain a postvoid radiograph to rule out posterior extravasation (**Fig. 7**). CT scanning can provide additional information and should be ordered in the ED. Patients with a suspected rectal injury should consult surgery for endoscopy to rule out rectal injury.

Class III Fractures (Potential Orthopedic Complication)

All pelvic fractures that include a double break in the ring are in this category. A double break in the pelvic ring usually causes instability of the pelvis. In addition, any displacement or dislocation of the pelvis, including the acetabulum, that requires external or internal fixation is also in this category.

Class III fractures include open pelvic fractures, and sacral, acetabular, open-book, straddle, Malgaigne, bucket handle, or other multiple displaced fractures. Although these fractures do not meet class I or II criteria, orthopedic consultation is required to consider admission for surgical fixation. Pelvic dislocations should be treated the same way as pelvic fractures because high energy is required to cause pelvic dislocation. It should be emphasized that, given the high risk of pelvic instability in pelvic dislocations, potential hemorrhagic, GU/GI complications, or any other associated injuries should be ruled out initially before considering orthopedic complication.

Emergency department management of class III fractures (potential orthopedic complications)

The stability of the pelvic ring is compromised in the presence of a class III fracture. CT scanning is usually necessary, and surgical fixation is done at the discretion of the orthopedic surgeon.

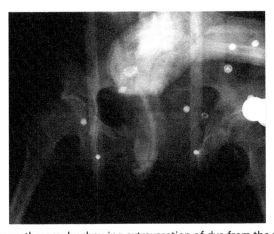

Fig. 6. Retrograde urethrography showing extravasation of dye from the posterior urethra.

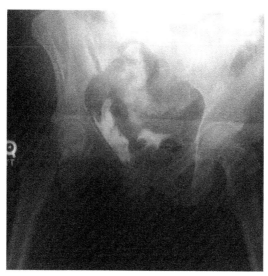

Fig. 7. Extraperitoneal extravasation on postvoid cystography.

Class IV Fractures (Potential Neurologic Complications)

Neurologic injury after pelvic fractures can be a cause of significant long-term morbidity. It can occur because of the proximity of nerves to the sacrum and acetabulum, especially with posterior ring disruption. EPs must consider the potential for neurologic complications in the fractures listed here.

Sacral fractures

Neurologic deficits can be found in about 15% to 40% of sacral fractures.[15,17,68,69] These deficits include cauda equina injuries, radiculopathies, or plexopathies. The sacral roots, obturator nerve, and fifth lumbar roots can be damaged by sacral fracture.

The incidence of these neurologic injuries varies depending on the fracture types and location. A study has reported that the incidence of neurologic injuries increased from 1.5% in Tile type A to 14.4% in Tile type C fractures (Tile classification is mainly based on the integrity of posterior SI complex as mentioned earlier. Briefly, type A is intact SI complex, type B is partial disruption of posterior SI complex, and type C is complete disruption of posterior SI complex).[70] Sabiston and Wing's[71] classified sacral fractures into 3 categories (**Fig. 8**). The first category consists of sacral fractures occurring in conjunction with another pelvic fracture, and these account for approximately 90% of sacral fractures.[69] The sacrum usually is fractured in a vertical, transforaminal orientation. Vertical fractures are less likely to be associated with neurologic damage.[69,72] Sabiston and Wing's[71] second category is made up of isolated sacral fractures below the S2 level. These fractures usually are caused by direct blow to the sacrum. Although these fractures are commonly oriented transversely, they are not usually associated with significant neurologic injury owing to their position on the sacrum. Sabiston and Wing's[71] third category includes isolated sacral fractures above the S2 level. These fractures are the least common, but potentially the most serious because there is a high incidence of neurologic deficit associated with these fractures.[71] Nicoll[73] proposed that these fractures occur as a result of forced flexion at the sacrum when the patient is in a position of hip flexion with knee extension. These

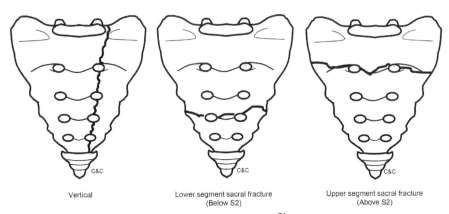

Fig. 8. Sacral fractures according to Sabiston and Wing.[71]

fractures are often associated with fractures of the lumbar transverse processes. The Denis classification is another classification system that identifies the severity of sacral fractures with the main focus being to predict the neurologic injuries. As mentioned earlier, zone 2 involves the neural foramen and zone 3 involves the spinal canal. It is reported that the incidence of neurologic injuries increased with the higher zone injuries. Zone 2 injuries have a 28% neurologic injury rate, usually involving L5, S1, and S2 nerve roots. Zone 3 injuries have a 56% incidence of neurologic injury. Such injuries frequently involve the bowel and bladder and may also cause sexual dysfunction. In addition, higher risk of neurologic injuries (46%) can be seen if injury patterns involve the SI area of the pelvic ring.[74] All these classifications of sacral fractures predict neurologic injuries to certain degrees but they are varied and inconsistent. It is challenging for EPs to remember and identify the type of sacral fractures based on plain films or CT images. It also has less practical value for EPs to predict the potential neurological injuries in these trauma patients. Therefore, any patients with SI disruptions, SI dislocations, widening SI joint, associated pelvic ring fractures, spinopelvic dissociation, or transverse sacral fractures potentially have neurologic injuries that the EP should consider.

It is sometimes difficult to predict potential neurologic complications of sacral fractures based on findings on routine radiographs. In general, transverse sacral fractures are associated with more extensive neurologic injuries than other types of fractures that are identified on plain films.[72] If sacral fractures are not identified on routine pelvic radiographs, EPs should pay special attention to the physical examination. Perianal pain, buttock pain, localized bruising, decreased anal sphincter tone, or loss of perineal sensation are all clinical clues to a sacral fracture. When physical examination has suspicious signs of sacral fracture, further CT of abdomen and pelvis is warranted. Although the literature differs on classification methods and incidence of sacral fractures, it supports an aggressive approach to diagnosis and a conservative approach to treatment.[71,72,75,76]

Acetabular fractures

Acetabular fractures account for 20% of all pelvic fractures (**Fig. 9**).[39] The prevalence of injury to the sciatic nerve after acetabular fracture or fracture-dislocation of the hip has been reported to be between 10% and 25%.[77,78] Previous studies also showed that the displaced fracture of the posterior column and fractures with posterior dislocation of the femoral head were more commonly associated with sciatic nerve

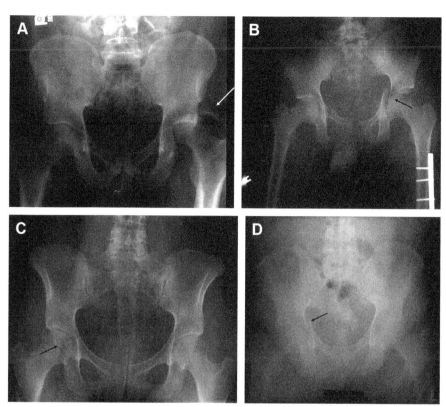

Fig. 9. (*A*) Posterior acetabular rim fracture (*arrow*). (*B*) Complex acetabular fracture (*arrow*). Note disrupted ilioischial line indicating ilioischial column fracture. Also note iliopubic line disruption, posterior rim fracture, and contralateral comminuted ischiopubic rami fracture. (*C*) Transverse fracture of the acetabulum (*arrow*). Note separation of innominate bone into superior iliac and inferior ischiopubic segments. (*D*) Iliopubic column fracture of the acetabulum (*arrow*). Note disruption of the iliopubic line. The ilioischial line remains intact.

injuries.[79–81] Another study on both anterior and posterior column acetabular fractures showed nearly 9% of occurrence of sciatic nerve injury preoperatively and the same investigator later reported that more than 20% of sciatic nerve injuries occurred if the fracture was on the posterior wall.[82–84] Therefore, the type of acetabular fracture might influence the incidence of neurologic injury to a different degree. Although the risk of sciatic nerve damage is high in acetabular fractures regardless of the type, 60% to 75% of patients with neurologic injuries recover well after surgery. Letournel and Judet reported 60% complete neurologic recovery after surgically treated acetabular fractures and Tile[22] reported 75% recovery, including both traumatic and iatrogenic injuries. In addition, studies have found that severe involvement of the peroneal nerve is usually associated with a poor prognosis.[22,79] Taken together, different classifications of acetabular fractures have been reported with different foci and rarely have practical value for EPs in terms of management. Therefore, because of the high risk of neurologic damage in patients with acetabular fractures, EPs must consult trauma and orthopedic surgeons emergently for potential neurologic injury and these patients should be admitted for further observation.

Sciatic nerve injury may present with a wide range of clinical findings, including sensation and motor changes, such as posterior thigh pain, radiculopathy along the nerve distribution, or paralysis of muscles. If the peroneal division of the sciatic nerve is involved, it can also result in weakness of the lower extremity. Sometimes, these signs and symptoms mimic impinged spinal nerve symptoms. Therefore, EPs should perform a thorough neurologic examination in these patients. The sciatic nerve is also sensitive to longitudinal stretching and the impairment in the axonal flow proximally could also make the distal nerve more vulnerable. Some of these initial neurologic signs and symptoms can predict the long-term neurologic outcome. Giannoudis and colleagues[85] reported a simple classification based on the initial clinical presentations in patients with acetabular fracture. Class A was defined as patients with complete foot drop. Class B referred to weakness of the foot dorsiflexors, and class C referred to altered feeling in the foot with burning pain, diminished feeling, and dysesthesia or hyperesthesia. Patients in class A showed poor clinical prognosis, whereas patients in classes B and C showed significant neurologic recovery. Therefore, patients with acetabular fractures and complete foot drop with no movement should have immediate trauma and orthopedic surgery consultation for potential severe sciatic nerve damage.

Emergency department management of class IV fractures (potential neurologic complications)

Neurologic injury can occur secondary to the proximity of nerves to the sacrum and acetabulum. Sacral fractures below the S2 level rarely result in neurologic injury.[71] These patients are treated symptomatically with bed rest and analgesia for 4 to 5 weeks. Patients with neurologic deficit or fracture above the S2 level must be referred to neurosurgery or orthopedics for follow-up care. Unless displaced, these fractures rarely require surgical fixation. Acetabular fractures can result in injury to the sciatic nerve, especially with fractures of SI complex and signs of complete foot drop.[86] In the ED, these fractures are managed with immobilization and orthopedic consultation. Surgical management is the preferred treatment, with better long-term clinical outcome.[87]

Class V Fractures (Uncomplicated)

These fractures are simple and stable, and include avulsion fractures of the pelvis, single pubic and ischial rami fractures and unilateral double rami fractures, ischial body fractures, iliac wing fracture (Duverney fracture), and coccyx fractures. They can result in a single break in the pelvic ring and usually do not require extensive orthopedic repair. These fractures are usually not associated with serious complications and can be managed on an outpatient basis.[88]

Avulsion fractures

The muscle attachments to the pelvis serve a dual purpose of support and mobility (**Fig. 10**). Forceful contraction of these muscles in areas where apophyseal centers are not yet fused can cause avulsion fractures. There are usually no associated injuries with these fractures, and they can be treated symptomatically. The current literature confirms that the highest prevalence of avulsion fractures occur among adolescents, and most pelvic avulsion fractures occur during the phase of a sporting activity because of the higher forces generated when muscles are contracted. However, avulsion pelvic fractures do occur in older populations because of osteoporosis or some pathologic bone changes.[89–92] In general, avulsion fractures of the pelvis can be treated with bed rest and rehabilitation, which usually has a satisfactory outcome. However, if significant avulsion fractures occur with more than 1.5 cm to 2 cm of

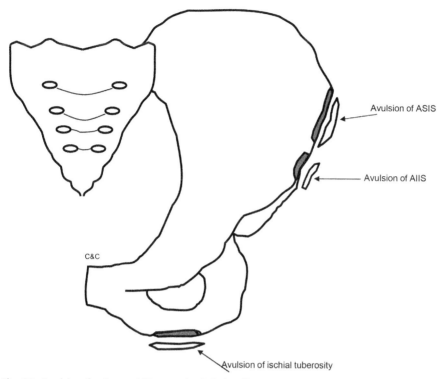

Fig. 10. Avulsion fractures. AIIS, anterior inferior iliac spine.

displacement, cutaneous nerve entrapment, or severe rotational deformity, surgical operation can be considered, especially in athlete populations.[93–96]

The most commonly reported sites of avulsion fracture in the pelvis are the ASIS, anterior inferior iliac spine (AIIS), and ischial tuberosity (IT).[26,97] Avulsion of the ASIS can occur with forceful contraction of the sartorius muscle. These fractures are usually seen in athletic male patients in their midteens, classically in sprinters and soccer players.[98] These injuries present with pain and tenderness over the ASIS. The pain is worsened on flexion and abduction of the hip (use of the sartorius muscle). ASIS avulsion fracture can be managed conservatively or by operative fixation (OF). OF is preferred if significant displacement of avulsion fracture occurred or if the patient is an athlete who requires rapid return to sport activities.[99] However, there is still disagreement about which approach is better.[100] Conservative treatment involves bed rest, analgesia, and graded mobilization and weight bearing. These patients should be prescribed analgesics and bed rest for 3 to 4 weeks. The hip should remain in a flexed, abducted position as much as possible. Patients can usually resume vigorous activity in about 8 weeks. Reported complications of ASIS avulsion include nonunion of the fracture, clinical deformity at the ASIS with exostosis formation, and entrapment of the lateral cutaneous nerve of the thigh causing sensory symptoms.[101]

Forceful contraction of the rectus femoris may cause avulsion of the AIIS. This injury is classically seen in field-goal kickers or soccer players and is less common than ASIS avulsions. Patients present with pain and tenderness in the groin and with pain on active hip flexion. If there is no significant displacement or nerve entrapment, patients with AIIS avulsion generally should be treated conservatively. The goal of the treatment is returning to daily life and maintaining regular sporting activities. Analgesics and bed rest for 3 to 4 weeks with the hip in flexion are recommended. Patients usually can resume full activity in 8 weeks.[102]

IT avulsion fractures are injuries resulting from forceful contraction of the hamstrings or less commonly, the adductor magnus. Athletes such as hurdlers, pole vaulters, and cheerleaders are typically at risk. Because the apophyseal center at the IT does not fuse until the age of 25 years, these injuries can be seen in older patients (compared with the previously discussed avulsion fractures). Patients present with sudden buttock or thigh pain during strenuous activities, or chronic tenderness over the IT or pain when in the seated position. Because the sacrotuberous ligament antagonizes displacement of the IT, palpation of this ligament on rectal examination may cause pain. Sometimes a gap is palpable in the area of the ischial apophysis. Hamstring stretching elicits pain as well. Treatment of these fractures can be conservative in most cases and includes analgesics and bed rest with the hip in extension, external rotation, and slight abduction for 3 to 4 weeks. Surgical intervention may only be considered in athlete population requiring rapid recovery or having substantial displacement.[94,103–106]

Single pubic and ischial rami fractures and unilateral double rami fractures

Fractures of the pubic and ischial rami are the most commonly seen pelvic fractures, especially in the geriatric population (**Fig. 11**).[2,105–107] In elderly patients, these fractures are typically caused by falls from a standing or seated position. The EP must examine the ipsilateral hip to rule out associated fracture. When seen in younger patients, these fractures can occur as stress fractures secondary to strenuous exercise or persistent pelvic tension, as in the third trimester of pregnancy.[88] Patients present with pain to deep palpation or on walking. Treatment consists of bed rest and

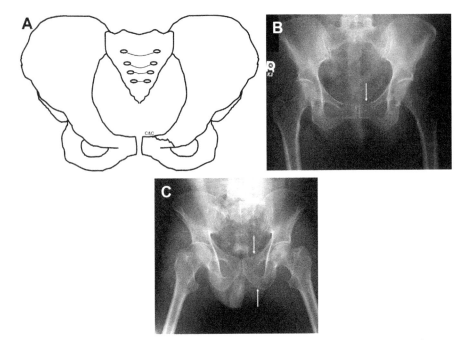

Fig. 11. (A, B) Single pubic rami fracture (arrow). (C) Unilateral double rami fracture (arrows).

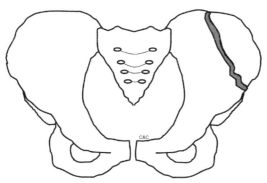

Fig. 12. Iliac wing fracture (Duverney fracture).

analgesics. Patients may begin crutch walking and weight bearing as tolerated. Normal activity usually can be resumed in 8 weeks. Ischial rami fractures are usually stable fractures with fewer complications and better clinical outcome. A previous study showed good prognosis, with 95% return of normal performance of daily activities.[108] However, if pain control and progressive mobilization are required, hospital admission or home care service may be recommended, especially in geriatric patients.[108,109] In addition, EPs should pay special attention to patients with multiple preexisting comorbidities because of higher in-hospital and 1-year mortalities.[109,110]

Iliac wing fracture (Duverney fracture)

Isolated fractures of the iliac wing are caused by direct trauma, usually a medially directed force (**Figs. 12** and **13**). They are rotationally and vertically stable. Because the abductors of the hip insert on the iliac wing, pain is elicited with walking or hip abduction. Previous studies showed that multiple additional injuries could occur along with iliac wing fractures and acetabular fractures.[88,111] Comminuted iliac wing fractures are extremely rare and occur with high-energy mechanisms. Comminuted iliac wing fractures require surgical intervention but have good clinical prognosis afterward.[112] Although Rockwood and Green[55] suggest strapping of the pelvis below the iliac crest, most patients heal well with bed rest and analgesics until weight bearing is tolerated.

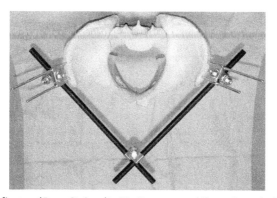

Fig. 13. External fixator. (*From* Steinsultz KL. Trauma, mobile and surgical radiography. In: Bontrager KL, Lampignano JP, editors. Textbook of: radiographic positioning and related anatomy. 7th edition. St Louis (MO): Mosby; Elsevier; 2010, p. 589–643; with permission.)

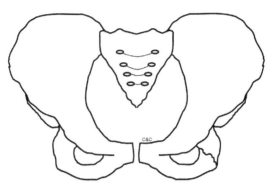

Fig. 14. Ischial body fracture.

Coccyx fractures
Fractures of the coccyx can occur as a result of falls in the seated position, following childbirth, or from iatrogenic injury during surgery. Patients present complaining of localized tenderness. Pain is exacerbated while sitting or defecating owing to the use of the levator ani and the anococcygeal muscles. Because part of the gluteus maximus inserts on the coccyx, pain can also occur when rising from a seated position. The diagnosis can be made by history and external tenderness, and rectal examination and radiographs are not necessary. Because many muscles insert at the coccyx, immobilization is difficult at best. Treatment is limited to analgesics, air cushions, stool softeners, and time, and patients must be informed of the extended time of healing. However, if chronic pain persists, coccygectomy is an option.[113] Coccygeoplasty, injection of polymethylmethacrylate cement, results in immediate relief of symptoms.[114]

Ischial body fractures
Ischial body fractures are the least common of all pelvic fractures (**Fig. 14**),[88] usually resulting from falls in which the patient lands in the seated position. Patients complain of pain to deep palpation and on flexion of the hips while the knee is extended. The lumbar and thoracic spine should be examined for associated fractures. Treatment includes 4 to 6 weeks of bed rest and analgesics.

Emergency department management of class V fractures (uncomplicated)
The management of these injuries has been discussed previously. Most of these fractures can be treated conservatively with bed rest and analgesics.

SUMMARY

The diagnosis and treatment of pelvic fractures are problems fraught with challenges and nuances for EPs and the trauma teams. This article discusses pelvic fractures and classifies them into an organized and simplified schema (US-VAGON classification). This ED classification of pelvic fractures provides EPs with a practical guideline to initiate the necessary evaluation and treatment of these patients. In addition, algorithms recommending a general approach are proposed for patients with both hemodynamically stable and hemodynamically unstable pelvic fractures.

REFERENCES

1. Pereira SJ, O'Brien DP, Luchette FA, et al. Dynamic helical computed tomography scan accurately detects hemorrhage in patients with pelvic fracture. Surgery 2000;128:678–85.

2. Trunkey DD, Chapman MW, Lim RC Jr, et al. Management of pelvic fractures in blunt trauma injury. J Trauma 1974;14:912–23.
3. Gurevitz S, Bender B, Tytiun Y, et al. The role of pelvic fractures in the course of treatment and outcome of trauma patients. Isr Med Assoc J 2005;7:623–6.
4. Jerrard DA. Pelvic fractures. Emerg Med Clin North Am 1993;11:147–63.
5. Moreno C, Moore EE, Rosenberger A, et al. Hemorrhage associated with major pelvic fracture: a multispecialty challenge. J Trauma 1986;26:987–94.
6. Gustavo PJ, Coimbra R, Rasslan S, et al. The role of associated injuries on outcome of blunt trauma patients sustaining pelvic fractures. Injury 2000;31: 677–82.
7. Starr AJ, Walter JC, Harris RW, et al. Percutaneous screw fixation of fractures of the iliac wing and fracture-dislocations of the sacro-iliac joint (OTA Types 61-B2.2 and 61-B2.3, or Young-Burgess "lateral compression type II" pelvic fractures). J Orthop Trauma 2002;16:116–23.
8. Balogh Z, King KL, Mackay P, et al. The epidemiology of pelvic ring fractures: a population-based study. J Trauma 2007;63:1066–73.
9. Rothenberger DA, Fischer RP, Strate RG, et al. The mortality associated with pelvic fractures. Surgery 1978;84:356–61.
10. Mucha P Jr, Welch TJ. Hemorrhage in major pelvic fractures. Surg Clin North Am 1988;68:757–73.
11. Sarin EL, Moore JB, Moore EE, et al. Pelvic fracture pattern does not always predict the need for urgent embolization. J Trauma 2005;58:973–7.
12. Manson T, O'Toole RV, Whitney A, et al. Young-Burgess classification of pelvic ring fractures: does it predict mortality, transfusion requirements, and non-orthopaedic injuries? J Orthop Trauma 2010;24:603–9.
13. Pennal GF, Davidson J, Garside H, et al. Results of treatment of acetabular fractures. Clin Orthop Relat Res 1980;(151):115–23.
14. Burgess AR, Eastridge BJ, Young JW, et al. Pelvic ring disruptions: effective classification system and treatment protocols. J Trauma 1990;30:848–56.
15. Gibbons KJ, Soloniuk DS, Razack N. Neurological injury and patterns of sacral fractures. J Neurosurg 1990;72:889–93.
16. Mehta S, Auerbach JD, Born CT, et al. Sacral fractures. J Am Acad Orthop Surg 2006;14:656–65.
17. Denis F, Davis S, Comfort T. Sacral fractures: an important problem. Retrospective analysis of 236 cases. Clin Orthop Relat Res 1988;227:67–81.
18. Isler B. Lumbosacral lesions associated with pelvic ring injuries. J Orthop Trauma 1990;4:1–6.
19. Hak D, Baran S, Stahel P. Sacral fractures: current strategies in diagnosis and management. Orthopedics 2009;32.
20. Capaul M, Zollinger H, Satz N, et al. Analyses of 94 consecutive spinal cord injury patients using ASIA definition and modified Frankel score classification. Paraplegia 1994;32:583–7.
21. Judet R, Judet J, Letournel E. Fractures of the acetabulum: classification and surgical approaches for open reduction. preliminary report. J Bone Joint Surg Am 1964;46:1615–46.
22. Tile M. Fractures of the acetabulum. Orthop Clin North Am 1980;11:481–506.
23. Harris JH, Coupe KJ, Lee JS, et al. Acetabular fractures revisited: a new CT-based classification. Semin Musculoskelet Radiol 2005;9:150–60.
24. Davis JW. The relationship of base deficit to lactate in porcine hemorrhagic shock and resuscitation. J Trauma 1994;36:168–72.

25. Mattox KL, Bickell WH, Pepe PE, et al. Prospective randomized evaluation of antishock MAST in post-traumatic hypotension. J Trauma 1986;26:779–86.

26. Bickell WH, Pepe PE, Bailey ML, et al. Randomized trial of pneumatic antishock garments in the prehospital management of penetrating abdominal injuries. Ann Emerg Med 1987;16:653–8.

27. Mattox KL, Bickell W, Pepe PE, et al. Prospective MAST study in 911 patients. J Trauma 1989;29:1104–11.

28. Aprahamian C, Gessert G, Bandyk DF, et al. MAST-associated compartment syndrome (MACS): a review. J Trauma 1989;29:549–55.

29. Brown JJ, Greene FL, McMillin RD. Vascular injuries associated with pelvic fractures. Am Surg 1984;50:150–4.

30. Fang JF, Shih LY, Wong YC, et al. Repeat transcatheter arterial embolization for the management of pelvic arterial hemorrhage. J Trauma 2009;66:429–35.

31. Shapiro M, McDonald AA, Knight D, et al. The role of repeat angiography in the management of pelvic fractures. J Trauma 2005;58:227–31.

32. Cothren CC, Osborn PM, Moore EE, et al. Preperitonal pelvic packing for hemodynamically unstable pelvic fractures: a paradigm shift. J Trauma 2007;62:834–9.

33. Rothenberger DA, Fischer RP, Perry JF Jr. Major vascular injuries secondary to pelvic fractures: an unsolved clinical problem. Am J Surg 1978;136:660–2.

34. Cryer HM, Miller FB, Evers BM, et al. Pelvic fracture classification: correlation with hemorrhage. J Trauma 1988;28:973–80.

35. Rainer TH, Ho AM, Yeung JH, et al. Early risk stratification of patients with major trauma requiring massive blood transfusion. Resuscitation 2011;82:724–9.

36. Sagi HC, Coniglione FM, Stanford JH. Examination under anesthetic for occult pelvic ring instability. J Orthop Trauma 2011;25:529–36.

37. Weaver MJ, Bruinsma W, Toney E, et al. What are the patterns of injury and displacement seen in lateral compression pelvic fractures? Clin Orthop Relat Res 2012;470:2104–10.

38. Blackmore CC, Cummings P, Jurkovich GJ, et al. Predicting major hemorrhage in patients with pelvic fracture. J Trauma 2006;61:346–52.

39. Kricun ME. Fractures of the pelvis. Orthop Clin North Am 1990;21:573–90.

40. Bucholz RW. The pathological anatomy of Malgaigne fracture-dislocations of the pelvis. J Bone Joint Surg Am 1981;63:400–4.

41. Salim A, Teixeira PG, DuBose J, et al. Predictors of positive angiography in pelvic fractures: a prospective study. J Am Coll Surg 2008;207:656–62.

42. Elzik ME, Dirschl DR, Dahners LE. Hemorrhage in pelvic fractures does not correlate with fracture length. J Trauma 2008;65:436–41.

43. Tseng S, Tornetta P III. Percutaneous management of Morel-Lavallee lesions. J Bone Joint Surg Am 2006;88:92–6.

44. Day AC, Kinmont C, Bircher MD, et al. Crescent fracture-dislocation of the sacroiliac joint: a functional classification. J Bone Joint Surg Br 2007;89:651–8.

45. Collinge C, Tornetta P III. Soft tissue injuries associated with pelvic fractures. Orthop Clin North Am 2004;35:451–6, v.

46. Richardson JD, Harty J, Amin M, et al. Open pelvic fractures. J Trauma 1982;22:533–8.

47. Black EA, Lawson CM, Smith S, et al. Open pelvic fractures: the University of Tennessee Medical Center at Knoxville experience over ten years. Iowa Orthop J 2011;31:193–8.

48. Morey AF, Metro MJ, Carney KJ, et al. Consensus on genitourinary trauma: external genitalia. BJU Int 2004;94:507–15.

49. Bjurlin MA, Fantus RJ, Mellett MM, et al. Genitourinary injuries in pelvic fracture morbidity and mortality using the National Trauma Data Bank. J Trauma 2009;67: 1033–9.

50. Gansslen A, Hildebrand F, Heidari N, et al. Pelvic ring injuries in children. Part I: epidemiology and primary evaluation. A review of the literature. Acta Chir Orthop Traumatol Cech 2012;79:493–8.

51. Morehouse DD. Injuries to the urethra and urinary bladder associated with fractures of the pelvis. Can J Surg 1988;31:85–8.

52. Colapinto V. Trauma to the pelvis: urethral injury. Clin Orthop Relat Res 1980;(151):46–55.

53. Ellison M, Timberlake GA, Kerstein MD. Impotence following pelvic fracture. J Trauma 1988;28:695–6.

54. Koraitim MM. Pelvic fracture urethral injuries: the unresolved controversy. J Urol 1999;161:1433–41.

55. Rockwood C, Green D. Fractures in adults. Philadelphia: JB Lippincott; 1984. p. 1093–209.

56. Conolly WB, Hedberg EA. Observations on fractures of the pelvis. J Trauma 1969;9:104–11.

57. Neser CP, Lindeque BG. Bladder interposition in traumatic diastasis of the symphysis pubis. A case report. S Afr Med J 1986;69:640–1.

58. Finnan RP, Herbenick MA, Prayson MJ, et al. Bladder incarceration following anterior external fixation of a traumatic pubic symphysis diastasis treated with immediate open reduction and internal fixation. Patient Saf Surg 2008;2:26.

59. Koraitim MM, Marzouk ME, Atta MA, et al. Risk factors and mechanism of urethral injury in pelvic fractures. Br J Urol 1996;77:876–80.

60. Brandes S, Borrelli J Jr. Pelvic fracture and associated urologic injuries. World J Surg 2001;25:1578–87.

61. Tile M. Acute pelvic fractures: I. Causation and classification. J Am Acad Orthop Surg 1996;4:143–51.

62. Tile M. Acute pelvic fractures: II. Principles of management. J Am Acad Orthop Surg 1996;4:152–61.

63. Monahan PR, Taylor RG. Dislocation and fracture-dislocation of the pelvis. Injury 1975;6:325–33.

64. Andrich DE, Day AC, Mundy AR. Proposed mechanisms of lower urinary tract injury in fractures of the pelvic ring. BJU Int 2007;100:567–73.

65. Mundy AR, Andrich DE. Pelvic fracture-related injuries of the bladder neck and prostate: their nature, cause and management. BJU Int 2010;105:1302–8.

66. Tsugawa K, Koyanagi N, Hashizume M, et al. New therapeutic strategy of open pelvic fracture associated with rectal injury in 43 patients over 60 years of age. Hepatogastroenterology 2002;49:1275–80.

67. Esposito TJ, Ingraham A, Luchette FA, et al. Reasons to omit digital rectal exam in trauma patients: no fingers, no rectum, no useful additional information. J Trauma 2005;59:1314–9.

68. Pohlemann T, Gansslen A, Tscherne H. The problem of the sacrum fracture. Clinical analysis of 377 cases. Orthopade 1992;21:400–12 [in German].

69. Bonin JG. Sacral fractures and injuries to the cauda equina. J Bone Joint Surg Am 1945;27:113–27.

70. Schmal H, Hauschild O, Culemann U, et al. Identification of risk factors for neurological deficits in patients with pelvic fractures. Orthopedics 2010;33.

71. Sabiston CP, Wing PC. Sacral fractures: classification and neurologic implications. J Trauma 1986;26:1113–5.

72. Schmidek HH, Smith DA, Kristiansen TK. Sacral fractures. Neurosurgery 1984; 15:735–46.

73. Nicoll EA. Fractures of the dorso-lumbar spine. J Bone Joint Surg Br 1949;31B: 376–94.

74. Conway RR, Hubbell SL. Electromyographic abnormalities in neurologic injury associated with pelvic fracture: case reports and literature review. Arch Phys Med Rehabil 1988;69:539–41.

75. Weis EB Jr. Subtle neurological injuries in pelvic fractures. J Trauma 1984;24: 983–5.

76. Fisher RG. Sacral fracture with compression of cauda equina: surgical treatment. J Trauma 1988;28:1678–80.

77. Jacob JR, Rao JP, Ciccarelli C. Traumatic dislocation and fracture dislocation of the hip. A long-term follow-up study. Clin Orthop Relat Res 1987;(214): 249–63.

78. Fassler PR, Swiontkowski MF, Kilroy AW, et al. Injury of the sciatic nerve associated with acetabular fracture. J Bone Joint Surg Am 1993;75:1157–66.

79. Issack PS, Helfet DL. Sciatic nerve injury associated with acetabular fractures. HSS J 2009;5:12–8.

80. Epstein NE, Epstein JA, Carras R. Unilateral S-1 root compression syndrome caused by fracture of the sacrum. Neurosurgery 1986;19:1025–7.

81. Epstein HC. Posterior fracture-dislocations of the hip; long-term follow-up. J Bone Joint Surg Am 1974;56:1103–27.

82. Gansslen A, Frink M, Hildebrand F, et al. Both column fractures of the acetabulum: epidemiology, operative management and long-term-results. Acta Chir Orthop Traumatol Cech 2012;79:107–13.

83. Gansslen A, Hildebrand F, Heidari N, et al. Acetabular fractures in children: a review of the literature. Acta Chir Orthop Traumatol Cech 2013;80:10–4.

84. Gansslen A, Hildebrand F, Kretek C. Transverse + posterior wall fractures of the acetabulum: epidemiology, operative management and long-term results. Acta Chir Orthop Traumatol Cech 2013;80:27–33.

85. Giannoudis PV, Da Costa AA, Raman R, et al. Double-crush syndrome after acetabular fractures. A sign of poor prognosis. J Bone Joint Surg Br 2005;87: 401–7.

86. Oxford CF, Stein A. Complicated crushing injuries of the pelvis. J Bone Joint Surg Br 1967;49:24–32.

87. Butler-Manuel PA, James SE, Shepperd JA. Pelvic underpinning: eight years' experience. J Bone Joint Surg Br 1992;74:74–7.

88. Simon RR, Koenigsknecht SJ. Emergency orthopedics: the extremities. 3rd edition. Norwalk (CT): Appleton & Lange; 1995.

89. Cannada LK, Taylor RM, Reddix R, et al. The Jones-Powell Classification of open pelvic fractures: a multicenter study evaluating mortality rates. J Trauma Acute Care Surg 2013;74:901–6.

90. Metzmaker JN, Pappas AM. Avulsion fractures of the pelvis. Am J Sports Med 1985;13:349–58.

91. Orava S, Ala-Ketola L. Avulsion fractures in athletes. Br J Sports Med 1977;11: 65–71.

92. Rossi F, Dragoni S. Acute avulsion fractures of the pelvis in adolescent competitive athletes: prevalence, location and sports distribution of 203 cases collected. Skeletal Radiol 2001;30:127–31.

93. Kaneyama S, Yoshida K, Matsushima S, et al. A surgical approach for an avulsion fracture of the ischial tuberosity: a case report. J Orthop Trauma 2006;20:363–5.

94. Servant CT, Jones CB. Displaced avulsion of the ischial apophysis: a hamstring injury requiring internal fixation. Br J Sports Med 1998;32:255–7.
95. Buch KA, Campbell J. Acute onset meralgia paraesthetica after fracture of the anterior superior iliac spine. Injury 1993;24:569–70.
96. Yildiz C, Yildiz Y, Ozdemir MT, et al. Sequential avulsion of the anterior inferior iliac spine in an adolescent long jumper. Br J Sports Med 2005;39:e31.
97. Oldenburg FP, Smith MV, Thompson GH. Simultaneous ipsilateral avulsion of the anterior superior and anterior inferior iliac spines in an adolescent. J Pediatr Orthop 2009;29:29–30.
98. Pointinger H, Munk P, Poeschl GP. Avulsion fracture of the anterior superior iliac spine following apophysitis. Br J Sports Med 2003;37:361–2.
99. Doral MN, Aydog ST, Tetik O, et al. Multiple osteochondroses and avulsion fracture of anterior superior iliac spine in a soccer player. Br J Sports Med 2005;39:e16.
100. Veselko M, Smrkolj V. Avulsion of the anterior-superior iliac spine in athletes: case reports. J Trauma 1994;36:444–6.
101. Rosenberg N, Noiman M, Edelson G. Avulsion fractures of the anterior superior iliac spine in adolescents. J Orthop Trauma 1996;10:440–3.
102. Gomez JE. Bilateral anterior inferior iliac spine avulsion fractures. Med Sci Sports Exerc 1996;28:161–4.
103. Wootton JR, Cross MJ, Holt KW. Avulsion of the ischial apophysis. The case for open reduction and internal fixation. J Bone Joint Surg Br 1990;72:625–7.
104. Kujala UM, Orava S. Ischial apophysis injuries in athletes. Sports Med 1993;16:290–4.
105. Coppola PT, Coppola M. Emergency department evaluation and treatment of pelvic fractures. Emerg Med Clin North Am 2000;18(1):1–27.
106. Gidwani S, Jagiello J, Bircher M. Avulsion fracture of the ischial tuberosity in adolescents–an easily missed diagnosis. BMJ 2004;329:99–100.
107. Hill RM, Robinson CM, Keating JF. Fractures of the pubic rami. Epidemiology and five-year survival. J Bone Joint Surg Br 2001;83:1141–4.
108. Koval KJ, Aharonoff GB, Schwartz MC, et al. Pubic rami fracture: a benign pelvic injury? J Orthop Trauma 1997;11:7–9.
109. van Dijk WA, Poeze M, van Helden SH, et al. Ten-year mortality among hospitalised patients with fractures of the pubic rami. Injury 2010;41:411–4.
110. Krappinger D, Struve P, Schmid R, et al. Fractures of the pubic rami: a retrospective review of 534 cases. Arch Orthop Trauma Surg 2009;129:1685–90.
111. Abrassart S, Stern R, Peter R. Morbidity associated with isolated iliac wing fractures. J Trauma 2009;66:200–3.
112. Switzer JA, Nork SE, Routt ML Jr. Comminuted fractures of the iliac wing. J Orthop Trauma 2000;14:270–6.
113. Cebesoy O, Guclu B, Kose KC, et al. Coccygectomy for coccygodynia: do we really have to wait? Injury 2007;38:1183–8.
114. Dean LM, Syed MI, Jan SA, et al. Coccygeoplasty: treatment for fractures of the coccyx. J Vasc Interv Radiol 2006;17:909–12.

Index

Note: Page numbers of article titles are in **boldface** type.

Emerg Med Clin N Am 33 (2015) 475–482
http://dx.doi.org/10.1016/S0733-8627(15)00018-8
0733-8627/15/$ – see front matter © 2015 Elsevier Inc. All rights reserved.

emed.theclinics.com

Moving?

Make sure your subscription moves with you!

To notify us of your new address, find your **Clinics Account Number** (located on your mailing label above your name), and contact customer service at:

Email: journalscustomerservice-usa@elsevier.com

800-654-2452 (subscribers in the U.S. & Canada)
314-447-8871 (subscribers outside of the U.S. & Canada)

Fax number: 314-447-8029

Elsevier Health Sciences Division
Subscription Customer Service
3251 Riverport Lane
Maryland Heights, MO 63043

*To ensure uninterrupted delivery of your subscription, please notify us at least 4 weeks in advance of move.

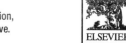

Printed and bound by CPI Group (UK) Ltd, Croydon, CR0 4YY

03/10/2024

01040495-0006